NATURAL CAUSES

NATURAL CAUSES

Death, Lies, and Politics in America's Vitamin and Herbal Supplement Industry

Dan Hurley

Broadway Books ⬭ New York

PUBLISHED BY BROADWAY BOOKS

Published in the United States by Broadway Books, an imprint of
The Doubleday Broadway Publishing Group, a division of Random House, Inc.,
New York.
www.broadwaybooks.com

BROADWAY BOOKS and its logo, a letter B bisected on the diagonal,
are trademarks of Random House, Inc.

Book design by Elizabeth Rendfleisch

Library of Congress Cataloging-in-Publication Data
Hurley, Dan.
    Natural causes : death, lies, and politics in America's vitamin and herbal
supplement industry / Dan Hurley.— 1st ed.
        p. cm.
    1. Herbs—Toxicology. 2. Dietary supplements—Toxicology. 3. Herb
industry—United States. 4. Dietary supplements industry—United States.
I. Title.

RA1250.H87 2006
338.4' 76151—dc22

                                                    2006047576

ISBN: 978-0-7679-2042-1

PRINTED IN THE UNITED STATES OF AMERICA

10   9   8   7   6   5   4   3   2   1

First Edition

For my mother, Mary,
and
in memory of
my father, David

CONTENTS

PROLOGUE   Sue Gilliatt's Nose   **1**

PART 1 A BRIEF HISTORY OF THYME

CHAPTER 1   The Rattlesnake King   **23**

CHAPTER 2   Mother Nature   **37**

CHAPTER 3   Wholesome as a Glass of Milk   **54**

CHAPTER 4   Kessler vs. Kessler   **72**

CHAPTER 5   Ancient Chinese Remedy   **104**

PART 2 ALTERNATIVE UNIVERSE

CHAPTER 6   What's Really in That Bottle?   **135**

CHAPTER 7   One a Day   **163**

CHAPTER 8   Women and Children First   **182**

CHAPTER 9   Shark Bait   **201**

CONTENTS
viii

CHAPTER 10 Looking for Mr. Natural **225**

CHAPTER 11 Proof **241**

CONCLUSION What We Can Do **262**

ACKNOWLEDGMENTS **273**
NOTES **275**
INDEX **309**

NATURAL CAUSES

PROLOGUE
SUE GILLIATT'S NOSE

Seen at a distance, from the sidewalk of her home on the south side of Indianapolis, Sue Gilliatt looks as pretty as ever. With a warm, shy smile, intelligent blue eyes, and shoulder-length chestnut hair, she appears younger than her forty-nine years. Not until you reach the steps of her wraparound porch and walk under the gingerbread trim adorning her 1869 home does it become clear that something has happened to her face. The bridge of her nose doesn't rise up from her face as one normally would, and the left nostril is misshapen, with a white scar below it.

"Most people assume I've been in a car wreck and went through the windshield," Sue says unselfconsciously.

Inside, the austerity of the hardwood floors and doors is heightened by the spare furnishings. The dining room has no dinner table. Antique lighting fixtures hang from the ceiling, incense fills the air, and two bookshelves in the corner of the living room are filled with Frank Herbert's *Dune*, the works of Lewis Carroll, a book on Einstein's theory of relativity, another on astrology, a copy of the Kabbalah, *The Gnostic Bible*, *The Herbal Drugstore*, and *Encyclopedia of Natural Medicine*. In the kitchen, three pumpkins grown in the backyard rest on the counter beside eight bottles of supplements: flaxseed oil, vitamin E, biotin, magnesium, Citrical Plus, folic acid, Coenzyme-q-10, and a multivitamin. Next to the kitchen is a room where Sue keeps ten cats and kittens she's rescued over the years from the street and local shelters.

Dressed in blue jeans, a blue wool sweater, and black slippers, Sue fixes a cup of tea and explains that it was concern about her looks—fear, really—that started everything. "I was trying to avoid disfigurement," she says. "And look what I got."

And so she begins telling her story.

⬭ ⬭ ⬭

The oldest of six, part Cherokee on her mother's side, Sue came of age in the late 1960s and early 1970s. Although she was something of a back-to-nature "flower child," in 1973 she obtained a degree as a licensed practical nurse. She married, then divorced, bought the house where she lives to this day, and worked as a nurse at a nearby hospital.

In mid-June of 2001, a few weeks after going fishing with her mother on Mother's Day, Sue noticed a pink area about the size of a pencil eraser on the left side of the bridge of her nose. Irregularly shaped and covered with flaky skin, it turned raw and red after she scratched at it—all worrisome signs of possible skin cancer, she knew. A few years earlier, she had developed a somewhat similar spot on her left hip, but that one had a regular oval shape, a better prognostic sign.

The treatment of the earlier spot on her hip had left Sue leery of her primary care doctor's judgment. He had diagnosed it as a cyst, but she felt certain it wasn't one. When he prepared to remove it in a simple outpatient procedure in his office, he first injected her with a local anesthetic, but did not prep the site with alcohol or any other sterilizer. Realizing he needed his nurse to assist him, he walked to the door with his sterile gloves on, opened the door, asked the nurse to come in, and returned to complete the procedure without changing his gloves. Sue ended up developing an infection at the site and needed three more office visits, and three rounds of antibiotics, to treat it. And the "cyst," as her doctor had called it, turned out to be a benign tumor called a dermatofibroma.

And so when Sue finally went to see the same doctor again for the spot on her nose—after waiting until the last day of August, hoping it would just go away and wishing she could head straight to a dermatologist rather than seeing her primary care doctor first, as required by her HMO—she did not entirely trust his diagnosis. Dermatitis, he called it: a mild irritation of the skin. A scab had formed over the sore and normal skin had begun to grow, but Sue could still see a subtle discoloration underneath. Peering in the mirror, she thought the "lesion," as she called it—some type of cancer, she felt certain—was moving deeper into the lower layers of her skin and spreading toward her left eye. But she had gotten what she wanted from the doctor: a referral to a dermatologist.

The first appointment she could get was not until October 1—a whole month away. Nervous and afraid that the cancer might spread and become untreatable by then, she found herself thinking about a traditional Native American salve for skin disorders: bloodroot. Vaguely recollecting that it was used to treat skin cancer, warts, and moles, she decided to investigate it.

That an educated person like Sue would consider using an herbal remedy to treat something as serious as cancer is hardly surprising; in fact, surveys show that she is precisely the typical kind of person to do so. A 1998 survey in the *Journal of the American Medical Association* found that usage of alternative medicine is most frequent among people between the ages of thirty-six and forty-nine with a college education and an income of over $50,000. Another survey published that same year in the *Journal of the American Dietetic Association* found that a staggering 80.9 percent of women who had been diagnosed with breast cancer in the past four years had used a dietary supplement, and that older, more educated white women were more likely to have done so than younger, less educated minorities. The more advanced the breast cancer had been, the survey found, the likelier the women were to have used "miscellaneous" products, such as shark cartilage. Desperate people, the survey seemed to suggest, are more willing to give anything a try.

Searching for information about bloodroot on Google in hopes of finding a reliable, credible source, she got a hit from the Web site of Andrew Weil, MD, director of the University of Arizona College of Medicine's interactive medicine program, former researcher at the Harvard Botanical Museum, and author of the best-selling books *Spontaneous Healing, Eight Weeks to Optimum Health*, and *Healthy Aging*. With his bald head and white beard, the smiling Weil had by then become the alternative medicine guru of his generation. There, published on his site on July 31, 1996 (and still there until it disappeared from the site by January 2005), was a short article about bloodroot.

"Bloodroot," he wrote, "or *Sanguinaria canadensis,* is a small woodland herb that grows in the North Central United States and Canada. The red juice from the root was a very popular remedy among Plains Indians—and later, the European settlers—for sore throats, respiratory problems, and growths on the skin." A few sentences later, he wrote: "Externally, it has a unique ability to dissolve abnormal growths without disturbing normal tissue. So people continue to use it for moles, warts, and some kinds of external cancers."

After citing a book that describes the use of bloodroot for cancer, he continued: "I've been overwhelmed with requests for information about the availability of bloodroot to dissolve skin growths since I published *Spontaneous Healing* (Fawcett Book Group, 1996). I want to emphasize that bloodroot paste is in a different league from the herbal remedies I usually recommend, since its actions are drastic. If you're interested in using it, please inform yourself carefully about its properties and risks. And use it with great caution." He then listed four companies that, he wrote, "supply information and bloodroot products." Third on the list was Alpha Omega Labs, with a post office box in Nassau, the Bahamas, and an 800 telephone number. At the bottom of the list was a digital reproduction of Dr. Weil's signature.

Searching again on Google, Sue found the official Web site for Alpha Omega Labs at www.altcancer.com, which remains up and running to this day. The information she found there indicated the kind of respect for traditional remedies shared by Dr. Weil. But whereas Dr. Weil has built his considerable reputation on bridging the gap between mainstream and alternative medicine, Alpha Omega took a decidedly hostile attitude toward what it called the "Medical Industrial Complex."

"The current orthodox system of treating illness," states Alpha Omega's welcome page, "is not only monopolistic, but it prevents safe, inexpensive, and often more effective treatments from reaching the mainstream." Using arguments remarkably reminiscent of those used by snake oil salesmen of a hundred years earlier, the company insists that the many scientific studies proving the worth of the company's products have been censored by the modern medical industry, which it says controls the media, politicians, academic researchers—everybody, apparently, except the good folks at Alpha Omega. The site spins a vision of a world conspiracy in which good medicines are being withheld from a hoodwinked public by a horde of money-loving doctors. As proof of their products' efficacy, Alpha Omega offers none of the studies it claims to know about but instead proffers the classic gimmick of snake oil ads from the nineteenth century: the money-back guarantee. "No doctor, hospital or pharmacy in the world, which we are aware of, offers this kind of guarantee," they assert.

Reading through the site, Sue quickly found that while it did offer bloodroot, it strongly recommended another product for skin cancer: Cansema, "the internationally recognized skin cancer treatment system." For a price of $49.95 per jar, the site proclaimed, Cansema was guaranteed to be 100 percent effective in removing any type of skin cancer, including the often fatal melanoma.

In detail, the site described how Cansema works, including graphic step-by-step photographs that lend an air of unflinching honesty. To achieve its miraculous result, the site stated, Cansema "necroses the aberrant tissue (i.e., kills the cancer cells), creates an 'eschar' (what would appear to the layman as a pus formation)—after which the body itself expels the 'scab,' leaving a pit ('decavitated area')." The pit heals over within a few weeks, according to the site, leaving behind a "depigmented area," which likewise heals over within a few months or years. While acknowledging that the product contains zinc chloride—a caustic that "will cause serious burns if applied in high concentrations"—Alpha Omega went on to say that the zinc chloride in Cansema is in quantities too small to cause such damage.

A page listing the side effects conveyed an even more dramatic sense of forthright truthfulness. For some who try it, the site conceded, reactions to Cansema "may even be a bit frightening." To begin with, the size of the "eschar" will usually be twice as big as the cancerous lesion appeared to be on the surface, but only because "many people have far more cancer activity 'beneath the skin' than is visible on the surface." Next, Cansema will cause pus to drain from the site. Larger tumors might develop heavy "weeping" requiring frequent bandage changes. Third, the surrounding skin and muscles, even joints, will almost always look inflamed after applying the product. And finally, there will usually be some pain associated with the treatment, "from mild . . . to considerable. Our experience is that at its worst, Cansema is rarely more painful than that to be endured in the healing process that follows surgery."

As to the question of whether or not Cansema could be legally sold in the United States, the site described the issue as "complex." It was not approved by the FDA, the site conceded, and no specific health claims could be made for it. One would wonder, then, why the FDA hadn't approved such an effective remedy. Because, the site claimed, the FDA is only looking out for the big pharmaceutical companies. "There can be no greater example of corruption in government," the site states, "than an instance of a federal body suppressing compounds that save lives just so a select group can milk the citizenry for the maximum amount of health dollars with second-rate, but 'approved' drugs and deadly, questionable therapies, such as chemotherapy."

Of course, there is a great deal of truth in the company's harsh indictment. Many drug companies *do* milk the citizenry. Many medicines *are* exorbitantly priced. Chemotherapy, not to mention many other approved drugs, *can* prove deadly. And since the 1990s, the FDA *has* come under increasing criticism for cozying up to the pharmaceutical companies it regulates. Such failings of the country's traditional healthcare system go a long way toward explaining why so many are drawn to alternative treatments that are less expensive and, their makers claim, perfectly safe because they are perfectly natural.

⊂⊃　⊂⊃　⊂⊃

Sue didn't stop with the Alpha Omega Web site. She also checked out www.skincanceranswer.com, run by a Reverend Dan Raber. "WARNING!" the site, still up and running in 2006, shouted in large red letters. Without aid of a proofreader, it continued: "The information offered in [sic] not approved by the F.D.A., AMA, FTC or any other Federal or State agency. If you believe you need protection or permission from the Government 'State and Federal ABC groups' please leave this site immediately."

What caught Sue's eye, as she considered the possibility that even minor outpatient surgery on her nose could leave a permanent scar, was the section where Rev. Raber stated that his bloodroot salve "was a very selective cancer and pathogen treatment, eradicating only the malignant tissue." The salve, he claimed, was "selective (destroying only malignant mass with a minimum of damage to surrounding tissue)."

On September 15, Sue picked up the telephone to call Rev. Raber's office but reached only an answering machine. Sue doesn't like answering machines, so she didn't leave a message. Instead, she went online and ordered a jar of Cansema over Alpha Omega's Web site. Three days later, on September 18, she called Raber's office again, got through this time, and ordered his bloodroot paste.

On Friday, September 21, the Cansema salve arrived from Alpha Omega Labs. The small jar contained a half ounce of a thick black paste with the consistency of peanut butter. After showering, she applied a small bit directly to the spot on her nose, covered it with a transparent Band-Aid, and went to work at Community Hospital East. It tingled, causing a mild pain all through her shift in the renal oncology ward, where she cared for patients suffering from renal failure or cancer. But the mild pain was exactly what she had expected, based on the stern warnings on Alpha Omega's Web site.

That night, after arriving back home, Sue removed the bandage and noticed a milky white-yellow scab—again, pretty much as predicted. She put on a second application, this time over her entire nose, from between her eyes to the base of the bridge, and some adjacent area on her left cheek. She wanted to be sure she got all of the "metastases," as she thought of them. And, after all, the Alpha Omega site had assured her that the salve would not harm healthy tissue.

She went to bed but woke up within a few hours. The tingling had turned to a painful burning. The brochure accompanying the salve had instructed her to keep it on for a full twenty-four hours to kill all the cancer, but at six a.m. she could stand it no longer. Sue got out of bed and washed the salve off.

The black paste now removed, the face Sue saw looking back at her in the mirror was not the one she had gone to bed with. Her nose was covered by a white scaly eruption with a clear discharge. The skin underneath was discolored a frightful yellow. It looked horrible, she thought—like something out of a freak show.

Still, she was not afraid. A stoic nurse who had seen far worse in her day, she knew the reaction was still following the description outlined in

Alpha Omega's Web site. In fact, her main concern was that she had not left the Cansema on long enough for it to destroy all the cancer cells. So she covered it with Vaseline and sat tight.

On Monday, when the bloodroot paste arrived from Rev. Raber's company, Sue followed the accompanying instructions and applied it to her nose. She covered it with a Band-Aid and went to work.

"Oh my God, what happened to you?" a coworker asked her that day. "Your face is all puffy and your eyes are nearly swollen shut."

She explained that she was using a treatment for a skin condition, and just kept working—despite growing side effects that had not been described by either Rev. Raber or Alpha Omega: nausea, profound tiredness, rapidly beating heart, and extreme thirst. But she didn't leave work early. She prided herself on being a tough bird.

First thing Tuesday morning, at 8:32 a.m., according to her phone bill, she called not her primary care doctor, not the dermatologist she was still scheduled to see in a week, but Rev. Raber in Abbeville, Georgia. That she, a nurse, would still not call to tell a doctor what was happening to her at this point may seem puzzling, but in fact it's typical for users of alternative medicines to hide what they're doing from physicians, in great part because they believe that traditional doctors will neither understand nor support their use of such products. A study presented in October 2005 at the annual meeting of the American Society for Therapeutic Radiology and Oncology found that 75 percent of cancer patients don't tell their doctors when they use alternative medicines.

Sue spoke with Rev. Raber for forty minutes. She told him that the skin on her nose was forming a scar. She told him that she'd used another product called Cansema, but it had burned so badly that she wasn't able to keep it on for the recommended twenty-four hours. She told him that she had used his bloodroot paste for twelve hours. She told him about the side effects. And then she told him, "I need you to advise me what to do next."

"Make another application," Rev. Raber said. "Cover it with Saran Wrap. Leave it on for twenty-four hours and then remove it."

So she did. Six days later, having spent the intervening days sterilizing her nose with hydrogen peroxide, soaking it in a mild saltwater solution, and covering it with Vaseline, Sue finally had her appointment with the dermatologist: Christopher G. Rehme, MD, a past president of the Indiana State Dermatology Society.

On her medical record, Dr. Rehme described her appearance: "There is a thick, yellow, necrotic eschar present on the nose with a serious drainage," he wrote. "The nose is severely necrotic." *Necrosis,* according to *Webster*'s, means "localized death of living tissue." And yet, he noted, "The patient appears to be tolerating this well."

He gave her a work excuse so as not to expose her face to any bacteria, advised her to stop taking any further bloodroot products and to continue the saltwater soaks and Vaseline, gave her a prescription for the painkiller Darvocet, and scheduled a follow-up visit for one week later.

Back home, Sue called Rev. Raber again. He insisted once more that everything was going as expected and suggested she buy two more supplements to be taken by mouth, to help the healing process. The first one was pancreatic enzymes, which, according to his Web site, are the body's natural way "to digest the malignant tumor cells." He also recommended she buy methyl sulphonyl methane, a form of sulfur advocated by many natural food sites to strengthen bones, toughen the immune system, build muscles, clear acne, heal scars, relieve arthritis, boost energy, improve memory, sharpen hearing and vision, and ease constipation. She ordered both products, but with no intention of using them, having begun to suspect that the reverend was a charlatan and that she might need to have evidence in the event of a lawsuit.

Then she called Alpha Omega's toll-free number and got a guy named George on the line. George didn't give her his last name, but he did tell her what her problem was: the pH level of her skin was too acidic, indicating the presence of cancer. And he knew just what would cure it: H3O and HRx.

According to Alpha Omega's brochure, H3O and HRx are the "backbone" of the company's research into pH "adjusting formulas." The brochure states:

When tested analytically, our H3O appears to be nothing more than a diluted form of sulphuric [sic] acid. In reality it exhibits none of the properties of sulphuric [sic] acid—regardless of . . . concentration. This is because it is, in reality, a stabilized form of "hydronium" (H3O). . . . When diluted by about 1:120 (1 fl. oz. to a gallon of distilled water), H3O can be used in countless applications with excellent results, according to our users: athlete's feet [sic], eczema, gastrointeritis [sic], halitosis (via gargling), herpes sores, insect bites, lice, conjunctivitis (pink eye), sunburns, cuts and bruises, etc. One reputable scientist with whom we work calls H3O "one of the single greatest medical finds of our time."

When George had said over the phone that her skin's pH level indicated the presence of cancer, she decided he was lying to her. With her twenty-nine years of experience as a nurse, she knew that no pH test, the sort used by gardeners to gauge whether their soil needs lime, had ever been used to diagnose cancer. So she ordered both the H3O and HRx, but only in case she might need them for a lawsuit.

Even then, however, the appearance of her nose was pretty much following the course described by the Alpha Omega Web site. A large scab would form. Check. Pus would drain out. Check. The surrounding skin would become inflamed. Check. And there would be some pain. Check, check, check, check. Rev. Raber's Web site had specifically warned, after all, that the two major obstacles to following the treatment course were fear and lack of persistence.

Three days after seeing Dr. Rehme and calling the offices of Rev. Raber and Alpha Omega to order the H3O, HRx, pancreatic enzymes, and methyl sulphonyl methane, Sue noticed that the edges of the scab around her nose were lifting up and off the rest of the surrounding skin. This would be the next stage, she figured, in which "the body itself expels the 'scab.' " At this point, the scab smelled foul. Looking carefully in her bathroom mirror, she saw that it was hanging on by only a thin strand at the top, between her eyes. Being a nurse, she knew what had to be done. She took out some scissors, snipped the strand, and pulled off the scab.

When she looked back up to inspect her face in the mirror again, she saw what Alpha Omega had described as the "decavitated area." Where her nostrils had been, two gaping holes remained. The tip and bridge of her nose were livid red, without skin. Turning to the side, she saw what had happened: her nose was gone.

She didn't scream. She didn't cry. She was, after all, a tough bird. And something was telling her that she could get through this. Not a voice, but a presence that calmed and supported her. She was not really religious, but she had a strong spirituality that, she felt, harkened back to her Native American ancestry. She knew that God has things happen for a reason.

She called Rev. Raber and told him that her entire nose had come off. He told her not to worry.

"It will grow back," he said.

At that point, Sue could no longer delude herself. *I've been had,* she thought. *These people have lied to me.*

$\bigcirc \ \bigcirc \ \bigcirc$

It wasn't the first time that the owner of Alpha Omega Labs, Gregory James Caton, had lied to someone. In 1990, the U.S. attorney for the western district of Louisiana went after him for his role in a conspiracy to print phony money at the printing press where he worked. Caton pled guilty to conspiracy to counterfeit, a felony punishable by imprisonment for a term exceeding one year.

But the résumé on his Web site doesn't mention that. From 1981 to 1983, it states, Caton was the "founder/president" of Richland Foods, which developed soy-based meat replacements. The next entry on the résumé reads: "Founder, Consumer Express, 1984," referring to a multilevel marketing company that later became Nutrition for Life International, "a multimillion-dollar company now traded on the NASDAQ." (The company, which sold homeopathic, skin care, herbal, and vitamin products, filed for bankruptcy on July 8, 2003, and went out of business.)

Also not mentioned on his Web site is that in February of 1997, a U.S. district court judge in Houston ordered him to pay $133.2 million in damages for libel and slander against Nutrition for Life. Apparently, he hadn't liked the direction the company had taken after it became Nutrition for Life and had strongly criticized it in a 1990 book he'd published, *MLM Fraud: A Practical Handbook for the Network Marketing Professional.* The company's libel lawsuit against him claimed that Caton had made false assertions about the company and its principal salesman, Kevin Trudeau. The judge ordered Caton to withdraw all copies of his book from store shelves, forbade him from producing or distributing any additional copies, and demanded he turn over all negatives and typesetting files used for the printing of it. And he ordered Caton never to discuss

Nutrition for Life again, negatively or positively. (Trudeau, another ex-con, went on to fame as the creator of the Coral Calcium infomercials and the author of the number one bestseller *Natural Cures "They" Don't Want You to Know About.*)

Greg Caton—burly, baby-faced, and just two years younger than Sue Gilliatt—has been in the herbal and alternative food world for most of his adult life. On his Web page listing "50 Reasons Why I Am a Vegetarian," which plays mellow New Age music when viewed on a Web browser, reason 18 is "cancer prevention." Reason 46 is "world peace." And reason 47 is "clear conscience." In 1986, according to Caton's résumé, he founded another manufacturer of soy-based meat replacements, Lumen Foods, based in Lake Charles, Louisiana. The company, according to its Web site, sells to "retail, commercial, industrial, military and government accounts. Packaged, bulk, and private label. Foreign and domestic." Its Web site has the enviable address www.soybean.com.

But by September of 2003, the U.S. Food and Drug Administration, as well as the Federal Trade Commission, was wondering if Caton was lying, again, this time about the true location of Alpha Omega Labs. Although its Web site cited the company's headquarters as being in Nassau, the Bahamas, the federal agencies believed that all its manufacturing and administrative activities were happening in Louisiana, on the same property where Caton ran Lumen Foods. Such deception, if true, could be a potential violation of federal labeling laws.

In addition, the FDA had begun to get wind of cases in which patients had suffered serious harm from Alpha Omega products. Sue's was one; another was that of Sharon Lee of Mexia, Texas. When the thirty-three-year-old mother of two underwent a hysterectomy at Parkview Regional Hospital in Mexia in January of 2002, the physician who performed the procedure used Alpha Omega's H3O to irrigate the wound and speed the healing process. After suffering nausea, fever, and vomiting postoperatively, she ended up with complications that kept her in the hospital for thirteen days. Two subsequent operations were eventually performed at another hospital to treat adhesions and a hematoma. The H3O was tested and found to contain 8 percent hydrochloric acid.

On Wednesday, September 17, 2003, agents of the FDA and FTC raided Alpha Omega's offices. In the midst of seizing products for which they believed Alpha Omega had made illegal health claims, they found some things that a convicted felon is not supposed to have: ten guns, ten thousand rounds of ammunition, and two full suits of body armor, including helmets, jackets, and leggings. Caton was arrested and jailed in Lafayette, Louisiana, initially on charges of possession of a firearm by a prior convicted felon, which carry a mandatory minimum prison sentence of five years.

By early 2004, Alpha Omega's Web site declared: "We have a legal fund set up at this time in hopes of donations... for representation against any charges that the FDA may bring against Alpha Omega in the near future." The Donation to the Caton Legal Fund could be mailed to a post office box. Or, "if you would like to donate with a credit card," the page stated, you could e-mail them or call their toll-free line.

In May of 2004, Caton pled guilty to two counts: devising a scheme to defraud victims via interstate commerce, and introducing unapproved new drugs (Cansema and H3O) into interstate commerce. On August 24, 2004, U.S. district judge Tucker Melancon of Lafayette, Louisiana, sentenced Caton to thirty-three months in prison, to be followed by three years of supervised release and forfeiture of the $950,000 in assets he'd earned from his scheme. Having already served more than a year, he was released in March of 2006. An announcement placed on his Web site the same month he was sentenced stated: "For the time being, Alpha Omega Labs remains an 'information site' only. Its manufacturing capabilities are currently being setup [sic] in Central America and Eastern Europe by a new ownership that will be fully operational sometime in the fall of 2004. We would have liked to have some vestige of the operation in the U.S., but the virulent opposition to alternative health care in that country makes this impossible."

⊂⊃ ⊂⊃ ⊂⊃

The summer of 2005 proved eventful for Rev. Dan Raber. He settled a lawsuit that Sue had brought against him; FDA agents raided his business; Dr. Lois March, an ear, nose, and throat specialist who worked with him to provide pain management medication to his patients, was charged by Georgia's Composite State Board of Medical Examiners of aiding and abetting Raber's practice; and Raber himself became the focus of an investigation by the same board for practicing medicine without a license.

The medical board said it knew of seven breast cancer patients who had been treated by Raber with Dr. March's assistance, and that the bloodroot paste had "mutilated their breasts and caused excruciating pain." Another patient, who had applied the paste to his shoulder, was burned so badly by it that bone was exposed. Both Rev. Raber and Dr. March denied the charges, and Raber's Web site, www.cancerx.org, continued to sell his products.

Raber lives in Abbeville, Georgia, a rural town of three square miles and some 2,300 residents. When asked about him, a clerk at the local police station said, "Oh, Lord—he's the type, one minute he's trying to preach to you about God, the next minute he'll be attending DUI class." Police chief Cory Parker confirmed that Raber has been convicted of driving under the influence. "He's had a few run-ins, but that's all," Chief Parker said. "He lives right up the street." Although he didn't know anything about Raber's business, he described him as "an unpredictable person. You don't know what he'll do from one minute to the next."

Reached by telephone at his home, Raber said, "You don't have to call me Reverend. I'm Dan. I do object to anyone calling me doctor. I don't want to make a medical claim that I have any medical expertise. What I have is twenty-twenty hindsight. I know this sounds a little anti-intellectual, and I am, to the point where if it don't work, we don't have nothing to do with it. The bottom line is, does it or does it not work?"

He works regularly with medical doctors, he said, which he keeps "top secret." "When people come here, before anything they go to a medical examination, which I'll pay for. Many doctors refer their patients to me. I've taken tumors off an oncologist."

Asked if he was truly a reverend, Raber answered, "I was ordained by a Lutheran minister back in 1972, but I don't trade on that much. I'm a spiritual person, not religious. I believe in God but I don't believe in the amenities the churches offer." Was he a practicing churchgoer? "Not really," he said. "But I practice my faith every minute." In fact, he said, he was going that evening to a meeting of what he called a "Bible-type community, in the middle of Georgia. We're survivalists. God has instructed us. We expect tough times coming: economic collapse of the system as we know it. But to prepare ourselves, we know how to take food and sustenance from the land. We know how to hunt. We have beef cattle. Plus we have seven ponds stocked full of fish, and we have twenty-five thousand gallons of diesel fuel."

Raber started selling his bloodroot salve in 1992, when he met a man who said that he'd found a hundred-year-old recipe in a barn with the residue of the product in a jar and had used it to cure his skin cancer. Raber and the man cured a couple other people of various skin ailments using the recipe, and then Raber's brother and another friend helped improve the formula. "We worked it over to make the molecules fit," Raber said. "We normalized it. We changed it into a formula that worked better and faster."

The bottom line, he said, was this: "We've helped over three to four thousand people in the thirteen years we've been doing this. And we're not dialing for dollars. The Bible teaches: Go to all the world and heal the sick, provide neither gold nor silver for your purse. I could be a really good hustler. I could be a con artist. To stay away from that, I stay away from the money aspect, so I'm not money driven. We've worked for many years helping people on a donation basis only. Nobody has ever been turned away."

As for Sue, she has so far undergone six operations to reconstruct her nose. Bone was removed from her sternum, cartilage from a rib, and flesh from her forehead to replace what had been lost. Further operations will be necessary to widen her nasal passages and lengthen the tip of her nose to a more normal appearance. She has received countless steroid injections and laser treatments to relieve scarring. A lawsuit she filed against Alpha Omega was settled for an undisclosed sum that resulted in no apparent improvement in her lifestyle.

"I think I was had by con men," Sue says, displaying remarkably little anger. "I'm a trusting person. They gave specific instructions and reassurances that it wouldn't harm healthy tissue. They had pictures and testimonials. And the fact that Alpha Omega's site was listed on Andrew Weil's site as a source for bloodroot made it appear to be legitimate."

⊂⊃ ⊂⊃ ⊂⊃

As horrible as Sue's story is, the bigger horror is how common the sale of similarly fraudulent supplements has become in the United States today, how fully the most educated of consumers believe in their worth, and how frequently injuries and deaths have followed. Today, a staggering 62 percent of Americans use some kind of dietary supplements—whether vitamins, herbs, or so-called specialty products like melatonin or glucosamine—according to a 2004 survey commissioned by the Council for Responsible Nutrition. One fourth of U.S. adults, a total of 50,613,000, have used an herb or other nonvitamin, nonmineral supplement, according to the 2002 National Health Interview Survey (NHIS) conducted by the Centers for Disease Control and Prevention. The same survey also found that 7,379,000 adults have taken a homeopathic treatment (or 3.6 percent of all adults), and that 7,935,000 (or 3.9 percent) have taken high-dose megavitamins. According to Grant Ferrier, editor of *Nutrition Business Journal,* consumers spent more than $21.2 billion on supplements of all kinds in 2005, "and the 2006 forecast is $22.0 billion, or growth of 3.5 to 4 percent, negative media notwithstanding."

Supplements today are simply everywhere: touted in best-selling books; ever present on cable TV infomercials; hawked by ex–Playboy models and respected radio newscasters alike; sold in their own aisles at CVS and Walgreens, in single-serving sizes at gas stations, and in economy-size containers at Wal-Mart and Costco; and reported on daily as important health aids by the country's newspapers and magazines. Herbs are now added to a beer sold by Anheuser-Busch; vitamins and other "heart-healthy nutrients" are in every bite of a new chocolate candy by the maker of Mars bars; herbs and vitamins are loaded into special syrups that anyone can have pumped into their shakes at Carvel ice cream shops. Parents give these substances with confidence to their children in chewable bear shapes to help them grow; athletes in high school, college, and professional sports take them to gain a competitive edge; middle-aged women take them to treat menopause; seniors take them to ward off arthritis and every other disease; the severely ill depend on them to save their lives.

Where does this confidence come from? Not from scientific studies. Contrary to the widespread belief that few vitamins or herbal remedies have undergone serious scientific scrutiny, in fact hundreds of millions of dollars have been spent since the early 1990s on carrying out thousands of reasonably well designed studies. One federal agency alone—the National Center for Complementary and Alternative Medicine (NCCAM), an arm of the National Institutes of Health—has already expended nearly a billion dollars since being established (originally as the Office of Unconventional Medicine) in 1991. President George W. Bush's 2005 budget request included $121.1 million for NCCAM, an increase of 3.3 percent over 2004, the biggest proposed percentage gain for any NIH center or institute that year—and its annual budget has remained steady since then through fiscal year 2007. Dozens of academic institutes devoted to the study of alternative therapies, including dietary supplements, have also sprung up at universities around the country in the past twelve years, including Columbia University's Rosenthal Center for Complementary and Alternative Medicine, the Program in Integrative Medicine at the University of Arizona, Duke University's Center for Integrative Medicine, and Harvard University's Division for Research and Education in Complementary and Integrative Medical Therapies. As of 2005, a search on the Web site of the National Library of Medicine pulls up 1,307 studies on the use of melatonin for sleep, 59 on echinacea for the common cold, 92 on zinc for the common cold, 147 on vitamin C for the common cold, 378 on chondroitin for osteoarthritis, 270 on St. John's wort for depression, 41 on saw palmetto for the prostate, 37 on black cohosh for menopause, 83 on gingko to sharpen cognition, 205 on garlic to lower cholesterol, and 2,098 on vitamin E for the prevention of heart disease. And the startling conclusion of all this work—sad, shocking, incomprehensible—is that, with the possible exception of fish oil and vitamin D, no other herb, vitamin or specialty product, not even a daily multivitamin, has been shown to be both safe and effective for improving or preserving the health of most men, women, and children. A few vitamins and minerals, it is true, have been proven beneficial, even lifesaving during particular stages of life, such as iron to prevent anemia in menstruating women, or folic acid to prevent birth defects. But most of these are already added to so many foods that taking them as supplements is unnecessary. And in any case, the vast majority of the supplements taken by Americans have been proven to be unsafe, ineffective, or both. Vitamin E has now been shown in many large studies to actually *raise* the risk of heart failure and death; "natural" sources of progesterone may raise women's risk of breast cancer; multivitamins have been shown to raise children's risk of developing asthma and food allergies, and iron supplements are the leading cause of pediatric poisoning in the United States.

Since it was formed in 1983, the American Association of Poison Control Centers has kept statistics on reports of poisonings for every type of substance, including for dietary supplements. That first year, there were 14,006 reports related to the use of vitamins, minerals, essential oils (widely sold in supplement stores for a variety of uses), and homeopathic remedies. Herbs didn't even have a category that year, as they were so rarely used then. Twenty two years later, in 2004, the AAPCC reported a staggering 126,507 incidents related to supplements, with almost as many for herbs alone—12,331, for everything from echinacea to ginseng and ginkgo biloba—as for the entire category of supplements back in 1983. In all, over the twenty-two-year span, AAPCC has received a total of 1,534,232 reports of adverse reaction to dietary supplements—more than a million and a half—including 236,879 that were serious enough to require hospitalization. Even numbers such as these, however, represent a gross undercount, as evidenced by the case of a single company, Metabolife, which in 2002 revealed that it alone had received 14,684 injury reports from its customers in the prior six years.

The number of deaths directly caused by supplements is harder to know, because doctors and families rarely suspect them as a cause of death and manufacturers have not been required to report the deaths to any government agency when they learn about them. For what it's worth, U.S. poison centers received a total of 203 reports of deaths due to supplements between 1983 and 2004, with the yearly numbers leaping from just 4 in 1994 to a record 23 in 2004. Another key source for assessing the numbers of deaths is the FDA. In April of 2004, the agency revealed that it had received a total of 260 reports of deaths associated with herbal remedies since 1989. But a March 2000 study prepared for the FDA by Alexander M. Walker, MD, then the chair of the department of epidemiology at the Harvard School of Public Health, concluded: "A best estimate is that less than one percent of serious adverse events caused by dietary supplements is reported to the FDA. The true proportion may well be smaller by an order of magnitude or more." This would mean that the true number of deaths due to supplements since 1989 is at least 26,000.

Yet faith in their benefits seems Teflon-coated, impervious to the results of scientific studies. So fully has the public embraced the view that doctors, scientists, giant pharmaceutical companies, (sometimes referred to as "Big Pharma"), government agencies, and even consumer-protection groups are engaged in a grand conspiracy to deny them wholesome, inexpensive life-saving treatments that a widely condemned book written by an ex-con supplement huckster, Kevin Trudeau, has become a best seller by offering up a fundamentally paranoiac view of the world: *Natural Cures "They" Don't Want You to Know About.* In 2004—the very year the FDA finally banned the herbal stimulant ephedra after more than 19,000 people had suffered strokes, heart attacks, convulsions, psychoses, and death—a survey of U.S. adults found that 78 percent were still somewhat or very confident in the safety, quality, and effectiveness of supplements in general, and that 66 percent believed in the safety of herbal remedies in particular.

Unbeknownst to the public, such views have been methodically manipulated by a powerful industry that in 1994 succeeded in strong-arming a law through Congress that turned the clock back a hundred years on the regulation of their products. That law, the Dietary Supplement Health and Education Act (DSHEA), left the FDA virtually powerless to regulate supplements, which explains why the agency took so long to ban ephedra, and why the ban was promptly overturned a year later by a Utah judge. Yet a recent Harris poll found that 68 percent of Americans believe the government requires herbal manufacturers to report potential side effects or dangers (untrue), 58 percent believe the FDA must approve herbal products before they can be sold (untrue), and 55 percent believe that manufacturers cannot make claims for their safety or efficacy without firm scientific evidence (untrue).

How has it come to this? How has the United States of America, at a time of unprecedented twenty-first-century scientific and medical advancement—and having survived the horrors of thalidomide and DDT—found itself plagued by remedies redolent of the snake oil era of a hundred years past? A search for the answer begins with a journey back to those days, indeed back to ancient times and practices, before an understanding can be had of why supplements were finally embraced by the mainstream in the age of Big Pharma and Big Macs.

PART 1

A BRIEF HISTORY OF THYME

CHAPTER 1

THE RATTLESNAKE KING

There really was a snake oil. A hundred years ago, during the great patent medicine era, American consumers could buy Tex Bailey's Rattle Snake Oil (made not in Texas but in Troy, N.Y.); Tex Allen's Rattlesnake Essential Oil Compound, recommended for "rheumatic pains, back pain, strains, sprains, bruises, sores, aching feet, stiff joints, sore muscles, throat irritation, headache, earache, and more" (manufactured in Newark, N.J.); Rattlesnake Bill's Liniment, "made from the fat of a real diamondback rattlesnake" (manufactured in exotic Belleville, N.J.); the Great Yaquis Snake-Oil Liniment; Blackhawks Indian Liniment Oil; Monster Brand Snake Oil; and Mack Mahon the Rattle Snake Oil King's Liniment for Rheumatism and Catarrh.

Far from having the negative connotation we give it today, snake oil in those days was sold on the basis of Americans' infatuation with cowboys, the Old West, and Indians. No one better exploited that fascination than Clark Stanley, another self-crowned "Rattle Snake King." In a fifty-page booklet he published in 1897, Stanley gave the first twenty-five pages over to the colorful life of cowboys before devoting the remaining pages to the wonders of snake oil. With handlebar mustache, goatee, broad-brimmed hat, boots, kerchief, and jeans, he certainly looked the part of a cowboy. The story he told of his life was a compelling one: Born in Abilene, Texas, around the time of the Civil War, he lived the life of a cowboy from the age of fourteen to twenty-five. Then, in the spring of 1879, he followed some of his father's friends to Walpi, Arizona, to see the snake dance of the Moki (now known as the Hopi) Indians.

"There I became acquainted with the medicine man of the Moki tribe," Stanley wrote in his booklet, "and as he liked the looks of my Colt's revolver and asked me to show him how it would shoot, I gave him an exhibition of my fancy shooting, which pleased him very much; he then asked me how I would like to stay there and live with him, I told him I would stay until the snake dance." After witnessing the dance, his father's friends left, but Stanley decided to stay on, and he lived with the Moki for two years and five months.

"I learned their language and dances and the secret of making their medicines," he wrote. "The medicine that interested me most was their Snake Oil Medicine as they called it. It is used for rheumatism, contracted cords and all aches and pains. As I was thought a great deal of by the medicine man, he gave me the secret of making the Snake Oil Medicine, which is now named Clark Stanley's Snake Oil Liniment. Snake Oil is not a new discovery, it has been in use by the Mokis and other Indian tribes for many generations, and I have made an improvement on the original formula."

There are no independent historic documents attesting to how much, if any, of Stanley's story is true. But he certainly seemed to know a great deal about the cowboy life, and it is accurate that the Hopi Indians held snake dances in Walpi, Arizona; President Teddy Roosevelt would attend one in the summer of 1913. But in any case, Stanley's story continued with the turning point that stories such as these almost always have: he tried it on some friends and neighbors back home, and it was such a great cure that soon he was manufacturing it and selling it with great success. By his account, Stanley traveled the West and Southwest for some ten years, selling his snake oil "with unbounded success."

Then came the 1893 World's Columbian Exhibition in Chicago—the largest public event in the history of the United States to date, where President Grover Cleveland threw an electric switch to open it, the Ferris wheel made its international debut, and more than 25 million people attended during its six-month course. Here, dressed in his colorful cowboy outfit, Stanley made a show of handling snakes.

In the only surviving interview of Stanley conducted by an independent source, he described his routine this way: "The audience see [sic] me kill the snakes, draw out the oil and put it into a glass dish. Then I walk down among them and show it to them. Then, I go back and here is a big glass jar, like you make orangeade in. First, I put the snake oil in, and then I put nine other oils in which have previously been mixed in a can, so that they don't see all of what my formula is. I pour that in on top of the snake oil, turn the mixture around, and if it doesn't mix thoroughly, looks a little cloudy, I stir it again. Then I let it set for just a moment, and it becomes clear."

Then he would sell the freshly prepared snake oil liniment, along with many other bottles previously made. As the months passed, he met druggists from across the United States, including one from Boston who persuaded him to move there and open a manufacturing plant.

So it was that, according to a copy of a *Boston Transcript* article reprinted in Stanley's booklet, a reporter found him at his office at 67 Park Street in nearby Beverly with a house full of snakes. "The snake man took the reporter up to his bedroom, and opening a light wooden box, with a wire window in the side, dove his hand into it with as much unconcern as if he were taking an egg out of a basket, and brought it out again with a snake seven feet long writhing in it." Eventually he pulled out two more large venomous snakes and allowed them to twine themselves around his body, their forked black tongues flicking in and out against his skin.

"The bite of any one of these snakes is absolutely deadly," Stanley told the reporter. "No, I am not the least afraid of being bitten. In fact, I have been bitten hundreds of times. Look here!" He showed his hands, which were covered to the wrists in tiny white scars. Not all were from poisonous snakes, he said, but he continued, "I have also been bitten by snakes which had their glands full of poison, and meant business. The reason I am not dead is because I have what I believe is the only remedy for snakebite, and there is no question that it is a perfect one."

While it is possible that Stanley gradually built up a limited immunity to venomous snake bites, as other snake handlers have done, there was not any effective "remedy" for such bites in those days. Today, the only treatment is antivenom, made by injecting small amounts of venom into an animal and then harvesting the immune cells that the animal's blood generates.

By 1901, Stanley had moved to a bigger manufacturing plant in Providence, Rhode Island, where he claimed to have killed three thousand snakes for his snake oil the previous year, as well as two thousand more at his "snake farm" in Texas. "In covered pens may be seen thousands of snakes fattened ready to be killed for their oil," a reporter wrote. "Clark Stanley says that the world is just beginning to realize the actual value of snake oil and that there are hundreds of uses to which it might be applied that are not yet recognized."

His labeling, as well as the accompanying booklet, attempted to scratch the surface of those hundreds of uses: "For Rheumatism, Neuralgia, Sciatica, Lame Back, Contracted Muscles, Sprains, Swellings, Frost Bites, Chilblains, Bruises, Sore Throat, Bites of Animals, Insects and Reptiles. Good for Man and Beast. A Liniment that penetrates Muscle, Membrane and Tissue to the very bone itself, and banishing pain with a power that has astonished the Medical Profession." Two figures illustrated the "best method for curing Partial Paralysis of the Arms." Another figure illustrated "the way to bathe the head for Neuralgia, Headache, Tic Douloureux." For the bites of animals, insects, or reptiles, Clark Stanley's Snake Oil Liniment was to "be applied as soon as possible. It kills the poison, relieves the pain, reduces the swelling and heals the wound."

⌐⌐⌐ ⌐⌐ ⌐⌐⌐

On the day Columbus first set foot in the New World at San Salvador in 1492, he wrote in his journal, "The natives brought fruit, wooden spears, and certain dried leaves which gave off a distinct fragrance." The dried leaves, it turned out, were tobacco, the first pharmacologically active herb (due to its nicotine content) brought back to Europe—not that tobacco would ever be regulated as a drug, despite being an addictive stimulant.

"When we discovered the New World, the Old World was looking for cures for diseases," says Michael R. Harris, who served as the historian of pharmacy at the Smithsonian Institution for twenty-six years before becoming the historian and curator at the Drug Enforcement Administration Museum. He also consulted as a historian to the television show *Dr. Quinn, Medicine Woman.* Beyond cures, Harris says, people wanted stimulants. That's why when tobacco, coffee, and tea all hit world markets in the sixteenth century, "they became instant hits worldwide. No drugs, except later for the amphetamines, have spread around the world so quickly."

In 1632, Catholic Jesuits who had gone to Peru brought back a powder from the cinchona tree, which natives used to bring down the fevers of malaria. In Europe, no effective treatment had been known for malaria, and physicians were soon calling the "Jesuit bark" as important a development in medicine as gunpowder was to warfare. The powder, French scientists would determine nearly two centuries later, contained quinine. When it cured the malarial fevers of King Charles II of England, it confirmed the view that great medicines could be found in the forests of the New World.

Indeed, today it is estimated that more than one fourth of modern medicines are derived from botanicals, including aspirin, from willow bark, and the cancer-fighting compound paclitaxel (Taxol), from the Pacific yew tree. Digitalis likewise is derived from foxglove, but the plant was originally used for everything from treating wounds to, as one herbalist put it, curing a "scabby head," and had developed a reputation by the eighteenth century for being poisonous. Then, in 1775, the Scottish physician William Withering was asked his opinion of a folk remedy for "dropsy," what is now known as congestive heart failure, a condition for which mainstream medicine then had no cure. Dr. Withering described the remedy in his 1785 book, *Account of the Foxglove and Some of Its Medical Uses:* "I was told that it had long been kept a secret by an old woman in Shropshire, who had sometimes made cures after the more regular practitioners had failed. I was informed also, that the effects produced were violent vomiting and purging....This medicine was composed of twenty or more different herbs; but it was not very difficult for one conversant in these subjects, to perceive, that the active herb could be no other than the Foxglove."

As a medical student, Dr. Withering had hated his classes on the identification and preparation of herbs, thinking them dreadfully boring. But he developed a passion for them after meeting the beautiful Helena Cooke, who just happened to be an amateur painter of botanical specimens; they married in 1772. After witnessing a patient's remarkable recovery from dropsy after taking the old woman's remedy, Dr. Withering proceeded to test different formulations of foxglove extract on 158 patients, settling on a green powder made from the dried flowers harvested just before blossoming. Although only 101 of his patients experienced relief after receiving the foxglove treatment, Dr. Withering described all 158 cases in detail. As he wrote: "It would have been an easy task to have given select cases, whose successful treatment would have spoken strongly in favour of the medicine, and perhaps been flattering to my own reputation. But Truth and Science would condemn the procedure. I have therefore mentioned every case . . . proper or improper, successful or otherwise." Even then, he emphasized the provisional nature of his observations, insisted that doctors use care in selecting which patients to treat with it, and gave instructions on how to titrate the dosage. The synthetic versions, digitoxin and digoxin, remain widely used to treat heart failure to this day.

With the New World's medicines, however, came the snake oil. In 1630, Nicholas Knapp of Massachusetts Bay was sentenced to pay five pounds, or be whipped, for selling a would-be cure for scurvy that turned out to be nothing more than "a water of no worth nor value," which he "solde att a very deare rate." But it was often difficult to tell mainstream doctors from the quacks. Ben Franklin's own mother-in-law developed a salve for lice and itching called Widow Read's Ointment, which Franklin advertised before the Revolution in his *Pennsylvania Gazette*. And George Washington himself died in 1799 after a throat infection led his doctors to bleed him—a practice dating back to Hippocrates in the fifth century B.C.—reportedly draining about half of the seven liters of blood in his body in twenty-four hours, which, in the view of some doctors, may be what actually caused his death. Even in the nineteenth century, while the emerging science of chemistry gave medical doctors an aura of respectability, precious little of value made its way from the laboratory to the bedside. The most eminent physician of the early 1800s, Benjamin Rush of Philadelphia, developed a theory that the cause of fevers and most other illnesses was "excitability" of the blood vessels, or high blood pressure. He lowered the pressure by bleeding patients, removing up to 80 percent of their blood, and purging their bowels. His purgative of choice was calomel, or mercury chloride, a tasteless mineral so powerful that patients sometimes ended up losing their teeth and jawbones. Even a useful remedy like quinine was turned into an all-purpose "tonic" and used for just about anything. The other two popular tonics of the nineteenth century were iron and—in small amounts—strychnine, derived from the nux vomica plant, and better known these days as a poison.

With "cures" like these, it isn't surprising that other theories no odder than those of mainstream medicine's would arise and find support. One came from a German chemist, Dr. Samuel Hahnemann, who in 1796 developed his hair-of-the-dog-that-bit-me theory. "Let likes be treated with likes," he said, proposing that a substance causing certain unpleasant symptoms in a healthy person could, if given in minuscule amounts, cure a person who was suffering those very same symptoms due to an illness. He called his method homeopathy, from the Greek *homoios* (similar) and *pathos* (suffering or disease). Another of his counterintuitive beliefs was that the less of a substance he gave to patients, the more powerful it became. In fact, he claimed, the substances worked best when diluted until no discernible trace remained. A spiritlike essence, he believed, was left behind that would revive the body's vital force. Although not supported by modern science, homeopathy did have one great thing going for it: it didn't injure patients like bloodletting and calomel did. Many doctors began using homeopathic treatments, and eventually many schools of homeopathy were opened in the United States.

Another challenger to what passed for mainstream medicine was an unschooled frontier farmer, Samuel Thomson, who attacked the doctors' harsh medicines and championed the healing qualities of simple herbs, particularly lobelia (its prime effect implied by its folk name, pukeweed). His theory was that all illness was caused by "cold," and that the cure was "heat," which he achieved with steam baths, sweat-inducing herbs like red pepper, and other herbs that would cause people to vomit or move their bowels in an attempt to remove "obstructions" to the body's natural heat balance. Doctors derided his simple theories and overemphasis on lobelia, and he was jailed on murder charges after one of his patients died. But Thomson succeeded in setting off a historic cultural swing away from "scientific" medicine overseen by experts who emphasized chemically derived medicines to "natural" medicine overseen by individuals using herbs on themselves.

Far from quieting him, the trial on murder charges spurred Thomson to fight even harder against the medical establishment. He was found innocent and began traveling across the country to spread his views. Just as Andrew Jackson was being carried to victory in the 1828 presidential election on the shoulders of the common man, Thomson was proclaiming that uneducated, ordinary people were perfectly capable of being their own physicians. Herbs, free for the picking, were all anyone needed. What could be more in keeping with America's spirit of self-reliance? Championing a democratization of medicine, he sold families a twenty-dollar book on how to use his herbal remedies, and by 1839 he claimed to have sold 100,000 copies. As one New York doctor wrote of the growing self-treatment movement: "The people regard it among their vested interests to buy and swallow such physick as they in their sovereign will and pleasure shall determine." The movement gained such popularity that by 1850, most states had overturned the laws that had once reserved the practice of medicine to trained physicians. According to the historian James Harvey Young's authoritative work *The Toadstool Millionaires: A Social History of Patent Medicines in America Before Federal Regulation:* "The governor of Mississippi asserted that half the people of his state were treated according to Thomsonian principles, and in Ohio the regular physicians admitted botanical recruits to be at least a third of the population."

The swing toward self-treatment would not go on forever, of course. "It's a pendulum," says Harris, "because we've tended to wind up with extremes. We've gone through this cycles several times now." But even after Thomson's death in 1843, the pendulum of history kept going in the direction Thomson had pushed it. Spurred by increasingly florid ads, the self-medication movement shifted its focus from simple botanicals to fanciful patent medicines. According to Young's book, the patent medicine industry grew from gross sales of $3.5 million in 1859 to $74.5 million in 1904. He even credited the industry's enormous outlays on advertising with bankrolling the growth of newspapers during the Civil War, which saw the average number of copies sold per person jump from 29.5 before the war to 107.5 after. In 1905, Young noted, a pharmacy journal listed the names of more than 28,000 patent medicines. The next year, a congressional committee put the figure at 50,000.

The claims of the patent medicines were as astonishing as their numbers. Boston Drug, it was said, cured drunkenness. Hydrozone was a "positive preventive" for yellow fever. Liquozone could cure asthma, bronchitis, cancer, dysentery, eczema, fevers, gallstones, hay fever, malaria, tuberculosis, and tumors. Pond's Extract (a witch hazel preparation that became the forerunner of today's personal-care products still sold under the Pond's name) ran an advertisement in the early 1900s under the headline "Meningitis," stating "Pond's Extract is the oldest, best known and most effective remedy for all diseased conditions of the mucus membranes." Peruna, one of the most popular medicines sold at the turn of the century, healed one woman's "inflammation of ovaries and womb," and saved another's daughter from the grave. And a "miraculous cure" could be achieved with a product called Dr. Williams' Pink Pills for Pale People.

When he analyzed the ploys used to appeal to buyers, Young discovered no lure more effective than that of the exotic. "Millions of bottles," Young wrote, "have been vended on the authority of faraway places and ancient times." If they were both ancient and far away, like Chinese cures, so much the better. And if they were embodied in the country's own Native Americans, living way out West with their supposedly age-old cures, better still. "The romanticizing process represented in the novels of James Fenimore Cooper took place . . . at about the same time, on a lower literary level, in patent medicine promotion," Young wrote. "Unspoiled creature of Nature's original domain, the Indian was strong, virile, healthy. From the 1820s onward for a century the Indian strode nobly through the American patent medicine wilderness. Hiawatha helped a hair restorative and Pocahontas blessed a bitters. Dr. Fall spent twelve years with the Creeks to discover why no Indian had ever perished of consumptions. Edwin Eastman found a blood syrup among the Comanches, Texas Charles discovered a Kickapoo cure-all, and Frank Cushing pried the secret of a stomach renovator from the Zuni."

And then, inevitably, the pendulum swung back against the patent medicines. Attacks from medical societies, pharmacists, and a handful of periodicals—including, in particular, the *Ladies' Home Journal*—had been growing for years when, on October 7, 1905, *Collier's Weekly* launched a series of muckraking articles under the title "The Great American Fraud." The freelance reporter Samuel Hopkins Adams went at the patent medicines with enormous energy and careful research. He sent samples of popular remedies to chemists, who found that Peruna was 28 percent alcohol, Paine's Celery Compound was 21 percent alcohol, and Hotsetter's

Stomach Bitters was 44.3 percent alcohol. Dozens more, he reported, contained nothing more medicinal than morphine or cocaine (the most famous example of which would turn out to be Coca-Cola, originally promoted as a patent medicine "offering the virtues of coca without the vices of alcohol"). He discovered that middlemen were selling stock testimonial letters to the owners of patent medicines, who only had to fill in their products' names in the prewritten letters to use them in advertisements. He published copies of advertising contracts signed by newspapers that had agreed not only to run "news" articles promoting the advertisers' remedies, but also to never run any unflattering news about the product.

Most important, he named names. "Pond's Extract," he wrote, "could afford to restrict itself to decent methods, but in the recent epidemic scare in New York it traded on the public alarm by putting forth display advertisements headed, in heavy black type, 'Meningitis,' a disease in which witch-hazel is about as effective as molasses."

The key figure in the turn against patent medicines was not Adams, however, but an Indiana farm boy who grew into the tall, imposing chief of the Bureau of Chemistry of the U.S. Department of Agriculture. In 1903, Dr. Harvey W. Wiley declared that he wanted to require all producers of medicines to print their exact ingredients on their label, and to permit no medicines containing alcohol or cocaine to be sold without a prescription. "Such a law," the Propriety Association of America quickly concluded, "would practically destroy the sale of proprietary medicines in the United States."

But laws proposing to regulate the sale of both patent medicines and foods on related standards of purity had been dying ignominious deaths in the Congress for years. When the Pure Food and Drugs Act, spearheaded by Dr. Wiley, passed the Senate on February 21, 1906, it looked to be heading toward doom in the House. Then came the publication of *The Jungle*, Upton Sinclair's novel dramatizing the squalid conditions in the meatpacking industry. Meat sales fell by half, and President Roosevelt demanded that Congress act. On June 23 the bill passed the House, and Roosevelt signed it on June 30. Popularly known as the Wiley Act, the law empowered the USDA (the FDA would not be established for another twenty-one years) to ensure that all patent medicines list the presence and amount of any dangerous drugs, including alcohol and opiates, and to see that any other ingredients or claims on the label were accurate. For many patent medicines, the mere requirement for truth in labeling was enough to spell their end.

⊂⊃ ⊂⊃ ⊂⊃

On January 9, 1915, a shipment of twenty-five bottles of Clark Stanley Snake Oil Liniment was seized by the USDA on suspicion of violating the new drug laws. Ten months later, Dr. Francis P. Morgan, a medical expert retained by the USDA, stated that he was "prepared to furnish an affidavit that the product, in view of its composition, is not effective for the relief or cure of all pain and lameness, or effective as a remedy for rheumatism, sciatica, sprains, bunions, sore throat or bites of animals or reptiles; it does not make 'the declining years of life free from the pains that come as the days go by' . . . it is not effective as a remedy for paralysis or partial paralysis . . . it is not a perfect antidote to pain and inflammation. The statement 'a liniment that penetrates muscle, membrane and tissue to the very bone itself' is false and misleading and indicates fraud. The representations that the product 'oils dry joints' and 'banishes pain with a power that has astonished the medical profession' is of the same complexion."

Upon chemical analysis, Channing W. Harrison of the USDA concluded in an affidavit signed on April 19, 1916: "The sample consists principally of a light mineral oil (petroleum product) mixed with about 1 percent of fatty oil, probably beef fat, capsicum and possibly a trace of camphor and turpentine."

On May 20 of that year, the United States attorney for the District of Rhode Island filed an action against Stanley, charging that his snake oil was misbranded and in violation of the Pure Food and Drugs Act. On June 15, Stanley entered a plea of nolo contendere, and the court imposed a fine of twenty dollars. The very next day, on his company letterhead, Stanley sent a letter to the USDA with a revised circular stating only that the snake oil was "used with good results for pains, rheumatism, lame shoulders and lame back." He requested of the department, "Mark anything objectionable and return copy so marked to me, so that I may conform in every respect to the laws governing Interstate Commerce." But the agency's Bureau of Chemistry wasn't done with him yet. The assistant chief W. P. Jones wrote back to Stanley: "You are advised that until the pending case . . . has been disposed of, the Bureau prefers not to enter into a discussion of your revised circular."

Three months later, on August 23, 1916, Stanley was deposed by a Mr. Shanley at the USDA's Boston laboratory. "The charge here is that the sample of the product shipped is misbranded because the name Snake Oil Liniment is misleading in that the product contains little if any snake oil," Shanley said, according to a transcript on file in the Library of Congress. "What have you to say to that?"

"I say that it contains all the snake oil that I have been putting in according to my formula," Stanley replied.

"That is not definite," insisted his inquisitor. "Do you think there is enough snake oil in your preparation for effect?"

"Yes, I do," replied Stanley. "I have been selling this for about thirty-two years and all my testimonials I take from the letters that are sent in, stating that it has done so and so. I get letters reading 'the liniment helps my knee, and the pain is relieved or stopped.' Well, naturally, I take that as testimony of the efficacy of my preparation."

"Would you like to make a statement that you do put snake oil in your liniment?"

"Yes, by all means," Stanley said, adding a description of his preparation of the liniment during public demonstrations: "I kill the snakes in the presence of the public and manufacture the snake oil in full view of the public." Asked whether he made the liniment the same way in private as he did in public, Stanley conceded that sometimes he used a little more of the actual snake oil during the public demonstrations than he did when manufacturing it at his factory.

"What is the relative proportion of snake oil in the preparation?" he was asked. "What percentage of snake oil is there in the preparation?"

"Between 3 and 4 percent of snake oil in the final product," he testified.

Asked to comment on the label's claims, he said that he had discarded the old label and replaced it with the new one claiming it had been "used with good results for pains, rheumatism, lame shoulders and lame back."

"You have testimonials to the effect that this liniment has been used with good results?"

"Yes sir," said Stanley. "I can give it to you in the same letters that were sent to me."

What became of Clark Stanley and his snake oil after that deposition is unknown, as no further records remain in his file. It is safe to say, however, that the Bureau of Chemistry was not about to let him sell a product called Snake Oil that did not demonstrably contain snake oil, or to claim that it could achieve "good results" on "lame shoulders and lame back" when no such effect of even 100 percent snake oil had ever been demonstrated. And so, thirty-two years after he had begun selling it, Clark Stanley's Snake Oil Liniment slipped into history as nothing more than . . . snake oil.

⊂⊃ ⊂⊃ ⊂⊃

The swing of the pendulum toward ever-tightening drug regulation and respect for scientific medicine gained momentum with the extraordinary advances in treating age-old ailments that marked the first sixty years of the twentieth century: the discovery of insulin in 1921, penicillin in 1928, and the Salk polio vaccine in 1952. Revisions to the original Wiley Act came every few years. By 1914, it was not enough for manufacturers to simply list morphine on the label; the Harrison Narcotics Act required a prescription for any narcotic beyond an allowable low level, as well as increased record keeping for the doctors who prescribed them and pharmacists who dispensed them. In 1927, Congress established the Food, Drug, and Insecticide Administration as its own agency; three years later it shortened the name to the Food and Drug Administration.

But the FDA as we know it today did not really come into its own until 1938, following a great tragedy. "The story of drug regulation," notes Michael Harris, "is built on tombstones." In 1937, a manufacturer devised a new way to make the new antibiotic sulfanilamide, using the delicious-tasting solvent diethylene glycol—which is the chemical name for antifreeze. After 107 people, many of them children, died horrible, prolonged, and painful deaths, the Federal Food, Drug, and Cosmetic Act of 1938 was passed, requiring new drugs to be shown to be safe before they went on sale. The law also extended the agency's control to include cosmetics and medical devices, authorized it to conduct factory inspections, and gave it, for the first time, power to obtain court injunctions.

The FDA grew with the food and drug industries it regulated. In 1941, the Insulin Amendment required the agency to test and certify the pancreatic hormone's potency and purity. The 1945 Penicillin Amendment extended a similar requirement for all penicillin products, later extended to include all antibiotics. Then, in 1962, thousands of babies were born in Europe with serious birth defects after their mothers had taken the sleeping pill thalidomide, but none in the United States, because the FDA had refused to approve the drug. On the strength of public goodwill, Congress passed the Kefauver-Harris Amendments to require that all new drugs be shown to be not only safe but effective. A few years later, in 1966, the FDA contracted with the National Academy of Sciences to review the efficacy of the four thousand drugs that had been approved prior to 1962, and began implementing the academy's recommendations in 1968.

But by then, the respect and awe for science and medicine that had characterized the first six decades of the century were already beginning to ebb at the liberal fringes of American society. Doctors were criticized for indiscriminately prescribing "mothers' little helpers"—amphetamines and barbiturates for unhappy housewives. Rachel Carson's 1962 best-seller, *Silent Spring,* showed that the pesticides used by farmers and home-owners were far more harmful to people and the environment than the government had acknowledged. Tang and TV dinners, and their laundry list of chemical ingredients, might be fine for astronauts headed to the moon, but could they really be healthy for those of us here on Earth?

Slowly, the great pendulum of history began swinging back again.

CHAPTER 2
MOTHER NATURE

"**You could say** my interest in nutrition began when I was ten days old."

Daisie Davis was born in an Indiana farmhouse at three in the morning on February 25, 1904. Ten days later, her mother suffered a paralyzing stroke. Daisie, the last of five daughters, was taken away from her mother and wasn't fed for several days, "for the simple reason that there was a blizzard and bottles weren't sold in our small town." Seventeen months later, her mother died.

Daisie's lifelong obsession with food, she came to believe, derived from that early traumatic loss of maternal sustenance. "My interest in nutrition was neurotic," she conceded. "I spent all my time making up for the mother I didn't have." Even before she could read, she was carrying around a copy of Fannie Farmer's 1896 *Boston Cooking-School Cook Book*, begging her older sisters to read the recipes to her so she could cook them. Soon she was winning ribbons at the state and county fairs "for baking bread and canning things."

By the time she reached Indiana's Purdue University, she had stopped going by Daisie, thinking it sounded like the name of a cow, and begun using her middle name, Adelle. Her fellow students, however, gave her another name. "Vitamin Davis," they called her, because she never stopped talking about those newfangled substances supposedly associated with health. In the early decades of the twentieth century, vitamins were as hot a medical subject as genetic engineering would be by century's end.

The very notion of vitamins—that there are minuscule parts of food that could be isolated and shown to be essential to health—was barely older than Davis herself. Though the Scottish naval surgeon James Lind had discovered back in 1747 that citrus fruits prevented scurvy, he had no idea what it was about the citrus fruits that achieved the effect. Not until 1905, when the English scientist William Fletcher first observed that the disease beriberi would develop if a person ate only polished rice, but not if he ate unpolished rice, did the theory develop—and it was still only a theory—that some ingredient in the rice husk was important to maintaining health. Seven years later, the Polish scientist Casimir Funk found that ingredient by isolating thiamine from rice husks, the first vitamin to be isolated. It was Funk, in fact, who coined the word *vitamine* (later shortened to *vitamin*) to describe what he correctly guessed would be a whole group of essential nutrients; he combined *vita* from the Latin *life* with *amine* from *thiamine* (soon to be known as vitamin B_1). In the four short years between 1912 and 1916, vitamins A, B, B_1, and C were all discovered; the necessity of dietary minerals, such as calcium and iron, was also quickly established.

After two years at Purdue, Adelle Davis switched schools, heading north to the University of Wisconsin, then west to the University of California at Berkeley, where in 1922, the researchers Herbert Evans and Katherine Bishop discovered vitamin E in green, leafy vegetables. It was at UC Berkeley, the premier vitamin research institution in the nation, that Davis finally obtained her bachelor's degree in nutrition.

Brimming with enthusiasm for the young science, Davis moved to New York to become a dietician at Bellevue Hospital and a supervising nutritionist to the Yonkers public school system. Beginning in 1931, she also worked as a consulting nutritionist to three New York obstetricians. Finally, in 1935, the Indiana farm girl who couldn't stop talking about vitamins found an outlet in print, when a London publisher, Stationers' Hall, published her first small book, *Optimum Health*.

Although most leading researchers of the day took a circumspect view of vitamins' worth, Davis's perspective was as wide as an Indiana corn-field. Studies published in medical journals showed their value to be gen-erally limited to preventing a handful of diseases, which could be easily avoided by eating an ordinary balanced diet. Yet Davis believed that, taken in sufficient quantities, vitamins could improve mood, increase en-ergy, extend longevity—in short, that they assured "optimum" health. She shared this view with the marketers of vitamin pills and foods that were touted for their vitamin and mineral content, from bread to choco-late bars to even Popeye's favorite food ("I'm strong to the finich 'cause I eats my spinach"). Indeed, the phrase "health foods" was already being so widely exploited that Walter Campbell, commissioner of the nascent FDA, issued a warning to the American public in 1929. The phrase, he said in a press release, "implies that these products have health-giving or curative properties, when, in general, they merely possess some of the nutritive qualities to be expected in any wholesome food product. The la-bel claims on these products are such that the consumer is led to believe that our ordinary diet is sorely deficient in such vital substances as vita-mins and minerals, and that these so-called 'health foods' are absolutely necessary to conserve life and health."

Although health food stores were popping up in major cities across the country, devotees like Davis were still considered by most ordinary peo-ple to be a bit nutty, and were decidedly out of step with the cultural cli-mate of the Great Depression, when many counted themselves lucky to get any kind of food to eat. In those days, as she recalled years later, "I'd get so discouraged, I'd cry. For years people thought I was a kooky crank. I know how it feels to be sneered at."

Davis soon returned to California, where she graduated with a master's degree in biochemistry in 1939 from the University of Southern Califor-nia. That year, she published a ninety-page booklet with the same Lon-don publisher, *You Can Stay Well.* As her practice as a consulting nutritionist grew, she settled down and made Southern California her lifelong home. It was there that she wrote her next book, published in 1942 by Macmillan, *Vitality Through Planned Nutrition.*

In 1947, Harcourt Brace Jovanovich published the first of Davis's books to reach a wider audience: *Let's Cook It Right,* which Davis described as "not intended to be merely a cookbook. A cookbook has as its sole pur-pose showing how delicious foods may be prepared; my purpose is to help build health through applied nutrition which, if successfully applied, makes good cooking a necessity." Many of the recipes, it turned out, resembled that of an Indiana farm family's, with plenty of unpasteurized whole milk, eggs, and meat. (Cholesterol from egg and dairy products, she insisted throughout her life, is actually good for you, which is why her daily "pep-up" drink—which became the basis for the commercially sold Tigers Milk—included raw egg yolk. "It's impossible to get a high cholesterol level if your diet is right," she said. And whole milk was so beneficial, she believed, that "I have yet to know of a single adult to develop cancer who has habitually drunk a quart of milk a day.") At the same time, however, she began preaching a gospel that would seem remarkably au courant more than half a century later: stay away from the packaged, processed foods pushed by America's food industry; eat whole-grain wheat and rice; cook vegetables as briefly as possible, and keep sugar to an absolute minimum. The book did well enough to remain in print, and Davis's reputation grew.

In the early 1950s, Davis married George Leisey, adopting his two young children, a girl named Barbara and a boy also named George. (Davis never had children of her own.) With them, she could at last try out the nutritional methods she'd been teaching her clients and readers for years. One day, young George came home with a bottle of cola that a friend had given him. Davis, who was strictly against sugar-filled soft drinks, coyly suggested he place it in the refrigerator to chill it. Secretly, she emptied the can and refilled it with "the strongest possible instant coffee mix." After a few sips, she would proudly tell a reporter years later, neither of the children ever asked her for a soft drink again. It was only fair, then, that when she wrote her 1951 book, *Let's Have Healthy Children,* she dedicated it to George and Barbara, "without whose cooperation [it] never would have been written." (The 1972 paperback edition even featured Barbara's beautiful high school graduation photograph, with the caption: "The adequacy of the diet during the first six months largely determines the attractiveness of the adult.")

In 1954, Harcourt published what would become Davis's most popular book, *Let's Eat Right to Keep Fit.* In the second sentence of the first chapter, she stated her intoxicating thesis: "Your nutrition can determine how you look, act, and feel; whether you are grouchy or cheerful, homely or beautiful, physiologically and even psychologically young or old; whether you think clearly or are confused, enjoy your work or make it a drudgery, increase your earning power or stay in an economic rut." And the public responded. Here was a university-trained biochemist, described on the book jacket as "America's foremost nutrition authority," asserting that wealth, good looks, happiness, youthfulness, and mental clarity could all be found in a cookbook. And just in case anyone might miss the message, the 1970 Signet paperback edition reprinted most of that sentence on the back cover, in capital letters.

When reading through the book more than fifty years after Davis wrote it, it's easy to find many passages that have held up amazingly well, including well-deserved indictments of the fast food and prepared foods industries and perfectly sensible advice for how to eat better. In chapter 5, after railing against the classic hamburger-and-fries meal, she offered advice that few modern dieticians could find fault with: "Avoid hydrogenated fats such as hydrogenated peanut butter, processed cheeses, and solid cooking fats and the French-fried foods cooked in these solid fats; limit the solid, or saturated, animal fats obtained mostly from beef and lambs and increase your intake of fish and fowl having less saturated fat; eat no food containing coconut or palm oils.... Use unrefined, or cold-pressed, oils." On the sins of sugar, she wrote in chapter 6: "Our American diet has become largely one of sugar. The innocent victim is flooded by waves of sugar every time he entertains or is entertained, every time he eats at a restaurant, and often at every home meal and mid-meal."

But the farther one travels through the book's thirty-one chapters, the more one is likely to come upon passages, and whole chapters, devoted to the wonders of vitamins, and here the inaccuracies verge on the outlandish. Chapter 11, for instance, titled, "Are Blue Mondays Necessary?" puts forth the idea that grumpiness can be reduced, and happiness increased, by taking extra niacin, also known as vitamin B_3. "Persons whose diets are excellent not only are more mentally alert but usually find that blue Mondays can be largely avoided," Davis writes. In chapter 21, she tells us, "Calcium can be as soothing as a mother, as relaxing as a sedative, and as life-saving as an oxygen tent." Chapter 22, titled "Nature's Own Tranquilizer," states, "Persons only slightly deficient in magnesium become irritable, high-strung, sensitive to noise, hyperexcitable, apprehensive, and belligerent.... The principal reason physicians write millions of prescriptions for tranquilizers each year is the nervousness, grouchiness, and jitters largely brought on by inadequate diets lacking magnesium."

She went even farther in interviews, once saying, "Alcoholism, crime, insanity, suicide, divorce, drug addiction, and even impotence are often merely the results of bad eating." Even schizophrenia, the crippling mental illness, could be cured, she believed, with vitamin B_3.

By 1958, the hardcover book was in its seventeenth printing, and Davis was prosperous enough to build a new home in Palos Verdes with her second husband, Frank Sieglinger. Yet nutrition in general, and health foods in particular, remained decidedly marginal to the obsessions of the culture at large. It was, after all, the era of Eisenhower and Jell-O molds, of Elvis, milkshakes, and cheeseburgers. Health food "nuts" were still being popularly depicted as "little old ladies in tennis shoes."

And then came the sixties. Davis didn't change; the culture did. Viewed as eccentric in the Betty Crocker–infatuated fifties, she found herself swept up into the very vanguard of a social movement devoted to questioning authority. Davis wasn't just espousing good nutrition, after all, but attacking the country's entire food industry. Let others protest civil rights injustices or the Vietnam War; she stood on the front line of the righteous battle for good health. "The whole food industry is a cruel thing, a cruel, cruel, cruel, cruel thing," she once said. "You have to remember that I'm bucking a multibillion-dollar food-processing industry. This nutrition consciousness had better grow, or we're going under. We're watching the fall of Rome right now, very definitely, because Americans are getting more than half their calories from food with no nutrients."

The late 1960s and early 1970s brought her fame unlike that of any nutritionist before or since, and cultural influence equaled by few in any profession. With the rise of the antiestablishment, anticorporate, back-to-nature sixties, the youth generation discovered in Davis their "guru" (Associated Press), "oracle" (*New York Times*), "prophet" (*Washington Post*) and "high priestess" (*Life*). "Adelle Davis is to nutrition what Ralph Nader is to consumerism," the same Associated Press article declared in 1972. "Her early advocacy of wheat germ, yogurt and organic foods . . . would seem to have played a significant role in the development of the nation's billion-dollar-a-year health food business," the *Post* article stated. "Today she is the spokesperson and chief showwoman for health foods," pronounced another article in the *New York Times*. "Like Elijah, the Passover prophet, she is an unseen presence at the dinner table, advising us and admonishing us on every morsel we swallow. . . . As a celebrity she is almost as much a regular on television talk shows as Johnny Carson. . . . Her respectability is such that banks give away [her] books as promotional come-ons. She's highly regarded in the highest circles; Julie Nixon Eisenhower confided to Dinah Shore on the latter's talk show last year, 'I'm on an Adelle Davis diet. I think she's very good.' "

Perhaps it should not be surprising, however, that among nutritionists and physicians, the admiration Davis enjoyed from the 10 million buyers of her books was largely lacking. Some of these "establishment" figures, no doubt, simply scoffed at the idea that the American diet wasn't the finest in the world. But even those who applauded her emphasis on unrefined grains and fresh fruits and vegetables and backed her condemnation of sugar, saturated fats, and fast foods took issue with one fundamental problem in her books: their extraordinary lack of accuracy.

It was ironic, because her readers were drawn to her in part because of her credentials and apparent devotion to scientific studies. Festooned with 2,402 footnoted citations from prestigious medical journals, her 1965 book, *Let's Get Well*, exuded the erudition one would expect of a biochemist. In *Let's Have Healthy Children*, she wrote, "To gather the material for this book alone, I have spent approximately two years, eight hours a day, in a medical library; and I have taken 1,282 pages of closely written notes which, to make them usable, have had to be indexed and crossindexed." But researchers who checked her footnotes found them almost bizarrely inaccurate, given that she had gone to the trouble of making them.

Gordon Schectman, a researcher at Columbia University's Institute of Human Nutrition, noted that in *Let's Get Well*, almost every sentence had a footnoted reference. When he analyzed the 170 references in chapter 5, however, he found that 112 of them either did not relate whatsoever to the assertions Davis used them to back up, or actually contradicted them. Another 50 of the citations were taken out of context or misconstrued. Only 30 of the 170 citations accurately confirmed Davis's writings, Schectman concluded. The footnotes from two other chapters of *Let's Get Well* were reviewed by Rona Karny, a doctoral candidate in biochemistry at UCLA. She came to the same unfortunate conclusion that Schectman had.

Russell Randall, MD, who was a professor of medicine and chief of the division of renal diseases at the Medical College of Virginia in the early 1970s, said that a chapter on the kidneys in *Let's Get Well,* in which Davis had cited him as one of her sources, was "fraught with errors and inaccurate statements that are extremely dangerous and even potentially lethal, such as the suggestion that patients with nephrosis take potassium chloride."

"She's making people aware of the science of nutrition," said Leo Lutwak, MD, PhD, a professor of clinical nutrition at Cornell University, in a 1972 interview. "And she points out that nutrition is a science. But she misuses the science. Adelle Davis takes incomplete evidence and immediately extrapolates it to what are ridiculous conclusions from a clinical point of view."

Gladys Emerson, the UCLA researcher who in the 1930s had been the first to isolate pure vitamin E, signed a letter of protest when Davis was invited to speak at UC Berkeley. "She takes material out of context and her work has a great many inaccuracies," Emerson said. Ruth Huenemann, director of UC-Berkeley's School of Public Health nutrition program, wrote another letter of protest. Permitting Davis to speak there, Huenemann said, would "make the university at Berkeley the laughingstock of the scientific community in the field of nutrition throughout the country."

Edward Rynearson, MD, professor emeritus of medicine at the Mayo Clinic, said in a 1973 interview that Davis's books were "loaded with inaccuracies, misquotations, and unsubstantiated statements." He believed most were innocuous, but he said, "When she starts recommending things like taking huge doses of vitamin A and D, this can be potentially very dangerous. Both these vitamins are fat soluble and too much of either can produce all kinds of horrible symptoms."

Davis heard the accusations and fired back. "You tell that Dr. Rynearson," she said, "that overdosing with vitamin A and D is so rare that it is not even worth mentioning. Oh, these doctors with their mother problems. Let them call me anything they want. I have facts to back up everything I say. I'm very careful about my material."

That tart riposte echoed the view she had expressed in her 1942 book,

Vitality Through Planned Nutrition: "From a practical point of view, it is correct to say that it is impossible to obtain enough vitamin A to be harmful."

Unfortunately, the argument over whether it was possible to overdose on vitamins A and D was settled by two young girls whose mothers had followed Davis's advice. The first was Eliza Young, born in Maine on October 5, 1967. Her mother, Katherine Young, had bought a copy of *Let's Have Healthy Children* in August of that year and, following the advice in the book, began giving Eliza "generous amounts" of vitamin A in December. Prior to then, the baby had been perfectly healthy. But after the vitamin A treatments, Eliza "suffered certain irreversible and unalterable physiological changes; has been hospitalized on intermittent occasions for long periods of time; [and] her body has been so damaged, altered and impaired, that she will be . . . a dwarf for the remainder of her natural life." A lawsuit filed against Davis on behalf of Eliza in 1971 was settled five years later for $150,000.

The second child injured by Davis's advice was a four-year-old girl, hospitalized at the University of California Medical Center in San Francisco in 1971. Her symptoms at first seemed to indicate a brain tumor: diarrhea, vomiting, fever, hair loss, enlarged spleen, and enlarged liver. Her mother, said to be "a food faddist who read Adelle Davis religiously," had given her daughter large doses of vitamins A and D and calcium lactate. When the supplements were stopped, the child recovered. The mother chose not to file suit.

Another unfortunate event for the vitamin and health food movement occurred on June 8, 1971. That night, J. I. Rodale was scheduled to appear on a popular TV talk show hosted by Dick Cavett. Rodale, born Jerome Irving Cohen, was the founder of Rodale Press, publisher of the magazines *Prevention* and *Organic Farming and Gardening.* If Davis was the mother of the vitamin and health food movement, Rodale was its father. His magazines relentlessly pushed not only vitamins and minerals but herbal remedies and countless other products.

On a previous talk show appearance, Rodale had famously bragged, "I'm going to live to be a hundred unless I'm run down by a sugar-crazed taxi driver." During the afternoon taping of the Cavett show, Rodale said, "I'm so healthy that I expect to live on and on. I'm full of energy." Rodale remained on stage as Cavett welcomed his next guest, the writer Pete

Hamill. When Cavett and Hamill heard a sound like snoring coming from Rodale, they thought he might have fallen asleep, and touched him. He didn't respond. Upon inspection, Rodale turned out to be dead. The cause was an apparent heart attack. Rodale, born on August 16, 1898, was seventy-two years old.

But health food advocates weren't supposed to die at an ordinary age, and Rodale's death—premature only to those who really expected him to live "on and on"—posed an awkward problem for Davis. "I had the craziest letter," she told the *New York Times*, "from some man saying that Rodale had ruined the health food movement by dying." She laughed at the idea. "I don't know what I'm supposed to do about it if he did." The reporter replied that people were probably relying on her to live forever. She laughed again, and then there was an awkward pause. "Well," she said at last, "I sure as hell trust I won't die of pneumonia!"

Two years later, Davis began experiencing stabbing pains in her chest. Her doctor suggested it was pleurisy, an inflammation of the lungs. She thought that was wrong, and went first to a chiropractor and then to an acupuncturist. While she hadn't been known for advocating such alternative medical treatments, she also hadn't been known for relying on traditional medicine. But when she found no relief from the chiropractor or acupuncturist, she went to more doctors. Finally, the seventh doctor she saw gave her the diagnosis: she was suffering from multiple myeloma, cancer of the bone.

"I was shocked, absolutely shocked," she later wrote. "How did it happen to me? How could it happen in the face of my belief that cancer is a disease of people who eat a lot of processed and refined foods and drink a lot of soft drinks?" With remarkable grace and candor, she went on, "In one of my books I said I didn't know of a single adult developing cancer who drank a quart of milk daily, as I did. I have to admit I was wrong. But I doubt I will die of cancer. I have great hope."

After undergoing chemotherapy, Daisie Adelle Davis Sieglinger died at her home on May 31, 1974. She was seventy years old.

⌐⌐ ⌐⌐ ⌐⌐

The movement Davis had played a singular role in fostering did not die with her; indeed, it was just coming into its own. Between 1972 and 1974, sales of vitamins, minerals, and other supplements rose 40 percent from an estimated $500 million to $700 million. The Nobel Prize winner Linus Pauling, PhD, gained far more fame than his chemical research ever had by claiming that high doses of vitamin C (known in those days as "megadoses") could cure not only the common cold but cancer. Ernst T. Krebs, Jr., whose father had been selling one quack cure after another since the 1930s, also found fame in the 1970s when he started insisting that a cyanide-containing chemical derived from apricot pits, which he had been promoting for decades as a cancer cure called "laetrile," was in fact a vitamin—vitamin "B_{17}." With claims for vitamins (and pseudovitamins) growing ever more outrageous, officials at the FDA began getting nervous. By the time of Davis's death, a showdown between the FDA and the supplement industry had become inevitable.

The FDA had fired the first shot in December of 1972, when it announced its intent to issue a series of regulations that would limit the potency of any single vitamin pill to 150 percent of that vitamin's recommended daily allowance (RDA). At any higher dose, the agency would regard the vitamin as it would an over-the-counter drug and require manufacturers to provide the same kind of proof of safety and efficacy as demanded for other remedies. But even at the 150 percent dose, consumers would still be able to take as much as they liked; they would just have to gulp down more pills to do it. The regulations would also limit manufacturers' ability to mix together "irrational" combinations of supplements of varying strengths. By bringing such standards to a chaotic marketplace, the regulations would also make it easier for the FDA to take products illegally making false health claims off the market without having to spend years in court arguing over each and every violation.

Leading the fight against this measure was a group, composed primarily of manufacturers, called the National Health Federation. Of this group's past and present officers, six had been convicted of breaking medical and drug laws, and several had served prison sentences. In response to the FDA's announcement, the group had begun championing a law that would prohibit the agency from setting any limits on vitamin potency. As of the spring of 1973, the group's bill was considered obscure. A House staffer knowledgeable in health legislation used just two words to sum up its chances for passage: "No way."

But things had changed significantly by a year later, when Senator William Proxmire, the respected Democrat from Wisconsin, introduced Senate Bill 2801, giving the National Health Federation exactly what it had wanted: a ban on the FDA's ability to limit vitamin doses. That any Democrat would introduce a bill for *less* government oversight of public health and consumer affairs was extraordinary enough, but that it should be Proxmire—best known for his monthly Golden Fleece Award lampooning wasteful government spending, and widely seen as the Senate's voice of common sense—was an ominous signal for the FDA. So positive was the public's attitude toward vitamins, and so torrentially did they flood Congress with letters written in support of Proxmire's bill, that forty-four other senators—Democrats and Republicans alike—soon signed on as co-sponsors, including such luminaries as Bob Dole, J. William Fulbright, Barry Goldwater, Hubert H. Humphrey, George McGovern, and Sam Nunn.

By the morning of August 14, 1974—less than three months after Davis's death—much more than her lifelong advocacy of vitamins was in the air when Senator Edward M. Kennedy called to order the Senate Subcommittee on Health, of which he was chair, for the first of two days of hearings on Proxmire's bill. Five days earlier, President Richard M. Nixon had resigned from office in the wake of the Watergate scandal. Transcripts of Oval Office conversations had shown that he'd directed the cover-up of the break-in of Democratic Party headquarters. The House Judiciary Committee had recommended impeachment, charging him with obstruction of justice, contempt of Congress, and abuse of power. As a result, the public's cynicism toward government reached a historic high that would influence politics for decades to come. Whereas three quarters of the public had said in polls conducted in 1964 that they trusted their government to do the right thing, in the wake of Watergate the percentage plummeted to just 36 percent. The timing for anyone to defend the right of a federal agency to deprive people of seemingly life-saving vitamins could not have been worse.

But Kennedy, who had made health care a leading priority since first being elected to the Senate in 1962, gave it his best shot. "The Food and Drug Administration, in my opinion, has an obvious and important responsibility to protect the American consumer against foods and drugs, or combinations of foods and drugs, which are potentially harmful to their health," Kennedy declared in his opening remarks. "In addition, however, I believe the Food and Drug Administration has the responsibility to protect the American consumer against economic fraud. It must make certain that Americans are not led to believe that dietary products are therapeutic or in some other way beneficial when, in fact, they may be worthless and a waste of money. The subcommittee must determine whether enactment of any of the bills currently pending before Congress, which would strip the Food and Drug Administration of its authority to control the doses and combinations of drugs which could be legally marketed, [would] also strip the consumer of the protection against fraud he has a right to expect. It is the delicate balance between that protection and infringement upon the rights of individuals to purchase and consume whatever foods they wish that we hope will be examined during these hearings."

First up, to defend his bill, was Proxmire. His arguments seemed incontrovertible. The RDAs on which the agency intended to base its vitamin limits, he pointed out, had been changed repeatedly, and dramatically, over the past decade. Moreover, some leading nutritional authorities believed that the current RDAs remained way too low. "What the FDA wants to do," he said, "is to strike the views of its stable of orthodox nutritionists into 'tablets,' and bring them down from Mount Sinai where they will be used to regulate the rights of millions of Americans who believe they are getting a lousy diet to take vitamins and minerals. The real issue is whether the FDA is going to play God."

If vitamins were to be labeled and regulated like drugs on the basis of toxicity, he argued, then other potentially toxic foods should also be regulated as drugs. Sugar can be toxic to diabetics; salt, taken in large enough quantities, can kill a person; coffee, tea, and alcohol "have far more toxic effect than most vitamins," and even water in excessive amounts, he pointed out, can become toxic. "This is an upside-down world," Proxmire said. "There are more than one hundred deaths a day from drugs taken under medically supervised conditions. There are about two hundred deaths a year from overdoses of aspirin. There are virtually no deaths a year from taking excessive quantities of vitamins." On the contrary, millions of poor people, pregnant women, and "children who stuff themselves with candy and junk foods," he said, were in danger of suffering from the nutritional deficiencies that vitamins could correct.

Concluding his speech with a slam against the FDA, Proxmire attacked the agency in a way that would have been inconceivable a few years before: "This nutritional deficiency," he said, "is aided and abetted by a Food and Drug Administration which is reluctant to control [harmful prescription drugs]; an FDA which allows the wheat germ and other nutrients of bread to be discarded and fed to the pigs while humans are fed that white, watery, rubbery substance which they call bread; and an FDA which is up to its ears in cahoots with the producers of TV dinners, chemical additives, and non-nutritious breakfast food promoters."

Charged with countering Proxmire's arguments was the commissioner of the FDA, Alexander M. Schmidt, MD. He began by entering into the record a review of the agency's actions against supplement makers between the years 1960 and 1963. Running seventy-two single-spaced pages, the review covered hundreds of cases for products like Insta Pep, He-Man Hematinic Tonic, Red Rooster Pills, Hem-Glo Tablets, and Dixie Q Protein Wafers. "The current effective regulations dealing with vitamins and minerals are outdated by any standard and fail to set any real guidance for the composition and labeling of dietary supplements," Schmidt said. The last time the regulations had been updated, he pointed out, was in 1941. Since then, he said, "The promotion of such products has expanded to the point where the market now contains an almost endless variety of items which are offered to the public."

Playing devil's advocate, Kennedy asked him, "If it is not going to do them any harm, as Senator Proxmire has stated, and if no one has died of an overdose of vitamins, why should the federal government be establishing these regulations?"

"Well, the word *harm* is relative," answered Schmidt. "First of all, zinc in high doses is harmful. Second, what is overlooked by a great many people is that while there is not a lot of evidence that very large doses of water-soluble vitamins are harmful, there is not a lot of information that large doses of water-soluble vitamins are safe either."

Hoots of derisive laughter from the audience prompted Kennedy to say, "We will maintain order now, please."

When the second day of hearings began at 9:47 a.m. on Thursday, August 22, the second speaker was Senator Bob Dole of Kansas, who would one day become a spokesman for Viagra. "I would like to be on record as absolutely opposing any action by the Food and Drug Administration to regulate the retail sale of vitamin and mineral nutrients," he said. "In fact, it is a little inconceivable to me that such restrictions should ever have been promulgated in the first place."

Following Dole to the witness table were five representatives of the leading supplement trade organizations, including most prominently Milton Bass, the general counsel for the National Nutritional Foods Association (NNFA). Bass had devoted most of his many years of practice to defending manufacturers in court. He brought to his work an unmatched set of skills: a believer's passion, a general's tactics, a legislator's mastery of minutiae, and a master litigator's ability to win by setting the terms of the debate and then dashing his opponent's case with sheer bluster.

"Last Wednesday," Bass began, "we heard a great deal of testimony by Commissioner Schmidt, who told us that products were being sold with many claims. We must clarify that the Proxmire bill has nothing whatsoever to do with any claims which may be deemed false for any product. The Proxmire bill is designed for one purpose. It is designed to permit the consumer to buy a safe food product honestly labeled. Should the Food and Drug Administration be able to assert the power to tell the consumer, 'You cannot freely get the foods you want even though they are safe and honestly labeled because we think you do not need it'?"

To answer that question came Sidney Wolfe, MD, who a few years earlier had created the Health Research Group as part of Ralph Nader's consumer advocacy group, Public Citizen. Although he, like Nader, had devoted most of his health-care efforts to railing against the pharmaceutical industry, he refused to concede that "food supplements" were foods. "This is a drug industry," he said flatly. "The difference between large doses of vitamins . . . and over-the-counter [drugs] are nonexistent as far as I am concerned. Exploitation of genuine concerns people have for their health with easy vitamin pill-popping solutions is no better, although somewhat less expensive, than the fraud that is often the practice of medicine."

Wolfe then introduced Anita Johnson, an attorney with his organization. "Everything we have learned from environmental hazards," Johnson said, "shows us you cannot assume a product is safe if it has not been tested. For years, we have been living in our homes with polyvinyl chloride products, and finally somebody thinks to test them, and finds we have been living with a carcinogen. This was also true of the cyclamate [an artificial sweetener] ingested by perhaps three quarters of American households before somebody ran the proper tests [which found that it caused cancer in mice, leading the FDA to ban it in 1969]. And for these kinds of chronic hazards, there is no way the information can pop up as something that is dangerous unless you run the controlled studies." The Proxmire bill, she said, would "decimate" the FDA's power to regulate vitamins, by shifting the burden of proof entirely to the agency. She also pointed out a little-understood provision of the Proxmire bill that would make it apply not simply to vitamins and minerals but to any "special dietary foods and all ingredients of special dietary foods." By that definition, Johnson said, "Cyclamates would be back in health foods. Under this section, all the other things that we have been fighting to get out of the food supply will be ingested again."

Of all the witnesses to speak for or against the bill, perhaps none brought more independent and respected credentials than Marsha N. Cohen, an attorney with Consumers Union, the nonprofit organization founded in 1939 that publishes *Consumer Reports* and devotes itself to independently testing and rating the safety and usefulness of consumer products. And she had the best show-and-tell presentation of the day, setting eight cantaloupes on the table before her.

"Why should vitamin and mineral supplements be regulated if food itself, in which nutrients are found, is unregulated?" she asked. "I have here with me a little visual demonstration of our answer to that argument. We can safely rely upon the limited capacity of the human stomach to protect persons from overindulgence in any particular vitamin or mineral-rich food. For example, you would need to eat eight cantaloupes—a good source of vitamin C—to take in barely one thousand milligrams of vitamin C. But just these two little pills, easy to swallow, contain the same amount. A thirst-quenching two quarts of orange juice would have the same effect—and one thousand milligrams, it should be recalled, is on the low end of Dr. Pauling's recommended two hundred and fifty to ten thousand milligrams daily. If the proponents of the legislation before you succeed, one tablet could contain as much vitamin C as all these cantaloupes—or even twice, thrice, or twenty times that amount. And there would be no protective satiety level."

"Do you want those cantaloupes made part of the record?" Senator William Hathaway, Democrat of Maine, joked. "It is about lunchtime."

"If someone has a knife," Cohen replied.

But she and the other opponents of the bill, including the American Association of Retired Persons, the American Academy of Pediatrics, and the American Society of Clinical Nutrition, convinced no one. On September 24, 1974, Proxmire's bill passed the Senate by a vote of 81 to 10. On April 23, 1976, it became the law of the United States. Two months shy of the seventieth anniversary of the passage of the Pure Food and Drugs Act of 1906, Congress had made the decision to roll back the government's authority over the sale of foods or drugs for the first time in the twentieth century. So began an unprecedented experiment, to test whether the unbridled use of vitamins and other supplements would help or hinder health, with the American public as the guinea pigs.

CHAPTER 3

WHOLESOME AS A GLASS OF MILK

Paul L. Houts couldn't have been healthier. The editor in chief of the Congressional Budget Office, Washington's nonpartisan economic bureau, he walked as much as two miles a day to and from work, went to the gym regularly, and was out on the town with his wife as often as five or six nights a week. In the last weeks of 1987, while his office rushed to complete the annual economic forecast for the coming year, it was not unusual for Houts and his colleagues to pull all-nighters, working without sleep for sometimes two or three days in a row. When they did get a chance to sleep, many of them struggled with insomnia.

Word passed around the office about a natural remedy for insomnia that was all over the news, an over-the-counter amino acid called L-tryptophan. One of the essential amino acids necessary for health, tryptophan is a precursor to serotonin, used in the brain as a feel-good messenger. Tryptophan, studies suggested, could restock the shelves of the brain's serotonin supply, thereby easing pain and depression and inducing the peaceful feelings that could allow a frazzled adult to get to sleep. And, as almost every news story repeated, tryptophan was the ingredient in milk or turkey that made you feel sleepy after a turkey dinner or a glass of milk at bedtime. It was pure, the story went—wholesome as a glass of milk, and totally without side effects.

Along with three or four of his colleagues, Houts decided to give it a try. He began taking the suggested maximum dose, four tablets a day. But after a few weeks, he decided the L-tryptophan wasn't working, and stopped taking it.

Two months later, in February of 1988, his stomach began to hurt for no apparent reason. Then his legs and arms hurt. His doctor gave him a blood test and found he had a dramatically increased level of eosinophils, a type of white blood cell that typically proliferates in response to an allergy or infection. He was sent to a specialist in parasitic diseases, who took a month to declare him parasite-free. In April, a severe rash spread over his entire body. He began to have massive nosebleeds. While visiting his mother in Albany, he developed a fever of 105 and was diagnosed with the flu. All of these symptoms culminated in a two-day period in which his weight jumped from 145 to 195 pounds, impossible as it may seem, and his skin turned the color and texture of an orange peel. A colleague suggested to Houts's boss that he might need to go to a detox clinic for what she mistakenly assumed to be alcoholism. Eventually Houts's doctor prescribed large doses of prednisone, the anti-inflammatory steroid, and diuretics to help him expel water. By July of 1988, his hands were totally without feeling. And nobody could tell him why any of it was happening.

⊂⊃ ⊂⊃ ⊂⊃

In the single volume comprising the years 1900 through 1904, the *Readers' Guide to Periodical Literature* had no heading for "herbal medicine" or "dietary supplement." The *Readers' Guide*, an index of articles in major newspapers, magazines, and journals, had just one article in that volume listed under the heading of "botany, medical." Its title, from the August 2, 1902, issue of *Scientific American*, would prove prescient in the century to come: "Problems in the Chemistry and Toxicology of Plant Substances."

For the next seven decades, at most three or four articles in any given year would be listed under "botany, medical"; more often, there were none. "Dietary supplement" would not become a subject heading until 1980. So it was noteworthy when, in 1975, the first article in a popular magazine indexed by the *Readers' Guide* to tout the previously obscure amino acid L-tryptophan ran in *Newsweek* on October 13, 1975, under the title "Nature's Sleeping Pill?" The next story didn't come along until three years later, when *Psychology Today* published an article in December of 1978: "L-Tryptophan: The Sleeping Pill of the Future?" (The editors, it seemed, liked to hedge their bets with question marks.) In 1979, three articles ran, including one in *Psychology Today* ("The Promise of Drugless Pain Control: Increasing Beta-Endorphins with L-Tryptophan") and another in *Mademoiselle:* "L-Tryptophan: Is It the Magic Sleeping Pill?" In the next decade, the *Guide* listed another nine articles. The journals in which they were found ranged from *Health,* with an article in January of 1985 on the use of L-tryptophan to help infants sleep, to the venerable *Saturday Evening Post,* which in December of 1982 ran "Tryptophan for Depression." By 1986, the amino acid had been touted in the pages of *Prevention* for improving everything from cholesterol to blood pressure.

In addition to Paul Houts, another of the hundreds of thousands of Americans who tried L-tryptophan in the late 1980s was Frances L. Thompson. A divorced mother of two in her early forties, Thompson lived in Rockville, Maryland, and worked as a marketing assistant with the U.S. Pharmacopeial Convention. In December of 1987, she hurt her back in a car accident. A neurosurgeon at Johns Hopkins University Hospital recommended that she take L-tryptophan. He said it could help with sleep, pain relief, and stress symptoms, and that it had none of the potential complications of a narcotic.

In May of 1988, Dorothy C. Wilson's doctor prescribed her L-tryptophan for insomnia. She worked as a manager at Unisys in Philadelphia. She traveled regularly for both work and pleasure, walked two miles a day, swam, and enjoyed cooking, reading, movies, and restaurants. She had told her doctor she didn't want to take addictive medications with dangerous side effects. He explained that L-tryptophan was a naturally occurring amino acid found in turkey and milk—nonaddictive, with no side effects, and extremely safe. She took it for four months.

In September of 1989, Ruth Alterman, PhD, was enjoying the prime of her life. Slim and pretty, her three children grown and one of them married, Alterman lived with her husband, Carl, an engineer, in a townhouse in the tony northern suburbs of New York. Through their sliding glass back door, they could look out and see sailboats bobbing in the Long Island Sound. With a doctorate from New York University and a post-graduate degree in psychotherapy, she worked as director of special education at a public elementary school, jogged a couple miles nearly every day, and was looking forward to planning her second daughter's wedding. The one little problem was a bit of insomnia. She decided that rather than take sleeping pills to help her sleep, she was better off taking some natural substance like L-tryptophan. Although health conscious, Alterman wasn't a back-to-nature type who went to health food stores. But after reading about tryptophan in a magazine, she decided to buy some on her lunch hour at a health food store in nearby Greenwich, Connecticut.

After four months on L-tryptophan, Dorothy Wilson stopped taking it, her insomnia having gone away. But about that time, she began to feel a strange sensation in her legs during her daily walk. Soon she was feeling pain in her arms and legs, her torso, neck, and even her face and scalp. Painful muscle spasms attacked her body. Her doctor ordered blood work, which showed elevated liver enzymes, a high white blood cell count, and an extremely high count of something called an eosinophil. He knew of no single illness characterized by those symptoms.

Over the next few months, Wilson's pain worsened. She had difficulty getting up from chairs and walking up stairs. Her menstrual cycle stopped, her body hair thinned out, she lost her appetite, and she fell frequently. By December, she had weakened to the point where she was hospitalized. She was found to have extensive nerve damage and a suspicious breast mass, which turned out to be a breast cancer in a very early stage. Four months later, in April of 1989, she had a mastectomy. Soon after, her neurological symptoms stabilized. At that point, believing that L-tryptophan could in no way be related to her medical problems and, in fact, was as good for her as taking vitamin C, she resumed taking it.

By July, an itchy rash had appeared and the old weakness worsened dramatically. She had a fever and night sweats, and her skin became hard and tight. By August, she was unable to stand. Bedridden, she had to be picked up from a lying to a sitting position. Bedsores developed. She gave power of attorney to a friend because she could no longer sign her name. Her jaw locked and she had extreme difficulty eating. Her voice weakened. She couldn't cough or sneeze. She had unrelenting pain, spasms, and severe burning sensations. And nothing could explain her combination of symptoms.

That same summer, Frances Thompson was growing progressively weaker and more tired. In early August, she saw her doctor. In the middle of the month, he called and said the laboratory tests he had done were unremarkable, except for a higher percentage of eosinophils in her blood than normal. In September, he noticed that her skin appeared woody and dimpled on her forearms and, after a biopsy, diagnosed the disease as eosinophilic fasciitis. By the end of September, while she and her son were visiting during family weekend at her daughter's college, she was unable to walk any appreciable distance, and they were forced to rent a wheelchair. During this time, she also experienced fever, swelling, extreme muscle pain, skin tightness, and skin rashes. But no one could tell her why it was happening.

By late October, after a couple of weeks of taking L-tryptophan at bedtime, Ruth Alterman began to feel run down and achy. Other people in her office were coming down with the flu, and she figured she'd caught it too. She stopped taking the L-tryptophan, but after a few more weeks, everybody else in the office was getting better, and she was getting worse. As her breathing grew more labored, Alterman was diagnosed with pneumonia.

And then she started experiencing a host of other odd symptoms. Her heart pounded so hard at night that she was afraid to turn over in bed. She felt she might be about to have a heart attack. She started getting swollen hands, muscle aches and pains, nerve pain, and weakness. Her legs swelled. Then they turned orange and blue. She and her husband had no inkling of what was really happening. Certainly they did not connect it with L-tryptophan. No one did. After all, millions of people were taking it. And it was totally natural.

Tamar Stieber was nobody's idea of a journalist on the fast track. A college dropout in her midtwenties, she took a job in 1981 as a secretary for the San Francisco bureau of the Associated Press. Seeing the excitement of the reporters' pursuit of stories, she was bit by the journalism bug and decided she wanted to be out reporting stories, too. Encouraged by some of her colleagues, she quit after two years to return to college full-time at the University of California at Berkeley, finally obtaining her bachelor's degree in 1985. Two years later, she landed her first permanent reporting job, at the twice-weekly *Sonoma Index-Tribune*. It paid a pittance and was an hour commute from her home in Berkeley, but she loved it, and she was making her bones, as the saying goes. In November of 1988, she took a job as the city hall reporter for the *Vallejo Times-Herald,* circulation 26,000. In May of 1989, she accepted a job at *Journal North,* the Santa Fe bureau of the *Albuquerque Journal.*

Late that October, a part-time reporter mentioned to Tim Coder, Stieber's editor, that a friend was suffering from severe, unexplained muscle pain and had heard of another woman with the same condition. Nobody knew what was causing it, but Coder asked Stieber to check it out. She knew it was being given to her as just another throwaway story—otherwise one of the science reporters in Albuquerque would have gotten it. But for Stieber, hungry and determined, no story was a throwaway. Every assignment was a license to investigate and dig.

One woman, aged thirty-nine, turned out to be from Santa Fe. She had mouth sores and liver problems, in addition to severe muscle pain. A blood test also showed that she had remarkably high levels of certain white blood cells called eosinophils, a condition known as eosinophilia. The other woman, forty-four, from Los Alamos, had similar but milder symptoms. Both of the doctors had referred their patients to Dr. James W. Mayer, a rheumatologist from Santa Fe. When he reviewed their charts, Dr. Mayer discovered that both patients had been taking L-tryptophan. He told Stieber, "It seemed reasonable to raise the possibility that L-tryptophan might have a role in these problems."

Then, in a routine news meeting, Stieber casually mentioned the odd little story she was pursuing, and a fellow reporter piped up. He knew another Santa Fe woman hospitalized for severe pain and fluid in her lungs and her abdomen. She too had eosinophilia, and she too had been taking L-tryptophan. *What are the odds?* Stieber asked herself. Knowing in her gut that she was onto something, she called the woman's physician, Dr. Phillip Hertzman. As with the other two patients, the woman's level of eosinophils was off the charts. Where normal is up to 5 cells per cubic microliter of blood, one of the patients had 6,000 cells per microliter, while another had about 10,000.

"I've never seen anybody with a count like that, and I've been here for thirteen years," Dr. Hertzman told Stieber. "Now we have three in a thirty-mile radius." But he remained uncertain what to make of it. "I don't know of any reason why L-tryptophan per se would give someone eosinophilia," he said.

Stieber sought the expertise of Dr. Kathryn Keith, a physician with the Women's Health Services Family Care and Counseling Center in Santa Fe. Dr. Keith stressed that it was too early to know what role, if any, L-tryptophan played. Her boss, Dr. Mai Ting, director of the clinic, was even more outspoken against the possibility of a link. "I've spoken to other doctors in this town and in Albuquerque who feel the link between tryptophan and this particular situation is a red herring," she told Stieber. "A lot of people take tryptophan and nobody else has [reacted]."

Another doctor went still farther. Dr. Ron Voorhees, a medical investigator with the New Mexico Office of Epidemiology, told Stieber it would be "unethical" for the newspaper to publish speculation that L-tryptophan played a role.

But Stieber kept making calls. Finally she reached Dr. Gerald Gleich, chair of Immunology at the famed Mayo Clinic in Minnesota and an expert on eosinophilia. He told Stieber: "It could be a red herring, but a red herring in three people? I'm not willing to buy that. I'm trained to look for unexpected associations. Once is chance, twice is kind of interesting, but three and I say full speed ahead. It's too curious to be easily ignored."

Stieber's cautious story appeared on newsstands on the morning of Tuesday, November 7, 1989, under the headline, "Three N.M. Women Contract Unusual Medical Syndrome." Not until the fourth paragraph did she mention L-tryptophan as "the only common thread doctors have found so far."

The reaction was immediate. By the end of the day, alerted to the condition by Stieber's story, doctors reported nine more cases across the state. The next day, Wednesday, four more were reported, bringing the total to sixteen.

It was then that Stieber was told by the editors in Albuquerque that the story was being given to a science writer. She had been planning to go away for the weekend, but she immediately scrapped those plans and hunkered down to work harder. It was her story, and nobody was going to take it away from her.

On Saturday, she reported, the total number of cases had hit twenty-one, with patients now in Arizona, Missouri, Oregon, and Texas. CNN broadcasted a report, and Stieber realized that the story had gone national. Adrenaline pumping, she kept pursuing leads. That morning, the FDA issued a warning to consumers to temporarily stop taking L-tryptophan. Her Sunday front-page story reported that there were now fifty-five affected patients in eight states.

On Tuesday, November 14, New Mexico officials banned L-tryptophan's sale or display. Two days later, the number of cases nationwide hit 250. A couple more days after that, with 287 cases reported, the FDA called for a national voluntary recall of all L-tryptophan in the country, its hazard assessment committee having judged the supplement to be "a moderate to severe hazard."

By the end of the month, Ron Voorhees, the health official who had warned Stieber that it would be "unethical" to publish her report, was telling the *New York Times* that the publicity caused by Stieber's report had saved a mere week in the identification of L-tryptophan's role. In truth, there is no evidence that anyone else was ever close to connecting the dots, with the possible exception of a government researcher in charge of an obscure laboratory at the National Institute of Mental Health.

It was Esther M. Sternberg's morning to drive the carpool of children to her daughter's elementary school in the suburbs outside Washington, D.C. On the radio, over the chattering of the children, she heard the first report on National Public Radio about the mysterious illness in New Mexico associated with L-tryptophan. Sternberg, a rheumatologist and head of the National Institute of Mental Health's Unit on Neuroendocrine Immunology and Behavior, instantly realized that what the doctors in New Mexico were seeing was the early, acute phase of a disease she had been studying for years. In that moment, she became perhaps the first person in the country to glimpse the terrible future that awaited the L-tryptophan patients.

Back in the Christmas season of 1978, in her final year of clinical rheumatology training at McGill University School of Medicine in Montreal, Sternberg had treated a seventy-year-old man who had developed severe scleroderma, a disease that attacks the blood vessels and connective tissues, causing symptoms similar to rheumatoid arthritis. Examining the man, she found unusual scarring, like third-degree burns, on his skin, lungs, and other internal organs. What was unique about his case was the speed with which he'd developed the symptoms. He'd been totally without the disease until given something called 5-hydroxy-tryptophan, or 5HTP, a natural derivative of L-tryptophan made by the body. Although used by doctors as a drug to treat a rare form of epilepsy, it was regulated, like L-tryptophan, as a dietary supplement because of its natural origin. Following standard practice, the man was given 5HTP to treat his epilepsy, and it had successfully stopped his seizures. Except now he had the severe, life-threatening scleroderma.

The case was unusual enough that Sternberg wrote it up into a study, and it was published as the lead article in the prestigious *New England Journal of Medicine* in October of 1980. She hypothesized at the time that the 5HTP had triggered the scleroderma-like illness due to an inborn error in the man's tryptophan metabolism.

The paper had launched her into a career in research and ultimately landed her at the National Institutes of Health. But she had gone on to study other things until, in April of 1989—six months before Tamar Stieber's article would reveal the nationwide outbreak—Sternberg received a telephone call from a fellow rheumatologist at the Medical University of South Carolina. Richard Silver was breathless with excitement. Two patients in his office had the exact same condition she had described in her 1980 paper. But instead of having taken 5HTP, they had taken L-tryptophan, a close chemical cousin.

"Would you be willing to help me put together a study?" he asked.

"Sure, why not?" Sternberg replied.

At that point, both doctors assumed, as Sternberg had ten years earlier, that the tryptophan-induced illness was exceedingly rare, requiring an unusual, inherited error of metabolism to develop. They proceeded, therefore, at an unhurried, deliberate pace. They spread the word among rheumatologists in the Southeast that they were looking for patients with the illness. Slowly, one by one, reports of patients with the illness began to filter back to them. By that morning in November when Sternberg heard the radio report about the national outbreak, they had a total of nine patients.

When she arrived at work, she hurriedly called Silver, who'd heard the same news report and likewise realized the sudden significance of their ongoing study. They decided that rather than wait for more patients to begin analyzing the biochemistry of the nine patients' blood samples, they would do it immediately—but not before calling both the FDA and the Centers for Disease Control. A team of scientists from the NIH, the CDC, and the FDA was quickly formed to focus on the outbreak, with Sternberg in charge of the NIH team.

○ ⊂⊃ ⊂⊃

Living not far from Sternberg in the D.C. suburbs, Paul Houts read a story in the *New York Times* about the strange epidemic. He sent copies of the news clippings to his primary doctor, explaining his brief experiment with L-tryptophan. Almost before he could put them in the mail, several other doctors he'd previously consulted called to ask if they could have permission to re-review his case file. But the new understanding of the source of his illness did little to change its course. Two months later he found himself in the emergency room at Georgetown Hospital with a raging fever and unbearable muscle spasms, like the pain of a leg cramp multiplied a hundredfold. But these spasms hit every part of his body, sometimes simultaneously, leaving him howling in pain or writhing on the floor.

In Maryland, Frances Thompson likewise found little comfort in the news of L-tryptophan's role. That December, living alone, determined to remain cheerful despite being confined to a wheelchair, she succeeded in decorating one third of a Christmas tree that a friend had kindly brought into her apartment. Then she lost the use of her arms and hands. Over Christmas, the tree remained forlornly one third decorated. And then came reports in the press that patients were dying.

○ ⊂⊃ ⊂⊃

The disease now had a name: L-tryptophan eosinophilia myalgia syndrome, or L-tryptophan EMS. (In an odd coincidence that Sternberg could not help but notice, EMS also happened to be the three initials of her name.) Within months, the CDC had determined that nearly all of the new cases involved a single batch of L-tryptophan that had been manufactured by a single company, Showa Denko KK, one of the largest chemical companies in Japan, shortly after it had substantially changed its manufacturing process. A report on the nine patients Sternberg and Silver had gathered was published in the *New England Journal of Medicine* in March 1990. By then, the NIH, CDC, and FDA teams had joined together, and Sternberg was already at work on an animal study involving rats, in which they gave the batch of L-tryptophan made by Showa Denko to half of them, and another brand to the other half. Those who'd received the Showa Denko batch developed some of the EMS symptoms. But the picture remained somewhat murky. Some patients, such as Paul Houts, never took the implicated batch made by Showa Denko. And tens of thousands of other patients who did take the bad batch never developed any symptoms. The emerging theory was that a genetically predisposed person could develop EMS in reaction to even pure L-tryptophan, but that something in the Showa Denko batch made such a reaction far more likely.

Facing what would soon amount to $2 billion in lawsuits, Showa Denko suddenly began funding all kinds of studies. Soon, most of the nongovernment scientists with an interest in the matter were receiving funds from the company to study it. The company tried to get Sternberg to participate as well. First they offered her $3,000 to spend two afternoons talking with Showa Denko's attorneys. She declined. Then they sent a young rheumatologist whom they'd placed on their advisory board to offer her money for research with no strings attached. She wouldn't even have to write a grant proposal. The company, he told her, would give her whatever she wanted. She told him no thank you. Then the game got ugly.

At a meeting of the Pan American Health Organization, a researcher who happened to be receiving grant money from Showa Denko asked Sternberg, before the entire panel, "What about rumors that your animal study couldn't be reproduced?"

Sternberg was shocked. "I don't discuss rumors," she answered. But where had the rumors come from? Her animal study implicating the

Showa Denko batch had in fact been reproduced in two other peer-reviewed journals.

On July 18, 1991, Sternberg testified before a congressional hearing on the outbreak and the government's response to it held by the Intergovernmental Relations Subcommittee of the Committee on Government Operations. "In order to determine whether the implicated tryptophan did, indeed, cause the disease, we fed it to a special strain of rats," she said. "It did cause scarring of the connective tissue surrounding the muscle in these rats. That is the hallmark of the human syndrome. The purer, non-case-associated tryptophan did not."

She felt justly proud of the work her team had done in uncovering the cause of the outbreak. But when the hearing was over, the first person who came up to her was a young woman who worked as a reporter for *Forbes*.

"What about rumors that your studies couldn't be replicated?" the woman asked.

The rumors, it turned out, were based on one study, funded by Showa Denko, in which only two male and two female rats completed the full course of treatment. When the FDA had offered to confirm that the test material was in fact the implicated batch from Showa Denko, the company's attorneys refused. Eventually the study was published, although it took the authors five years to pass peer review, and then only in a supplement to the *Journal of Rheumatology* that was sponsored entirely by Showa Denko. The editors and most of the authors in the supplement had received grants and consulting fees from the company.

Soon, Showa Denko filed Freedom of Information requests for files on everything the government teams were doing. When Sternberg refused, the company filed a lawsuit seeking the information. All the studies coming from Sternberg's team members at the CDC, the NIH, and the FDA were held up from publication. Editors of the journals to whom they'd submitted the papers were deposed. A cloud loomed over Sternberg's work and reputation.

"Why is all this happening to me?" she asked a friend in the midst of the lawsuits.

"How much did you say that Showa Denko is being sued for?" he asked in reply.

"Two billion dollars."

"That's two billion reasons."

⊂⊃ ⊂⊃ ⊂⊃

By the morning of the 1991 hearing at which Sternberg testified, Ruth Alterman was slowly recovering, although she would eventually have to take an early retirement. And Tamar Stieber, the onetime college dropout who'd broken the story, had won the 1990 Pulitzer Prize for Specialized Reporting. Others were not doing so well. Some 5,000 cases of L-tryptophan EMS were eventually reported to the FDA, including 38 deaths.

The July 18 hearing convened at 10 a.m. at the Rayburn House Office Building, in room 2154, where the walnut paneling on the walls climbs as high as a house. Ted Weiss, the New York congressman who chaired the subcommittee, sat with four of his fellow members and four of the subcommittee's staff at the front of the room. Sitting at the witness table before them were Dorothy Wilson, Frances Thompson, and Paul Houts. Wilson, sitting in a wheelchair, was first to testify.

She began by reading from the label of a bottle of L-tryptophan, which claimed not only that the substance within was "pure" and "well tolerated by the most highly allergic individuals," but that it was manufactured in the United States, when in fact it had been manufactured in Japan by Showa Denko.

"Where was the FDA when this label was on a readily available product?" she asked. "Why didn't the FDA require a warning of possible side effects? I am irreversibly paralyzed. The excruciating pain, spasms, electric shocks, burning, and aching muscles have grown worse. I cannot work and am restricted to a house with thirteen steps. I suffer from exhaustion, weakness, and muscle fatigue, which often makes it impossible to undress, transfer from the wheelchair, or even move the wheelchair by myself. I need an aide to help me shower and do the basic things that most people take for granted. And the story's obviously not finished."

The next speaker was Frances Thompson, likewise in a wheelchair. "EMS has ravaged my life and left it pointless," she told the congressmen. "I sit before you helpless, broke, alone, and in unyielding, relentless pain. Not only has the government or Showa Denko failed on all fronts, but I also have no adequate medical insurance and remain deeply in debt with no hope."

Mitch Zeller, counsel to the subcommittee, noticed that some of the congressmen with whom he was sitting were crying. Zeller had sat through more hearings in his career than he cared to remember, but never one that caused congressmen to cry. Neither had he ever seen members of Congress applauding at the end of a witness's testimony, even if secretly, with their hands under the dais so that the public wouldn't see their personal reaction.

The last of the three patients to testify was Paul Houts. Although not in a wheelchair, he told how the endless muscle spasms, pain, and other symptoms had finally led him to be hospitalized for depression in June of 1990. "How did Dante put it?" he asked, and then paraphrased the first line of the *Inferno:* " 'In the middle of the journey of our life, I found my-self in a dark wood, for I had lost the right path.' For myself and many others in this room, our dark wood has been EMS. What do I face each morning? Certainly a day of unrelenting and, at times, unbearable pain. I continue to black out, just as the nosebleeds are a daily feature of my life. And so I zigzag from physical to mental anguish like so many EMS patients, carrying my own desolation as I do my walking stick wherever I go."

The three patients made their way to the back of the room, and the next round of speakers was called forth: Sternberg, a collaborator of hers, and the doctor who had first discovered tryptophan's mood-altering role. Their testimony lacked the drama and pathos of the victims'. They made nobody cry. But what they had to say was no less important, for no one in the country could better explain why the lives of Wilson, Thompson, Houts, and some 5,000 other Americans had been ruined.

First up was Sternberg, who explained how her team had figured out the role of Showa Denko. Next to speak was Dr. Richard J. Wurtman, a professor of basic neuroscience at the Massachusetts Institute of Tech-nology, a physician at Harvard Medical School, and director of MIT's Clinical Research Center. Over the prior two decades, he'd coauthored some four hundred scientific papers on L-tryptophan and other amino acids. Sadly, he appeared to be apologizing for discovering tryptophan's effects.

"I feel a small amount of responsibility for what we've heard described here today," he began, "because one of the things my laboratory did, twenty years ago, was to discover that tryptophan levels normally controlled the production of a brain chemical, serotonin. This brain chemical is involved in sleep, mood, appetite, et cetera. And so my associates and I proposed at that time that perhaps someday tryptophan would become a legitimate drug that could be used to help people sleep, diminish pain, control mood and appetite, and so forth. I had assumed pharmaceutical companies might take this discovery and invest the ten or twenty million dollars, whatever it took then, to do appropriate safety and efficacy studies. But it didn't work out that way."

His regret for what might have been—had tryptophan been regulated as a drug, had its true benefits and dangers been clearly defined, had its manufacturing process been closely regulated like other drugs'—was overshadowed only by anger. Not only had so many people suffered needlessly, but now, even were it not already banned, no drug company would ever dare attempt to go back and develop it as a drug. A simple legal classification and the havoc it caused had forever lost to humanity's patrimony a potentially important medicine.

For a scientist, Wurtman made his case in remarkably clear, direct language. "Tryptophan in dietary protein is an important nutrient," he said. "When you have it in protein it comes along with twenty-one other amino acids, and you need the pattern, all of them, in order to utilize them to make your own protein. When you take pure tryptophan in pills or in a bottle, it's not natural. Never in man's evolutionary history did he or she take an individual amino acid. The body does not handle it the same way the body handles tryptophan in protein. The body cannot use it, for instance, to make its own protein. So tryptophan, in spite of being called a nutritional supplement, has nothing whatsoever to do with nutrition. Tryptophan is a drug. Apart from the amino acids and protein, its administration in pills does change the chemistry of the brain. It's probably safe to say that ninety-nine percent, ninety-nine point nine percent of the people who bought tryptophan when it was for sale in catalogs and health food stores bought it precisely because they knew that it was a drug, that it would have useful effects, they thought, upon sleep or pain." But, he went on, "there are extremely important implications involved in whether you call it a drug or call it a nutritional supplement. Things that we call drugs must be safe, and we have criteria for establishing safety. They have to be efficacious and they have to be of adequate purity and the impurities have to be known."

The question that Dorothy Wilson had asked—"Where was the FDA?"—still echoed in the room as the third and final panel of the day sat down at the witness table: a group of FDA officials, including Douglas L. Archer, PhD, the agency's deputy director of the Center for Food Safety and Applied Nutrition. He explained that the FDA had, in fact, tried and failed to bring L-tryptophan under tighter regulations. But, he said, "the FDA has been deterred from moving against the illegal sales of L-tryptophan as a dietary supplement because we were twice rebuffed in the courts."

The problem, he explained, could be tracked back to 1972—the same year the FDA's decision to set limits on the potency of vitamins had set in motion the reactionary movement that resulted in the passage of the Proxmire bill. As part of the agency's generally stepped-up effort toward clamping down on the booming supplement industry, the FDA had also decided to remove L-tryptophan from its official list of dietary supplements that are generally recognized as safe (GRAS). On July 26, 1973, in the Federal Register it was officially removed from the GRAS list, which should have required companies from then on to submit detailed safety studies if they wanted to sell it. Then came an almost absurd bit of bureaucratic bungling: on March 15, 1977, when an updated Code of Federal Regulations was published with a GRAS list, L-tryptophan was mistakenly included. The error was corrected by a notice in the Federal Register on October 28, 1977, but it was too late. Ridiculous as it may sound, with that one error, attributable to some unknown gnome in the bowels of the agency, manufacturers could now claim an excuse for selling it—which is exactly what a company called Schiff Vitamins did that year when the FDA seized a shipment of its L-tryptophan tablets. In court, the FDA insisted that it was an unapproved food additive. Schiff insisted it had merely relied on the mistaken GRAS listing. The judge sided with Schiff, saying it was entitled to rely on the published regulations, even if the regulations were in error. Schiff and other manufacturers were now free to continue selling L-tryptophan.

But the agency kept fighting. The same year it had seized the Schiff product, it seized another one called L-Tryptophan-Rest. Back in the

1960s, seizing products like this had been routine. But after five long years of litigating what became known as the "Trypto-Rest" case, the FDA concluded in September of 1982 that the case was hopeless and agreed to drop it. And unlike with the Schiff case, in which the judge's ruling was based on a mere technicality, this time the FDA saw that the judge appeared to be convinced that Trypto-Rest was truly safe and viewed the FDA's attempt to prove otherwise with marked suspicion. "It was clear that the court was inclined to agree with the defendant's position that the product was generally recognized as safe," Archer testified. "This litigation is indicative of the resource-intensive nature of this type of case and became a significant factor in deciding whether to pursue additional cases."

Another factor in the FDA's decision in the early 1980s to stop trying to regulate sales of L-tryptophan, Archer added, was the Proxmire Amendment. "The amendment was passed in direct response to an FDA rule-making effort," Archer said, "and it seemed to signal congressional intent that supplement-type products not be regulated without indications of real danger to health."

What Archer was saying, in sum, was that agency officials had finally gotten the message that the courts and the Congress had been sending them: that they should keep their hands off supplements unless they could be plainly shown to kill or injure people—not just theoretically, but in actuality, with dead bodies or people in wheelchairs. *That* was why they hadn't prevented the L-tryptophan tragedy: they were just following orders to wait until the proverbial shit hit the fan.

Now that the awful price of such a policy had been paid, no one leaving the hearing room that morning doubted that the FDA, with the help of Congress, would have to do something to avoid a similar disaster. Finally, the warnings of everyone who had opposed the Proxmire amendment had come true. After all, every time a medical catastrophe like this had occurred in the twentieth century, the power and authority of the FDA to prevent similar tragedies had been expanded. The death of 107 people due to a contaminated batch of the antibiotic sulfanilamide had led to the passage of the Federal Food, Drug, and Cosmetic Act of 1938. The thousands of birth defects due to the sleeping pill thalidomide had led to the Kefauver-Harris Amendments of 1962. To repeat the words of historian Michael Harris: "The history of drug regulation is built on tombstones." Now that more tombstones had been planted in the name of L-tryptophan, surely new regulations could not be far behind. And sure enough, the FDA did commence a battle for expanded powers—one of the biggest battles in the agency's history, led by one of the strongest commissioners it had ever known. He could only hope that his effort would fare better than the two heroines of the L-tryptophan story.

For years, Esther Sternberg fought the industry-fed rumors that her research couldn't be duplicated, as well as the perception that she had strayed too far from her job description as a unit head at the National Institute of Mental Health—no matter that she had spearheaded an extraordinarily fast and effective national response to a public health crisis. Hounded by government officials to "just do her job" instead of testifying in public about the dangers of supplements, she was repeatedly told to stay quiet—and refused. Denied a promotion, she hired a lawyer and eventually won the new job. Yet her experience was considered harrowing enough that when the American Association for the Advancement of Science held a special session titled "Manipulation of Science by Vested Interests: Money and Power Versus Public Health," Sternberg co-chaired the session and was one of the speakers, along with Dr. Victor DeNobel, a cigarette industry scientist whose research was stopped short when he proved both that nicotine was addictive and that one of the additives in cigarettes greatly increased their addictiveness.

Tamar Stieber, after winning the first Pulitzer ever received by a New Mexico journalist, was promised by her newspaper a beat pursuing special projects, but instead she was given minor assignments about the weather and such and was paid some $10,000 less than the next lowest-paid investigative reporter. She finally sued for sex discrimination, and lost both the case and her life savings in the process of paying her lawyer. She resigned, made a brief effort at freelancing, and finally left journalism forever to become a hospice worker. For years her Pulitzer certificate sat in a box, a bitter reminder of a career she had loved and lost, despite having single-handedly uncovered the first great calamity of the supplement boom.

CHAPTER 4
KESSLER vs. KESSLER

Born in New York on May 31, 1951, David A. Kessler pursued an education and career that could hardly have been more perfect to prepare him to lead the Food and Drug Administration. After graduating from Oberlin College in the spring of 1973, he enrolled at Harvard Medical School. Not finding that to be enough of a challenge, he simultaneously pursued a law degree at the University of Chicago. By 1979 he had an MD from Harvard and a JD from Chicago. After a few years as a consultant to Senator Ted Kennedy's Committee on Labor and Human Resources, he became special assistant to the president of Montefiore Medical Center in New York. In 1984, still in his early thirties, he became medical director of the hospital of the Albert Einstein College of Medicine, a job that men twice his age would find a fitting capstone to a career. On the side, he taught food and drug law at Columbia University School of Medicine.

But when, on Thursday, October 11, 1990, the first President George Bush nominated Kessler to be the new commissioner of the FDA, the agency he was being handed was widely seen as facing the worst crisis in its history, with challenges going well beyond dietary supplements. The previous full-time commissioner, Frank E. Young, had resigned a year earlier, just around the time of the L-tryptophan outbreak, in the wake of a bribery scandal that saw several FDA officials convicted of helping generic drug manufacturers fake their safety and efficacy data. And even though its staff was smaller than it had been a decade earlier, its responsibilities were growing amid a flood of new drug applications for AIDS treatments. Ted Kennedy said at the time, "The Food and Drug Administration is caught in a downward spiral of declining resources, credibility, and morale," while Dr. Sidney Wolfe, head of the Public Citizen Health Research Group, told the *New York Times*, "[Now is a] key time, after the worst leadership in FDA history, which demoralized the agency unlike anything I have ever seen."

It was with remarkable enthusiasm, therefore, that Kessler's nomination was greeted by virtually every official and commentator of the day. Wolfe called the appointment "promising." Peter B. Hutt, a lawyer and consultant to the agency who sat on several of its advisory panels, said Kessler's résumé was perfect for the challenges facing the agency, adding, "If he can't do it, nobody can." Senator Orrin Hatch, the Republican from Utah who sat on Kennedy's Committee on Labor and Human Resources, thought so highly of the committee's former employee that he urged his colleagues to confirm Kessler without delay. "I do not think we ought to wait the regular time," Hatch told Senator Howard M. Metzenbaum, the Democrat of Ohio who also sat on the committee. "I think he is absolutely superb. He is qualified. He has a tremendous background. He is intelligent. He understands the issues as far as safety for the American people are concerned. There could not be a better choice for the position, and instead of going through the normal procedures, Howard, I would appreciate it if you would just sign off and we could confirm him promptly."

Having been implored and entreated by such a persuasive and respected member of the Senate, Metzenbaum and his colleagues confirmed the nominee after a quick midnight vote on Saturday night, October 27. On Thursday, November 8, Kessler took office at the age of thirty-nine, vowing that the FDA would no longer be just a "paper tiger" on enforcement of the food and drug laws. That very same day, as chance would have it, President Bush signed into law a bill meant to give the agency new powers in the regulation of supplements. At least, that was the idea.

⊂⊃ ⊂⊃ ⊂⊃

Written partly in response to L-tryptophan, the Nutrition Labeling and Education Act (NLEA) took aim at the increasingly outrageous claims being made not only for supplements, but also for ordinary foods. "The magnitude of the death and permanent injury that took place from unregulated tryptophan happened because of the claims," said Mitchell Zeller, who served as counsel to the House subcommittee that held the hearings on L-tryptophan. "There wouldn't have been such widespread use of the product and there wouldn't have been so many deaths and injuries without the claims."

False label claims, after all, were what put Clark Stanley and his snake oil out of business back in 1916. But while drug claims remained under the tightest oversight of any consumer product in the country, by the early 1990s food and supplement claims had grown increasingly outrageous. In the view of Representative Henry Waxman, who chaired the House Subcommittee on Health and the Environment, "Food labeling was out of control. Consumers could not possibly understand terms such as 'light' or 'low fat' since their meaning varied from product to product. Manufacturers were allowed to make claims such as 'fiber prevents cancer' without having first presented their scientific evidence to the Food and Drug Administration."

The NLEA, which Waxman had introduced, was designed to set clear new rules for what could be claimed both for foods and for supplements. The bill brought into being the now familiar Nutrition Facts box placed on the label of every food or supplement, describing the serving size, servings per container, and percentage of daily recommended values contained in each serving. The law also stipulated that before any food or supplement could make a health claim, the FDA would first have to find that there was evidence to back the claim. So before milk manufacturers could claim that the calcium in milk prevents osteoporosis, or before supplement manufacturers could make the same claim for their products, the FDA would have to review the evidence. Such "pre-market review" put the burden of gathering the evidence on the manufacturers and freed the FDA from the Sisyphean task of checking the accuracy of thousands of individual label claims after they were already on the market—or, worse yet, from having to conduct its own studies to prove that a claim was *not* true.

Waxman had wanted the standard of proof for claims to be the same for both supplements and foods, since after all the same ingredients were usually at stake. And what Waxman wanted, Waxman usually got. Considered at the time one of the most powerful Democrats in Congress, he represented, as he does to this day, what the *Almanac of American Politics* describes as "the biggest and flashiest concentration of affluence in the world": the 30th Congressional District of California, encompassing Bel-Air, Brentwood, Beverly Hills, Malibu, Westwood, and West Hollywood. But he is also considered, as the *Almanac* put it, "one of the ablest members of the House, a shrewd political operator who is a skilled and idealistic policy entrepreneur." The standard he proposed seemed emblematic of his shrewd yet idealistic approach. On the one hand, it fell far short of the standard for a new drug, which requires multiple double-blind, placebo-controlled trials involving more than a thousand people before going on the market. On the other hand, he wanted something stricter than the "competent and reliable" evidence standard used by the Federal Trade Commission when reviewing health advertisements, since any food or supplement company could presumably scare up a few "competent" experts and a few "reliable" studies to prop up all but the most baseless claims. Seeking a middle path between those two extremes, Waxman proposed a standard of "significant scientific agreement"—meaning not just that a handful of little studies had found that vitamin D might do such and such, but that most studies, and most experts, had reached a similar conclusion.

"No one was saying that dietary supplements should be subjected to the drug standard of the FDA," said Zeller. "What got written into the NLEA was a more flexible standard. The food industry decided to work with Congress, work with the FDA, and ultimately be at the table on behalf of sensible public health legislation." Supplement manufacturers, however, believed the "significant scientific agreement" standard would seal their industry's doom, because so few of their products could live up to it. So they turned to the one senator they believed to be their most reliable advocate: Utah's Orrin Hatch.

Why him? For starters, dietary supplements are the third-largest industry in Hatch's state, now generating over $3 billion in sales per year from dozens of manufacturers, including four of the industry's top thirty (Weider, Nutraceutical Corp., Nature's Way, and Nu Skin International). Undeniably, Utah is viewed by many as being at the heart of the supplement industry. It is, after all, the only state in the country to have its very own supplement trade association, the Utah Natural Products Alliance. And the fact that 70 percent of its population is Mormon also plays an important role. According to Hatch, "Active Mormons abstain from alcohol, coffee, tea, and tobacco," whereas many of them use dietary supplements to "promote good health." He himself has been an avid user for more than three decades. He earned pocket money selling vitamins as a young man, and now takes a pack of vitamins every morning, according to the *Washington Monthly*. He has also said he takes saw palmetto, an herb believed to relieve the symptoms of an enlarged prostate, a condition that affects many men over the age of fifty. "I really believe in them," he has said on the Senate floor. "I use them daily. They make me feel better, as they make millions of Americans feel better. And I hope they give me that little added edge as we work around here."

The supplement industry has also given an added edge to Hatch's campaigns, his family, his bank account, and many of his former staff aides. One company, Herbalife International, gave more to Hatch's Senate campaigns between 1989 and 2004 than all but two other companies, totaling $49,250, according to the Center for Responsive Politics. His tenth-largest donor was Metabolife, which gave $31,500. Three other firms—Rexall Sundown, Nu Skin International, and Starlight International—gave a total of $88,550. In addition, according to Hatch's personal financial disclosure for 2003, he owns 35,621 shares of Pharmics Inc. through a limited partnership, representing 1.16 percent of the company, which deals in real estate and sells dietary supplements. When Hatch's interest in the company was raised by the *Los Angeles Times* in 1993, he wrote a huffy letter to the editor, complaining that the firm is "primarily a real estate company" and that it "sells only two products that would be potentially affected" by the legislation he sponsored on dietary supplements. Presently, however, the Web site for Pharmics lists six supplements for sale and describes itself as a "Utah based company that has been providing quality pharmaceutical nutritional products to the pediatric and obstetric market since 1970." In his 1993 letter, Hatch wrote that Pharmics's gross sales of supplements "have never exceeded

$42,000." But in 2002, according to the company's financial statement, the company's pharmaceutical operations had total sales of $422,491; six of its eleven pharmaceutical products are supplements, and together they accounted for 37 percent of the company's total sales that year.

What's more, Hatch's son Scott began working in the early 1990s for lobbying firms that counted supplement manufacturers among their top clients. In the decade that Scott worked for Parry, Romani (cofounded by Thomas Parry, Hatch's former chief of staff), the firm pulled in nearly $2 million in fees from supplement manufacturers, according to the *Los Angeles Times*. (Yet another former chief of staff for Hatch, Kevin McGuiness, is also now a lobbyist for supplement companies.) When Scott left in 2002 to start a new firm with fellow lobbyist and former Hatch aide Jack Martin, two of their first clients were the National Nutritional Foods Association, the supplement industry's largest trade group, which paid the firm $44,900 in 2002, and TwinLab Corporation, which paid $35,000. Both the senator and his son defended the relationship as perfectly ethical, however, and no law prevents the family of senators or members of Congress from lobbying. However, according to Bill Schultz, who wrote much of the NLEA as counsel to Waxman's Subcommittee on Health and the Environment, it was clear that "Hatch wanted a weaker standard for dietary supplements."

Unable to settle on a standard for label claims on supplements, Hatch and Waxman finally agreed to disagree. At Hatch's insistence, they opted to allow the FDA itself to come up with the label rules. Essentially, the two men punted, both of them trusting that the agency would figure out a compromise standard for supplements that everybody could live with. But that was before anyone realized just how uncompromising David Kessler could be.

○ ▭ ◯

Soon recognized around Washington for his round wire-rimmed glasses and closely trimmed red beard, Kessler quickly earned himself the nickname "Elliot Knessler" (a reference to the "untouchable" agent who put Al Capone behind bars) by dint of his dogged enforcement actions. In April of 1991, just two months after his appointment, he drew page one headlines by sending federal marshals to a Procter & Gamble warehouse to seize and destroy 40,000 cases of Citrus Hill Fresh Choice Orange Juice. P&G's crime: although the name said "fresh," the label noted in small type that the juice was, in fact, from concentrate. Days later, Kessler demanded that Unilever remove the words "means fresh taste" from its Ragu spaghetti sauce label because the tomatoes in the sauce were from concentrate.

By then, he had already appointed Gary Dykstra, his deputy associate commissioner for regulatory affairs, to head a Dietary Supplement Task Force to settle on the standard for supplement label claims, the job that Hatch and Waxman had left for the agency to figure out. As Kessler told a reporter, "In the district offices and in the consumer affairs office, the number one complaint is 'How can you allow these products to make these kinds of claims?' The public has to be aware that these products have not been regulated in any systematic way. We have not set any product standards, any manufacturing controls, nor required any safety testing. If you walk into a health food store, you have to recognize that we have not approved the safety of these products nor substantiated their claims."

Kessler knew, however, that the agency he'd taken control of lacked something that most other federal agencies took for granted: subpoena power. Waxman set out to fix that for him when on June 7 he introduced HR 3642: the Food, Drug, Cosmetic, and Device Enforcement Amendments of 1991. In addition to giving the FDA subpoena power to investigate potential violations of the law, it would "authorize any U.S. district court to order the recall of a food, drug, device, or cosmetic which is in violation of the [law] if the violation involves fraud or presents a significant risk to human or animal health," and would likewise authorize the secretary of health and human services to order such a recall. Without doubt, the "fraud" part was aimed directly at supplement claims, and the bill struck fear into the heart of any manufacturer wise enough to understand its potential impact.

Then, on November 27, 1991, the day before Thanksgiving, the Federal Register published the rules proposed by Dykstra's task force for regulating the label claims of supplements. To the shock of just about everybody, the proposed rules used the exact same "significant scientific agreement" standard that Waxman had wanted but Hatch had refused to accept, and that the industry considered ruinous. Apparently, Dykstra and others at the agency thought Waxman's logic flawless: what was the point, after all, of having one standard to justify touting the health benefits of vitamin D in milk, but a lesser standard to tout those benefits when the vitamin D, in more concentrated form, was in a pill? But the industry considered the proposed rules a threat to its existence, because if manufacturers couldn't claim benefits for their products without strong scientific support, why would consumers buy them? Soon Dykstra was receiving death threats, according to a report in the *National Journal.* "This issue tends to get more emotional than most," he dryly observed. Steadier heads, however, saw that the proper target was not Dykstra, and not even his boss, but Congress. And in a bit of irony too outlandish for any work of fiction, the man who would organize the industry campaign to fight back against Kessler's move to take control of the supplement marketplace, indeed to declare war upon the agency, would just happen to share his last name.

○ ⊂⊃ ⊂

Kessler's doppelganger lived much of the year on a spectacular ranch located half an hour inland from Santa Barbara, over the Santa Ynez Mountains, past vineyards and white-railed horse farms—not far, in fact, from Michael Jackson's Neverland estate. The 240-acre grounds of the Circle K Ranch boasted trumpeter swans in a man-made koi pond, a flock of exotic ostriches, a 17,000-square-foot main lodge built of massive stones, tennis courts, swimming pools, a dozen or so visitors' cabins, a fitness center, venerable oaks, elaborate gardens, and a fantastic pedigree: the place used to belong to Ray Kroc, founder of McDonald's, and was said to be where the Egg McMuffin was invented. Best yet, the 5,000-square-foot main house was round—like a hamburger.

Tall and handsome, with a deep voice, a mane of thick white hair brushed straight back, and a striking resemblance to the late actor James Coburn (who happened to be a good friend of his), Gerald A. Kessler embodies the classic rags-to-riches American success story. Born in the midst of the Great Depression, he lived with his parents until his father died unexpectedly when Gerry was six. His mother, with no means of support, placed him in a Florida orphanage. A Jewish child in an institution run by harsh Baptists, he realized that the only other Jew in the place was Jesus, who had been crucified. The Dickensian experience there would shape his life. He decided that he would never again let any other human being control him.

Once his mother remarried when Gerry was nine, he went back to live with her and his new stepfather. He shoveled snow, shoveled coal, did a paper route—anything for a buck, to his stepfather's puzzlement. When the family moved north to Forest Hills, Queens, Kessler went to high school there. Being six-foot-seven, he landed a spot on the basketball team, which went on to enjoy an undefeated season—a metaphor for how he intended to live his life. After graduating from New York University in the mid-1950s, he went to work as a salesman for Sandoz, a pharmaceutical company. He learned much about the business of selling medicines, but after some fourteen years, he began to suspect that he was selling products that only masked disease, whereas vitamins and other supplements, he believed, could actually eliminate or prevent diseases. When his son, Craig, was diagnosed with hyperactivity, a doctor wanted to put him on tranquilizers. A second doctor, however, suggested that the boy might be lactose intolerant and said he should take calcium supplements. It worked, and Gerry was sold on the power of supplements.

In 1970, he left Sandoz, and in 1972, at the height of Adelle Davis's fame, he started Nature's Plus. At first, he worked days at other jobs and nights on his new business, putting in sixteen hours a day, seven days a week. By the early 1990s, Nature's Plus was one of the top ten supplement manufacturers in the United States, and Gerry, as sole owner, was one of the richest men in the industry. But now he saw everything he had built threatened by David Kessler and his agency's proposed standard for regulating supplement claims, not to mention Waxman's bill to permit the recall of products making "fraudulent" claims.

Within days of the publication of the FDA's proposed rules, Gerry hit the phones. His idea was simple: to call together the industry's leaders and form a plan for fighting back. Hardly the most popular man in the business, Gerry at first found it hard to convince everybody of the need for a summit meeting. Forceful to a fault, witheringly direct, and lacking the patience for political wrangling, he held none of the leadership positions in industry organizations that many of those he called enjoyed. Then again, most of them treasured his bracing honesty and forthrightness, and recognized his high intelligence and fierce determination—even if he could be a pain in the ass, an unbearable bully who didn't know the meaning of compromise. "My dad's a very determined guy," his son, Craig, once told an interviewer. "When he sets his mind to do something, he does it." Said a local real estate businessman, Pete Robinson: "He doesn't like to lose." It also didn't hurt that he was richer than most of them, with that incredible ranch, tangible evidence of his business acumen. Finally Gerry convinced them, and everything was set for late February of 1992 at his ranch: a war council unlike any before or since in the history of the supplement industry.

○ ⊂⊃ ⊂

On the morning of February 22, nearly all seventy-two of the leather swivel chairs and mahogany desks in the auditorium of Gerry's ranch were filled with industry leaders. Little had changed from the way Kroc had kept the room for meetings of McDonald's executives. The brownish orange rug matched the seat of each chair. Mounted on the back wall was a buffalo head with a plaque reading, "To Ray A. Kroc. This Cape Buffalo taken by me in September 1970, on Safari at Victoria Falls, Rhodesia, South Africa. James C. Schindler."

Just as Gerry had envisioned it, the roster of attendees was a who's who of the supplement industry, including Allen Skolnick, president of Solgar Vitamins and Herbs (sold to Wyeth in 1998 for nearly half a billion dollars); Milton and Scott Bass, the father-and-son attorneys who represented the industry's largest trade group, the National Nutritional Foods Association; NNFA's president, Martie Whittekin; Sandy Gooch, founder of Mrs. Gooch's, the leading natural foods merchandiser in the western United States until it merged with Whole Foods in 1996; and Scott Rudolph of NBTY, the conglomerate that owns Nature's Bounty, Rexall Sundown, Puritan's Pride, and Vitamin World stores (and which Wal-Mart would name a "supplier of the year" in 2001, with sales of over $1 billion). Two top aides of Senator Hatch were also in attendance: Jack Martin (since gone on to become partners with Hatch's son, Scott, in a D.C. lobbying firm, some of whose clients are leading supplement manufacturers) and Patricia Knight, now Hatch's chief of staff.

The morning began in disarray, with many of the attendees questioning whether the FDA's actions formed any threat. During walks on the property, informal gatherings in front of the floor-to-ceiling stone fireplace, or sitting around their rooms, small groups debated what, if anything, should or could be done. Martie Whittekin, for instance, insisted that the NNFA already had everything under control. But by dinnertime of that first day, the view of those who thought the FDA's rule making would seriously hurt their industry if allowed to stand had won over almost everyone. No one, however, could agree on what to do about it.

The next morning, Gerry started off the day's proceedings by expressing his view: a new organization had to be formed, backed with big money from the industry and devoted to the single cause of fomenting a popular uprising against the FDA's proposed rules. Otherwise, he insisted, Armageddon awaited all their businesses. He was virtually shouted down, and the room went back to going in circles and debating various positions. Finally Gerry did something that would be vividly remembered years later by those in attendance.

"I remember that moment; I can see it right now," recalled Doug Greene, founder of *Natural Food Merchandiser* and *Nutrition Business Journal,* industry newspapers, and creator of the Natural Products Expo trade show—the industry's largest. "I have thought about it many times since. In fact, I used it just recently to explain to my son about the meaning of leadership. A huge contingency was against Gerry when he began speaking. There was clear, serious disagreement in the room. You could feel the lack of unity, the fear. But by the time he finished speaking, somehow, through the force of his personality and his leadership skills, Gerry had us all pointed in the same direction. I've never seen that before or since in my whole life."

Taller than anyone in the room, Gerry took the stage and began preaching in his basso profundo about the urgent need to act. "We've got to transcend industry politics," he said. "We've got to deal with this now. We've got to organize. We have to convince the grass roots, the consumers, to get on the bandwagon and fight."

As opinion in the room began to turn his way, some still took issue with his proposal that each of the major manufacturers pony up hundreds of thousands of dollars. "Maybe you can't afford it," Gerry answered them, "but you can't afford not to. Because if you don't do it now, we'll all be out of business."

By the end of the day, a decision had been reached: they would form not just another group but an umbrella organization of all the groups, with seven of the major manufacturers committed to being charter members of the Nutritional Health Alliance, or NHA. Their main strategy would be to use their thousands of stores as front-line campaign offices, to empower—some might say manipulate—the public into speaking out against the FDA. And Gerry himself agreed to devote himself full-time to the effort, even going so far as to hire someone else to run his company. He still wasn't the most popular guy in the room, but he clearly was the most committed to their cause.

"When people left that room," Greene remembered, "there were still some factions, but there was a more cohesive point of view. Things gelled. Gerry just gave us a lot of confidence that we had a strong guy helping out. We all left there more alert and aware that this had to happen. You could tell he was committed. If I ever needed a field general in a war, boy, I'd hire him."

In less than two months, Gerry had mounted a campaign that would have been the envy of Ulysses S. Grant. The April–May 1992 issue of *Health Store News,* which served as a virtual mouthpiece for the effort, demonstrated the discipline with which he'd already arrayed the troops. It included preprinted letters ready to sign and send to twenty-four representatives and senators, each one backed by advertisements sponsored by twenty-four companies and using a single slogan, compelling in its simplicity: "Omega Nutri-Pharm, Inc., Supports Freedom of Choice Regarding Natural Health Alternatives"; "Pep Products, Inc., Supports Freedom of Choice Regarding Natural Health Alternatives"; "Beehive Botanicals Supports Freedom of Choice Regarding Natural Health Alternatives." The front page of the paper had an inch-tall headline, in red, at the very top: "The Time to Act Is Now!!!" Another red headline proclaimed: "One Million Jobs Affected by FDA Regulations." At the bottom was a quote from Margaret Mead: "Never doubt that a small group of thoughtful, committed citizens can change the world: indeed, it's the only thing that ever has." During the mid-April Natural Products Expo in Anaheim, Gerry and Skolnick, who'd agreed to become the NHA's treasurer, pledged to raise $500,000 and to generate one million letters to Congress within six months. The fight was on.

Then, on May 6, while Gerry was suffering through unproductive meetings with aides to Waxman and Kennedy in Washington, D.C., the other Kessler, the one who ran the FDA, took an action that would ultimately prove as counterproductive to his mission as the attack on Pearl Harbor was, in the end, for Japan.

⌒ ⌒ ⌒

Within months of taking office, David Kessler had taken a keen interest in the For Your Health Pharmacy, located in Kent, Washington. The drugstore was located next to a medical clinic run by Jonathan V. Wright, MD, who practiced what he called "nutritional medicine." Despite the FDA's continuing ban on L-tryptophan, the drugstore was still selling it, with Wright insisting he had the right to prescribe it to his patients. It also sold high-dose vitamins designed to be injected. FDA agents who went to investigate found mold on some vials and were told that some of the products had been made at an adjacent laboratory. Wright, they discovered, was co-owner of both the laboratory and the clinic, and was in the process of building a clandestine manufacturing facility. When FDA investigators later showed up to inspect the laboratory, Wright refused them entry. Before the month was over, law enforcement agents had seized the drugstore's 103 bottles of L-tryptophan.

As part of a slow and thorough investigation, in early December of 1991 an FDA inspector went to Wright's clinic, posing as a patient. An employee of the clinic offered to examine him with something called an "Interro device," which could supposedly diagnose his allergies by measuring the electrical resistance on his fingers. Running a tiny probe over his fingers, she pointed to a computer screen and said that the height of the vertical bars on the screen represented the foods, chemicals, and other substances to which he was allergic. She printed out a list of his allergies, sold him several homeopathic remedies for them, and gave him instructions on their use and an article claiming he would find dramatic relief.

Apparently getting wind of the FDA's investigation, Wright then posted a notice on the door to his clinic. Licensed physicians, his notice stated, are "exempt from the restrictions and regulations of the federal Food and Drug Administration as a matter of federal law. No employee, agent or inspector of the FDA shall be permitted on these premises."

On May 4, 1992, the FDA obtained a warrant from a U.S. magistrate to conduct a criminal search of the clinic and pharmacy. According to an affidavit the agency had submitted, Wright's clinic was "receiving, using, and dispensing several unapproved and misbranded foreign-manufactured injectable drug products." Two days later, as it had done thousands of times since the days of Clark Stanley's Snake Oil Liniment, the agency raided the clinic and pharmacy. Because they had been previously refused entry by Wright when they had come to inspect the laboratory, and because the posted notice indicated they would be refused entry again, the FDA agents were accompanied by local sheriffs. When they knocked at the front door, they were indeed refused entry, so the sheriffs broke it down, and one of them drew his gun. They seized products, computer files, the Interro devices, and other materials. Two weeks later, the state pharmacy board suspended the pharmacy's license.

But Wright had something Clark Stanley didn't have: a video camera. A customer who'd been present during the raid had recorded the whole thing, and Wright soon began selling videos of what he called the "Vitamin-B Bust." The tape found its way onto TV news shows and quickly entered the media's echo chamber. In an editorial, for instance, the *Seattle Post-Intelligencer* wrote: "If there is any plausible excuse for the Gestapo-like tactics, it had better be forthcoming and fast." Then the *New York Times* weighed in with a front-page story on Sunday, August 9. The article, rife with inaccuracies, asserted that the FDA agents were armed and that the video showed them "dressed in bullet-proof vests, bursting into the clinic and commanding clinic employees to freeze." It went on: "Last year, the agency proposed regulations for the labeling law that would classify vitamins and minerals as drugs if dosages exceeded the daily recommended allowances; restrict or prevent the sales of most medicinal herbs like chamomile; prevent unsubstantiated health claims for most dietary supplements, and lower the recommended vitamin-intake levels for various age groups."

A week later, the *Times* ran a correction on page one, a location reserved for only the most heinous mistakes: "A front-page article last Sunday about Federal action on vitamins and other food supplements described new regulations incorrectly. The Food and Drug Administration has not proposed classifying vitamins as drugs if their potencies exceed recommended daily allowances." The correction further stated that no FDA employees had been armed during the raid, and quoted Kessler as saying: "The FDA is in no way interested in taking vitamins off the market. The agency is strongly in favor of availability of vitamins manufactured under safe and sterile conditions. Sterility is especially important in the case of injectable products."

But by then, the horse of public opinion had already galloped out the barn door. Senator Hatch and Representative Bill Richardson, Democrat of New Mexico (another state known for its love of alternative medicine), saw their chance and introduced a one-year moratorium preventing the FDA's proposed rules for supplements from going into effect. Hatch told the *Washington Post* that he wanted "a more intelligent approach" to the regulation of dietary supplements. The FDA, he said, "appears to be trying to impose severe prior restraints" on supplement manufacturers, he complained.

⊂⊃ ⊂⊃ ⊂⊃

As the two Kesslers' forces met on the legislative battlefield, it became evident that they were mismatched. The commissioner's side had science, evidence, and the facts—weak weapons, unfortunately, in political warfare. But the other Kessler had that one precious thing that every campaign manager knows the value of: a simple, resonant, intuitively compelling message. "Write to Congress today or kiss your supplements goodbye!" Gerry Kessler wrote on the cover of a brochure. "Don't let the FDA take your supplements away! Tell Congress to act now!" It little mattered that the FDA was trying to tamp down only on irresponsible advertising, and to limit only those supplements that were patently dangerous. In the coming campaign, Gerry Kessler would use his ingeniously simple message like a battering ram.

On August 15, 1992, his words were echoed by celebrities at a news conference in Beverly Hills. "Start screaming at Congress and the White House not to let the FDA take our vitamins away," said the actress Sissy Spacek, enunciating the lines as if from a script. Another actress, Mariel Hemingway, criticized the FDA's effort to limit the doses of certain vitamins and minerals. "It's easy to say, 'Just take more pills' if you want higher doses or potencies," Hemingway said. "But that means you'll go through a bottle of vitamins every week." Other actors, including Victoria Principal and James Coburn, appeared at trade shows and in industry-made videos.

A masterstroke of Gerry's campaign was to use each of the 10,000 or so health food stores in the United States as local political offices. "Making Your Retail Store a Political Action Center" was the title on one of the pages of the "Health Freedom Kit" he sent to every store. The kit recommended that retailers talk about the campaign with every customer, post information sheets and banners, have every employee write letters weekly, reach out to local media, give customers a 5 percent discount every time they brought in a handwritten letter to a politician, and "have envelopes, stamps, a table or counter space to work on, an instruction sheet, your local and other Congressional representative's name, address and telephone number." It included sample letters to editors and politicians, sample press releases, and information sheets on such topics as why the FDA had banned L-trytophan. According to an especially misleading brochure produced by the Nutritional Health Alliance, Gary Dykstra had supposedly said that the FDA intended to "classify herbs as drugs . . . lower potencies of vitamins and minerals to those found in food . . . [and] not allow truthful non-misleading health claims based upon the current state of scientific knowledge." Some stores went so far as to allow customers to use the store telephones to call Congress.

The result was an unprecedented avalanche of mail on Capitol Hill, estimated at the time to have exceeded 2 million letters—more, it was said, than Congress had received in ten years of controversy over the Vietnam War. ("No other law has ever received as much direct grassroots advocacy, with the number of supportive letters to Congress topping 2 million," wrote R. William Soller, PhD, director of the Center for Consumer Self Care at the University of California, San Francisco, School of Pharmacy, in an article in *HerbalGram*.)

"It was unlike any other lobbying campaign I've ever seen," remarked Henry Waxman, who first won election to Congress in 1974. "It was a very clever campaign, one that manipulated certain beliefs that many people have. When people are facing health insurance that they can't afford, and treatments for cancer that sometimes result in side effects that are just as awful as the cancer, they're ready for a cure—they're desperate for one. They would like to believe that there is some kind of conspiracy that's keeping them from knowing the true facts that could keep them healthy. And it must be the doctors, who never know about nutri-tion—for which there's some validity—or it must be the drug companies, or the government keeping them from getting what they need. People would say, 'Waxman is in the pocket of the pharmaceutical companies.' That's laughable. You could ask any lobbyist and they would point to me as the biggest critic of the pharmaceutical industry. But people believed what they were being told, because it fed into their view that doctors and pharmaceutical companies wanted to block alternative medicines that could keep people healthy. What they didn't understand, though, was that this view was manipulated by people who stood to make a lot of money, and did make a lot of money—billions of dollars."

On a Tuesday evening late in October of 1992, Waxman appeared at a debate in his Westside district of Los Angeles where he was lambasted over HR 3642, the bill he'd introduced to give the FDA subpoena power. "People have misread that legislation," he said. "We've put it on hold." But one of his opponents, the Republican Mark Robbins, criticized Waxman as being "by nature pro-regulation" and won enthusiastic applause from the audience of about 150. Afterward, Jarrow L. Rogovin, who owned a local supplement company, angrily confronted Waxman. In response to Wax-man's proposed bill, Rogovin said, "The whole industry has gone ballistic."

Perhaps it was Rogovin who, twelve years later, Waxman still remem-bered. "Some guy came up to me at a community meeting, arguing with me that a garlic supplement he was taking an enormous amount of was keeping him very healthy," said Waxman, sitting by his office's large win-dow overlooking the Capitol dome. "He looked like a healthy guy. But his breath smelled terrible." Waxman laughed. "It was awful. It was garlicky."

But there was nothing funny about the way Gerry Kessler's campaign began bussing in pro-supplement supporters to heckle Waxman at his public hearings. "They dominated the meetings," Waxman said. "One person after another would harangue me. The senior population who normally attended the meetings would be intimidated." His aides rou-tinely received calls to their direct lines, lambasting them over Waxman's position. Once their office windows were even pelted with tomatoes.

Just before the November election in which Bill Clinton would win the presidency, the one-year moratorium on the FDA's rules on supplements, which Hatch and Richardson had introduced, was signed into law by President Bush.

⌐⌐ ⌐⌐ ⌐⌐

On the strength of such remarkable political support, David Kessler could hardly refuse a meeting with his nemesis. At the first encounter of the two Kesslers, held at the FDA's office and arranged by industry lobbyists, Gerry put out his hand and joked, "I'll have to stop telling people you're my son." The other Kessler, however, didn't so much as smile. "Commissioner," Gerry continued, "I don't know whether you're for us or against us, but I will be here when you're gone, and so will this industry, so it would be good if you were for us."

David Kessler grew visibly upset. "Are you threatening me?" he asked.

"No," Gerry said, "I just hope you'll be for us."

During the many meetings that were to follow, the commissioner treated the manufacturer with great respect, sometimes giving him as much as a full day to hear his arguments. But there would be no bridging the Styx-like chasm that separated their worldviews. The commissioner saw his mission as safeguarding Americans' right to be protected from unproven, fraudulent, potentially dangerous snake oil; the manufacturer saw his mission as protecting Americans' access to innovative, God-given, life-saving natural remedies. Indeed, Gerry once said that he'd been picked by God to lead the industry's fight.

"I said it jokingly," he would later explain, "but I do think that at certain times, there are certain people standing in certain positions who can do certain things. There are many people on the bench. If you don't do it, someone else will get up and do it. The bench is full. But I was there, and I had the gazorts to stand up and do it."

Emboldened by his early success, by early 1993 Gerry began thinking beyond simply overturning the FDA's proposed rules to imagining what kind of pro-industry bill he could actually support. Hatch and Richardson both wanted to introduce a law aimed at getting the FDA off the industry's back, but they couldn't get Kennedy in the Senate, or Waxman in the House, to schedule hearings. Then one morning, when Gerry was at his ranch, he received a telephone call from Richardson, whom he had already met with many times. "You need a Democratic lobbyist," Richardson advised him. "I've got a guy in mind, and I'd like you to fly out to San Francisco to meet me for dinner tonight and I'll talk to you about it."

Until this point, Waxman had considered Gerry Kessler's lobbying efforts somewhat amateurish and ham-handed. At times, Gerry and the
young attorney he'd retained, Tony Martinez, would literally wander the
halls of Congress, going door to door, seeking to speak with representatives and senators. One such encounter turned out to be rather embar-
rassing, when Representative Mike Synar, Democrat of Oklahoma,
confronted them in the hallway. "Get out of my district!" Synar shouted.
"You're just a bunch of snake oil salesmen!" Gerry replied, "Sir, everything you are saying is incorrect. I wish you would stop shouting." But
Synar wouldn't calm down. They finally left, determined to let Synar's
constituents know his attitude toward supplements. (In the 1994 election, Synar did in fact go down to defeat, a result for which Gerry felt he
deserved partial credit.)

Eager to have more fruitful meetings on Capitol Hill, Gerry met
Richardson that evening in San Francisco. The person Richardson
wanted Gerry to hire was Tony Podesta, one of the most influential Democratic lobbyists in Washington and the brother of John Podesta. (In
1998, John would become Bill Clinton's chief of staff.) But Gerry thought
that Tony Podesta's fee was way too steep. Back at the ranch the next
morning, however, he received another phone call, this one from Orrin
Hatch.

"You need a Democratic lobbyist," Hatch pressed him.

"I just met with Bill Richardson last night," Gerry told him, "and he
suggested we hire Tony Podesta."

"Perfect," Hatch said.

Gerry followed Hatch and Richardson's advice, hiring Podesta and
paying him out of the considerable funds that he and other industry leaders had contributed to the NHA. The move quickly paid off, with Podesta
arranging a meeting with Kennedy to ask him to hold a hearing on
Hatch's bill.

"Look, I'm not on your side," Kennedy frankly told Gerry. "But I'll do
just about anything he asks me," he said, pointing to Podesta, who had
gone to the mat many times for Democratic causes cherished by Kennedy.
"What do you want?"

"Give us a date for a hearing," Kessler said.

What could it hurt to hold a hearing? An aide to Kennedy pulled out
an appointment book, and the Senate hearing was scheduled for October

21. A similar process took place with Waxman, and on July 29 at 10:06 a.m., the House hearing was called to order, with a list of politicians, experts, and citizens slated to testify, for and against.

The name of the matching bills introduced by Hatch and Richardson had been coined by Gerry in a meeting with Hatch and his aides. Like a father naming his child, Gerry called it the Dietary Supplement Health and Education Act of 1993. Its abbreviation, DSHEA, came to be pronounced as "dih-SHAY." Trish Knight and Jack Martin, the Hatch aides who'd attended the big meeting at Gerry's ranch, had a hand in crafting the bill. But more influential were Loren Israelson, another aide to Hatch, and Scott Bass, the attorney who represented the National Nutritional Foods Association. (Later honored along with Gerry by *Natural Foods Merchandiser* as among the "25 who fortified supplements," both Bass and Israelson listed the passage of DSHEA as the greatest accomplishment of their careers.) But exactly what the bills would actually accomplish became the subject of a heated debate at Waxman's hearing.

The first to testify was Hatch himself. "The Richardson-Hatch legislation makes clear that dietary supplements, which have been safely used for centuries, are essentially to be treated as what they are—foods," declared Hatch (ignoring the fact that most of the vitamins, minerals, and amino acids that concerned the FDA had been discovered only in the twentieth century). Hatch claimed that his bill used the same "significant scientific agreement" standard for permitting health claims that the FDA had proposed the year before. In truth, however, one section of his bill permitted claims based on a far looser standard than the FDA had ever proposed—"the totality of scientific evidence"—while another allowed "truthful and non-misleading information" to be placed on the label. But what does "truthful and non-misleading" mean? Is it "truthful and non-misleading" to prominently quote on the label a single small study that found supplement X to be safe and effective? A standard like that was wide enough for a manufacturer to drive a truckload of supplements through. Of most concern, however, was the provision that would bar the FDA from requiring that claims be approved before going on shelves.

Following Hatch came David Kessler. He began philosophically. "Americans view their government with a mixture of reliance and mistrust," he said. "We want to be free to choose whatever products we like until something goes wrong. Then we turn to our government and want to know why it happened and what the government is doing about it." The debate, he said, was not about the vast majority of vitamins, minerals, herbs, and other supplements that are safe. But, he said, "When supplements are really drugs in disguise, promoted to treat serious diseases, we have a problem."

He then released the results of an informal survey the agency had undertaken to quickly identify, in a few weeks, some 500 products making outrageous claims to treat or cure serious diseases such as cancer or AIDS. In a second survey reported by Kessler, FDA officials conducted 129 informal interviews with salespeople at health food stores, asking if they had any products that could treat such serious conditions as high blood pressure, cancer, or infections. Of those asked, 93 percent said their store did have products to treat those conditions. "Unsubstantiated claims are becoming more exaggerated, more products whose effects are unknown are available, and their use is escalating," Kessler said. "We are back at the turn of the century when snake oil salesmen could hawk their potions of promises that couldn't be kept."

He displayed a chart that listed serious side effects that had been caused by supplements. "Think about it," he said. "Half our prescription drugs are derived from plants, and no one doubts for a minute that drugs can have toxic effects. That is why we insist on rigorous testing to separate out those with unacceptable toxicity. We must not assume that all risk disappears when plants are sold as dietary supplements for therapeutic purposes."

If the FDA could not require premarket review of claims, he said, the agency would be put "in the position of chasing after problems after they have occurred. Furthermore, you are going to force the American taxpayer in the end to foot the bill to chase after the products and do the kind of testing to be able to make a case in court. The FDA is never going to have the resources. If you are going to sell a product, the burden should be on you to establish that the claims that you make are true. The burden shouldn't be put on the government."

When the other Kessler, the manufacturer, was called to the podium, he insisted, "We all want accurate labeling and safe products on the shelf. That is something both Kesslers agree upon." But later that day, Bruce Silverglade, director of legal affairs of the Center for Science in the Public

Interest, openly derided Gerry's statements. He pointed to the label of Ultra Male, a product manufactured by Kessler's company (and still sold to this day on many Web sites). "Who would buy Ultra Male if it was accurately labeled as bull prostate?" Silverglade asked the members of Waxman's subcommittee. (Apparently, more men than Silverglade would have expected, because today the product's label plainly states that it contains not only raw prostate concentrate but also raw eye concentrate, raw brain concentrate, and raw "orchic" concentrate—that is, bull testicles.) Silverglade went on to call DSHEA "a snake oil promotion act, because it would allow these types of health claims here and strip the FDA of its adequate, sufficient enforcement mechanism to keep these kinds of bogus health claims off the market."

"Well, you know, Mr. Silverglade," said Richardson, who had introduced the bill, "we are trying to resolve this issue. I think Dr. Kessler has shown an interest in doing so. I question whether you do by your statements relating to snake oil, statements that I consider to be impugning the good name of Gerald Kessler."

"At least we don't make death threats, which some segments of the industry made, as recorded in the *National Journal* last week," Silverglade fired back. "And I would hope that you would take this opportunity, Mr. Richardson, to condemn those tactics by whoever may support your bill. Those types of tactics have no place in our system of government, and they have no place, really, in our country."

If both Kesslers and their advocates on either side were guilty of sniping and intellectualizing, the patients they called to testify spoke with heartrending sincerity. "As a person living with AIDS, my very life depends on continued access to the supplements that the FDA apparently considers to be a threat to drug development," said Fred Bingham, executive director of a group called Direct AIDS Alternative Information Resources. He went on to say that the FDA's "paternalistic and prohibitionist solution to the supplement problem is a clear and present danger to our lives." The fact that no dietary supplement had ever been shown to slow the progression of AIDS made his testimony no less compelling. Equally moving, however, was Dorothy Wilson, one of the L-tryptophan victims who had spoken at Ted Weiss's hearing in 1991. "Mr. Chairman," she began, still wheelchair-bound, "it was difficult with my medical problems, but I had a burning desire to appear here. I wanted you to look at me condemned to a life of severe physical pain and disabilities and be reminded of the price I pay every day of my life due to L-tryptophan. What happened to me happened when the FDA had limited ability to control supplements. Before you weaken the statute and make it more difficult for the FDA to do the job, consider how my life was catastrophically and permanently changed. Think of my friend Donna, who died after a lung transplant; and Audrey, who took her life, not able to bear the physical pain; George, who served in Vietnam, now totally wheelchair-bound and dependent; and Chuck, a former psychiatrist who forgets where he lives. The Dietary Supplement Health and Education Act must not pass. Because the supplement industry misrepresented the public's ability to get vitamins and many uninformed consumers wrote letters is not the correct reason to pass it. Reject this act, because it is the right, courageous and honorable thing to do."

Also coming out against the bill that day was Consumers Union, the National Organization of Rare Disorders, the American Association of Retired Persons, the American Cancer Society, the American Heart Association, the American Nurses Association, and the American College of Physicians.

⬯ ⬯ ⬯

In August, the supplement industry pulled out its heavy artillery, when a one-minute commercial began airing on television stations across the country. The commercial began with white letters on a black background: "Los Angeles, 9:57 p.m." Police in black clothing, wearing night-vision goggles, burst out of a van holding rifles and began charging toward a house. They break in the door and go running upstairs. In the bathroom, they find a man wearing a robe taking a bottle from the medicine cabinet. The man turns around. It's Mel Gibson. "Hey, guys—guys!" he says. "It's only vitamins." Then, again in white letters on black: "The federal government is actually considering classifying most vitamins and other supplements as drugs. The FDA has already conducted raids on doctors' offices and health food stores. Could raids on individuals be next?" The picture then returns to Gibson, who says to the police, who are hand-cuffing him behind his back, "Vitamin C. You know, like in oranges?"

And then comes the final message: "Protect your rights to use vitamins and other supplements. Call Congress now."

The commercial had actually been made not by Gerry Kessler but by a San Francisco–based supplement manufacturer named Patrick Mooney. After attending a conference where Kessler had spoken, he became convinced of the threat to his business, but feared that Kessler's grassroots focus might not work. Then he had a brilliant idea. "Who does America listen to?" he asked himself. Although he had no Hollywood contacts, he placed an advertisement in the *Hollywood Reporter* asking for movie industry volunteers willing to make a commercial about the FDA's power grab. He soon had a writer, a director, electricians, set dressers, a couple dozen actors, and Mel Gibson, all happy to work for free. On the day of the shoot, held at an old estate that someone allowed them to use free of charge, forty-eight people showed up.

Once Gibson was in, other leading celebrities wanted to offer their services too. Mooney then organized a series of individual shoots into an hour-long video, which he sent to members of Congress in October of 1993. (The video has been virtually unseen since then, with no copy on record at any library or congressperson's office, and Mooney unwilling to share his remaining copy. The only tape of the commercial now available to the public is in the Archives of Appalachia at East Tennessee State University in Johnson City.)

After an earnest introduction from an unidentified woman, the video followed up the one-minute Mel Gibson commercial with a pitch by Eddie Albert, the onetime star of *Green Acres*. "That can actually happen," he began, referring to Gibson's fictional arrest. "The Food and Drug Administration recently stated that they plan to restrict herbs, amino acids, and high-potency vitamins from the open market because they say they're not safe. Safety records show that supplements are over two thousand times safer than over-the-counter drugs, and nearly one million times safer than prescription drugs. Don't let them take your supplements away."

The video then cut to Whoopi Goldberg: "A couple of us have gathered together to discuss . . . the right of American citizens to have free access to dietary supplements of their choice. But we're also here to talk about something else: the spirit of vitality and freedom that help make this country great."

The talk show host Jenny Jones declared: "We are certainly the greatest democracy on earth, but we're also struggling economically and spiritually and in terms of national health."

The actress Laura Dern continued: "And our national health has plummeted from about tenth among nations to somewhere between sixteenth and fortieth. We need help, but there's no one to give us help except ourselves."

Then came the country singer Randy Travis: "Right now Congress has the opportunity to reaffirm the spirit of vitality and freedom and give America a chance to revitalize itself."

"Congress," said the actor Wings Hauser, "is considering whether to allow the free enterprise system to continue growing in a new market and whether to reaffirm the commitment of Congress that the American public has the intelligence and the right to make its own choice when it comes to health."

"And in a larger sense," the actress Lesley Ann Warren said, "Congress is also deciding whether the entrepreneurs and small businesses who developed the market for dietary supplements should be allowed to continue to service the market as it grows, or to restrict that entrepreneurial sentiment and pave the way for the giant drug and pharmaceutical industry to take over this developing market."

As the video morphed into a parochial plea about business interests over safety, Jenny Jones finished up: "We need to ensure that Congress continues to give consumers the right to make intelligent choices about our health. Congress must stop the FDA from demanding expensive, drug-level proof-of-safety tests. At an average of two hundred million dollars per ingredient spent on testing, the small entrepreneurial companies which make up the dietary supplement industry will dry up."

The video apparently failed to work its magic on Senator Howard Metzenbaum. Speaking early in Kennedy's Senate hearing on October 21, he said, "The industry that has waged this campaign of misinformation wants to be able to make health claims without the approval of the Food and Drug Administration. Frankly, I am not sure that all of those manufacturers can be trusted. Some certainly cannot. If we are going to allow a manufacturer to make a health claim, then we need some independent review of the basis for that claim."

David Kessler reprised the testimony he had given before the House in July, and then Hatch began grilling him on some alleged inaccuracies in the report on fraudulent claims that Kessler had presented back then. "I think it will blow some of your minds that an agency of the federal government can be so incorrect in what they do and testify to before the Congress of the United States. Now, Dr. Kessler, it is very odd that the FDA sent employees undercover."

Kessler pointed out that the report had included 500 fraudulent claims. "I would like to submit to you another three hundred products with their claims," he said. "There is a problem out there. And you know it and I know it."

Senator Tom Harkin, Democrat of Iowa and a strong co-sponsor of Hatch's bill, then spoke about how bee pollen had recently cured his allergies. "I just do not believe that conventional wisdom is always right and that mainstream medicine meets the needs or demands of everyone," he said. "I started taking bee pollen. I have not had any allergies since." After receiving applause, he told a story about a constituent who had recently visited his office. "I told him I had a sore throat that day. He reached into his pocket, and he brought this [tree bark] out. He got it from some Native Americans in New Mexico. I don't remember what he called it. He said, 'Break off a piece and chew it,' and sure enough, it was the best anti–sore throat medicine I have ever used." More applause followed.

Picking back up his cudgel, Hatch demanded to know from Kessler why the agency had recently devoted energy to seizing supplies of evening primrose oil. "What safety hazard was the FDA addressing that warranted such intensive use of agency resources and personnel?"

"Senator, I can read you the claims made for oil of evening primrose," Kessler answered. "The list starts with cancer."

"Remember, the issue is safety I am talking about," Hatch said.

"My real concern," said Kessler, "is the types of diseases for which oil of evening primrose is promoted."

"But my question is: What proof do you have that this substance is unsafe?"

"This is being promoted for a lot of different diseases, anywhere from hypertension to atopic dermatitis."

"Safety, Doctor, safety. That is the question. Is an American citizen more likely to die from an adverse reaction to a drug approved by the FDA or a dietary supplement?"

"Senator, I am amazed. What do you think are in pharmaceuticals? I mean, half our pharmaceuticals come from plants. There are chemicals in pharmaceuticals, and those chemicals are found naturally. The issue is, I mean, they are molecules."

Awkwardly put though it was, Kessler's point went to the heart of his and every public health advocate's concern about supplements: that no matter how natural they may be, the ingredients can still have powerful effects for good or ill. In the words of Michael Harris, a historian of pharmacy: "It doesn't matter to your body if your caffeine comes from coffee beans or you get it from a tablet or from kava kava. It doesn't matter to your body whether ephedra is sold as an over-the-counter drug or as a natural supplement. It doesn't matter to your body how the FDA regulates something or what the dietary supplement label says. What matters to your body is what's inside the pill." That's why one of Harris's favorite sayings, borrowed from the slogan of the first Clinton campaign ("It's the economy, stupid") is this: "It's the molecule, stupid."

⬭ ⬭ ⬭

With both Kennedy and Waxman holding up the bills in their committees, refusing to let them out to the floors of the Senate and House for a final up-or-down vote, Hatch tried in November of 1993 to renew the one-year moratorium on the enactment of the FDA's proposed rules for regulating supplements. But Waxman managed to block the renewal, it expired, and on December 29, the FDA formally issued the regulations that the industry had been dreading.

Before they would take effect at the end of 1994, however, Gerry Kessler and friends worked hard to push a renewed version of DSHEA. On May 11, for the first time in memory, Kennedy was overruled by his own committee, when it voted twelve to five to approve Hatch's bill.

In July, having received 35,000 letters urging her to vote for the measure, Barbara Boxer, Democrat of California, became one of sixty-five senators to co-sponsor the bill. Donna V. Porter, a life science specialist for the Congressional Research Service, told the *Los Angeles Times:* "In fifteen years in this town, I've never dealt with anything as emotional as this issue. It's as volatile as abortion, gun control, and prayer in schools. People are irrational on this whole subject. They don't hear what they don't want to hear. They really believe FDA is out to get them."

By early October, the full Senate had passed the bill without a single dissent. But Waxman in the House refused to budge: exercising his prerogative, he would simply not allow the bill out of his subcommittee. Finally, late on Wednesday afternoon, October 5, with only about forty-eight hours until Congress's scheduled adjournment, Richardson, Harkin, and Hatch called a meeting with Gerry and other supplement industry leaders who had come to town in hopes of seeing it pass.

"You've done a great job," Hatch told them. "We came very close but we are not going to get the vote that you want, because it's not going to be brought up for a vote this year. We'll have to start again next year, so you all might as well go home."

To which Gerry replied, "Bullshit. We're not going home. We're not going to let this lie and we're going to get this bill through."

Ever the loose cannon, Gerry was ignored by the other manufacturers, who left the meeting, went back to their hotel rooms, packed up, and went home. Gerry, however, went into hyperdrive. He called up another lobbyist he happened to know and asked her if she could do anything to help.

"I'll make a phone call and you can go see Newt Gingrich," she said.

Sure enough, on Thursday morning, Gerry and his young attorney, Tony Martinez, found themselves sitting in Gingrich's office. Just one month before the 1994 election, Gingrich believed the Republicans to be on the verge of taking control of the House, with himself taking over Tom Foley's position as Speaker.

"Here's what I'm going to do," he told Gerry. "I'm going to write a letter to Foley, saying that we will not go out of session, Congress will not recess, until this bill is voted on."

"You don't have any control over them," said Gerry. "The Democrats are in charge."

"Listen, Gerry, Foley is in trouble, and he can't afford you guys to be screwing around in his election campaign."

On Friday morning, October 7, 1994, Gerry's lobbyist, Tony Podesta, received a call from Tom Foley's wife, Heather, who served as his chief of staff. Podesta implored her: "Work with us. Get this done. We're arguing about a few words and a few commas. People will be very upset if this doesn't happen. It's in your interest and Tom's interest to get this over."

She told Podesta that Foley had spoken to Waxman and John D. Dingell, the Democratic congressman of Michigan, and that they were all prepared to release the bill if an agreement could be reached. A meeting would be held that afternoon to work out the details.

At about seven o'clock that night, with Waxman, Dingell, Richardson, Hatch, Harkin, and their aides holed up in a meeting room, Gerry paced just outside the door on the marble floor, his footsteps echoing.

"Gerry, don't stand here," Podesta told him. "It's not right."

Podesta ushered him to a waiting room. By now, Gerry knew, the politicians in the meeting room had already cut from DSHEA one of his primary goals: to allow supplements to claim on their labels that they could treat, cure, or prevent a disease. Waxman just wouldn't go there. But a legalistic solution had been hammered out. The bill would now allow something called "structure/function" claims. Labels would be permitted to claim, for instance, that a product improves the function of the lungs, or strengthens the structure of bone cartilage. But the label could not claim that the product cures asthma or prevents arthritis. While Waxman thought it a useful distinction, it would prove virtually impossible for consumers to understand the difference, according to studies later carried out by both the FDA and the AARP. "Helps maintain normal cholesterol levels" would be allowed, but "lowers cholesterol" would not? It was a distinction without a difference. And although the law required that the claims be "truthful" and "nonmisleading," no means for judging those intentionally vague standards were included. The result was that for all practical purposes, so long as manufacturers stuck within the "structure/function" framework, they could claim whatever powers they wanted for their products.

But now Bill Schultz of the FDA, having carefully gone through the bill, was demanding some other seemingly innocuous changes: the replacement of an "and" with an "or"; the substitution of "inferred" for "implied," and so on. Gerry thought they had Waxman over a barrel now and should resist the changes, but Hatch felt they had to agree.

Finally, Tom Harkin came out with a final question for Gerry: "They want a warning on the label of every supplement, saying the FDA has not evaluated the claims. And they want the warning to say 'This product is not intended to diagnose, treat, cure, or prevent any disease.' Can you live with it?"

With passage of DSHEA on the line, Gerry replied, "You're asking me to make a decision for the entire industry. It's okay with me, but I have to make a couple of phone calls."

Gerry first tried calling Scott Rudolph of Nature's Bounty, but since it was well after business hours on a Friday night, nobody was in his office. Then Gerry tried calling Allen Skolnick of Solgar, and managed to reach him on his car phone. Skolnick and his wife, Connie, were driving to their home in central New Jersey.

Gerry told him what the label would say. "Can you tell me it's okay to go ahead?" he asked.

"Gerry, I can't make that kind of decision right now," Skolnick answered, using the speakerphone. "I'm in the car. It's Friday night. I haven't eaten. It's late."

"You have to make the decision," said Gerry. "Somebody has to."

Of course, Gerry could have made the decision on his own, having led the entire effort. At this final juncture, however, he felt the need for at least one voice of support. Yet no sound came from the other end of the phone as Skolnick tried to make up his mind. Finally, from the background, came the voice of Skolnick's wife. "Just tell him it's okay!" Connie yelled. Skolnick promptly echoed her: "It's okay, it's okay."

And so Gerry told Harkin it was okay, and minutes later, Waxman emerged from the meeting to shake Gerry's hand.

Before signing the bill into law a few weeks later, on October 25, 1994, President Clinton read from a statement, the first draft of which had been written by Gerry's lobbyist, Tony Podesta. "After several years of intense efforts," Clinton said, "manufacturers, experts in nutrition, and legislators acting in a conscientious alliance with consumers at the grassroots level have moved successfully to bring common sense to the treatment of dietary supplements. The passage of this legislation... speaks to the diligence with which an unofficial army of nutritionally conscious people worked democratically to change the laws in an area deeply important to them."

And so it was done. The onetime orphan boy, driven to succeed at all costs, had beaten the best efforts of some of the most powerful politicians in the United States, as well as one of the most powerful commissioners in the history of the FDA. In a stunning move of political jujitsu, DSHEA had taken the energy of Waxman's and Kennedy's and Dingell's and Dr. Kessler's efforts to clamp down on supplement claims and reversed it on them. Rather than suppressing claims, the bill would allow claims indistinguishable from those it forbade. Breathtaking in its dimensions, DSHEA would end forever the simple legal dichotomy between "food" and "drug" to create a third, hermaphroditic category that was both yet neither: the dietary supplement. And beyond the usual suspects—vitamins, minerals, herbs, and amino acids—the law would permit manufacturers to define a product as a "dietary supplement" merely by saying so, no matter if it were artificially derived. For this special, magical category of products, DSHEA would specifically exclude all their ingredients from the stringent laws used to guarantee the safety of food additives. Put lamb's brain in a drug or food, and prepare to spend millions of dollars and a few years on studies showing that it is safe and effective; put it in a supplement and you're good to go, no evidence necessary. And if the FDA ever wanted to remove a supplement from the market for safety reasons, DSHEA would require the agency to prove that the supplement was dangerous when used as directed, rather than the manufacturer ever having to prove that it was safe. Any risk from a supplement being used *other* than as directed would be specifically excluded from consideration; and in any enforcement procedure, a judge would have to decide each issue on a *de novo* basis, meaning that everything would have to be proven from scratch in the courtroom, without reference to prior cases or administrative records.

To add insult to injury, decades of precedents establishing that brochures and reading materials accompanying products in a store fall under the same strict standards as the products' labels would be tossed out, permitting such materials so long as they did not promote a particular manufacturer and were in a separate section of the store. So brochures and posters claiming that powdered apricot pits cure cancer would be perfectly okay—just put them in a different aisle than the powdered apricot pits you're selling. With a stroke of a pen, nearly ninety years' worth of laws dating back to Dr. Wiley's Pure Food and Drug Act of 1906 had been gutted for a huge category of products, and all because enough people had become absolutely convinced that nothing deemed "natural" could be unsafe.

Let the selling begin.

CHAPTER 5

ANCIENT CHINESE REMEDY

Julie Puett Howry may not have been the first person in the United States to die after taking ephedra for weight loss, but she was the first to come to the attention of Texas health officials. On April 14, 1994, six months before the Senate's passage of DSHEA, the healthy forty-three-year-old mother of two was playing doubles tennis with girl-friends at the elite Austin County Club in Austin, Texas. The daughter of Nelson H. Puett, a prominent Austin businessman who opened the coun-try's first twenty-four-hour laundromat in 1949, Julie had been married for twenty-two years to her college sweetheart when she collapsed on the court at around nine-thirty a.m. Paramedics from the Austin Emergency Medical Services arrived to find that her heart had stopped, but they managed to restart it and obtained a pulse. Flown by helicopter to Seton Medical Center, she clung to life for two more weeks but never regained consciousness. On April 28, she died.

Friends told health authorities that they suspected her death might have been caused by the supposedly safe and natural "pep pills" Julie had been taking to lose a few pounds. "They were vanity pounds," said Phil Howry, the husband left behind to raise their two teenagers after Julie's death. "She played tennis a few times a week in a competitive league. She was five foot, four inches and weighed about one twenty-five or one thirty. She just wanted to lose a few pounds." Nature's Nutrition Formula One, marketed by a Texas company called Alliance U.S.A., was labeled as containing ma huang, the Chinese name for the ephedra plant, and kola nuts, a source of caffeine. It was sold Amway-style by "independent distributors"—that is, by anyone willing to pay a $600 fee to sell the product to their friends and family, in return for getting a percent of each sale. The company estimated there were some 1,500 distributors in the Austin area alone, some 30,000 across all of Texas, and 85,000 nationwide. The Texas distributors were said by the company to be earning a combined $2 million each week. So popular was the supplement that a friend and neighbor of Julie's told the local newspaper, the *Austin American-Statesman,* "Out of a table of six at lunch the other day, four said they had taken it at one time or another. They said it made them feel peppy. They either hated the rush or they liked it. Most I knew were taking it because they wanted to lose weight."

Larry Cantrell, vice president for marketing for Alliance U.S.A., told the newspaper that his company's manufacturing process removed any negative effects of ephedra. "Using the whole Chinese herb ma huang, the components buffer each other and work synergistically," he said. "There's no credible scientific research that's ever shown the whole herb to have negative effects. When you isolate ephedrine from the whole herb, ephedrine in high doses and over the long term could have some bad effects, but we don't isolate ephedrine."

But for the Texas Department of Health, Julie's death was only the latest and worst incident in a remarkably sudden epidemic of more than thirty complaints about Formula One and other ephedra-containing products. "In the history of the department of health, never before had anything like this happened," said Cynthia T. Culmo, a pharmacist who served as director of the state health department's Drugs and Medical Devices division. "There had never been a situation like this, other than with a food-borne outbreak, where we had so many complaints so quickly for a specific product. It caused us great concern. We were wondering, 'What is going on and what is this?'"

By mid-May, Culmo's department had received reports of a woman hospitalized for atrial fibrillation (heart palpitations), two who suffered psychosis, one who went blind in an eye due to a stroke, and more than two dozen area students hospitalized—all after taking either Formula One or similar products made by other companies, such as Mini-Thins or Go Power. On May 12, just over two weeks after Howry's death, the state health commissioner (Culmo's boss) announced a statewide ban on sales of Formula One, and an immediate restriction on all ephedrine-containing products to anyone under eighteen. The reason for the ban on Formula One, he said, was because the label did not explain that both ma huang and kola nuts were stimulants, and that it falsely claimed to lower blood pressure, reduce cholesterol, and strengthen the heart. "Although our investigation is not yet finished, we have found that the unrestricted sale and use of ephedrine and related chemicals pose an immediate and serious threat to human life and health," said the commissioner, David R. Smith, MD. "Enough is enough. It really is time to stop this madness."

But the madness was only beginning. Five days later, in response to a lawsuit filed by the maker of Formula One, a Travis County district judge issued a temporary injunction, lifting the health department's ban pending a hearing to investigate whether it was justified. In the five days before the ban had been stayed, the company said, it had lost nearly a million dollars in income that it would have otherwise earned. But according to the distributor Barbara Whisenant of Lakeway, Texas, the brief ban had actually boosted sales. Although she had offered to buy back the pills from dissatisfied customers, she didn't seem to have any. "None wanted to give [the pills] back," she said. "That's the ironic part. They're wired on them." Women in her area, she said, had lost "twenty, forty, sixty pounds with this. They get up in the morning and clean house all day. They're higher than a kite."

Then, on May 30, while watching television at her home in Georgetown, Texas, fifty-four-year-old Judith Whisenhunt, a mother of two grown sons, lost consciousness and, after a day in the hospital, died on June 1. She too had been taking Nature's Nutrition Formula One to lose a few pounds. A week later, the state department of health introduced an amended version of the ban on Formula One, and this time Dr. Smith thought it would stick. But it took only a few minutes for the manufacturer to persuade a judge in Austin to issue another injunction.

Mark Blumenthal, executive director of an industry-funded group called the American Botanical Council, which happened to be based in Austin, told the *Austin American-Statesman* that he hoped ma huang would continue to remain available. The Chinese, he said, had used it safely for five thousand years. A similar sentiment was expressed by the callers who jammed Culmo's phone line, most of them among the 30,000 distributors who were furious with her department's attempted bans. "I can't tell you how many times I heard people say it had been safely used by the Chinese for five thousand years," she said. Senator Hatch had said much the same during the prior year's hearings over DSHEA. Herbal remedies, Hatch said, "have been on the market for centuries, to be honest with you. In fact, most of these have been on the market for four thousand years, and the real issue is risk. And there is not much risk in any of these products."

○ ▭ ⊂⊃

The discovery of ma huang—the Chinese name for the ephedra plant—is attributed to Shen Nong, the second of China's mythical emperors, said to have ruled circa 2800 BC. Also known as the Blazing Emperor, the Lord of the Burning Wind, and the Holy Ploughman, he is credited with inventing the cart, the plow, and slash-and-burn agriculture. He tamed the ox, yoked the horse, and was mythologized as having the head of a bull. All this, and he personally tested and described the 365 herbs listed in his *Ben Ca Jing,* once managing to poison himself seventy-two times in a single day in the course of his botanical research. In the oldest surviving editions of the *Ben Ca Jing,* ma huang is described as useful for coughs, colds, fever, sweating, congestion, shortness of breath, and water retention.

In 1887, while working in Germany, a Japanese chemist named Nagajoshi Nagai became the first to isolate and name ephedrine as the main active ingredient of ma huang. *(Ephedra* is the plant; *ephedrine* is the primary active chemical ingredient in the plant.) But he tested it at such high doses that he concluded it was toxic. Thirty-five years later, in the summer of 1922, Carl Frederic Schmidt, MD—the first graduate of the new Department of Pharmacology at the University of Pennsylvania School of Medicine—arrived in Beijing to teach and conduct research for two years at Peking Union Medical College. According to a memoir written ten years later by a colleague of Schmidt's: "It had been suggested that he investigate the drugs in the Chinese pharmacopoeia to find any that might be of particular value. There were approximately 4,000. As a basis for starting this awesome project, he and his young Chinese colleague, K. K. Chen, selected the drugs, mostly of botanical origin, that were prescribed most frequently." After testing a half dozen and finding nothing that seemed useful, Chen's uncle, a Chinese pharmacist, suggested they investigate ma huang. Chen prepared a liquid extract and injected it into a dog. The dog's blood pressure rose dramatically, a clear sign that something in the ma huang was pharmacologically active. After isolating the active ingredient, Chen researched the medical literature and found Nagai's brief description. Chen and Schmidt then carried out extensive tests of their own. They found that ephedrine appeared to be useful as a bronchodilator, clearing stuffy noses and easing congested breathing, much as the ancient Chinese had employed it. Ephedrine, however, turned out to be just one of a group of six related chemicals active in the ephedra plant. The others were pseudoephedrine, methyl ephedrine, methyl pseudoephedrine, norephedrine, and norpseudoephedrine. Together, the six were called the ephedrine alkaloids.

After completing their research in China, the two men parted ways: Chen went on to work for Eli Lilly & Co., which by 1927 was manufacturing ephedrine on a large scale, and Schmidt returned to the University of Pennsylvania, where he eventually became the second chairman of the Department of Pharmacology. But their great discovery slowly fell out of favor with the medical community. Even at recommended doses, pure ephedrine caused sweating, jitteriness, tremors, insomnia, headaches, and heart palpitations. It worked, after all, by stimulating the sympathetic nervous system, jacking up the body's flight-or-fight reaction in the same way that amphetamines do. Doctors and drug companies gradually switched to pseudoephedrine, which, while less potent, still effectively cleared stuffy noses. To this day, pseudoephedrine remains the active ingredient in Sudafed and many other over-the-counter nasal decongestants.

The story of ephedrine might have ended there, were it not for a Dr. Eriksen from Elsinore, Denmark—the hometown of Shakespeare's Hamlet. In 1972, Dr. Eriksen, a general practitioner, noticed unintentional loss of appetite and weight in his asthmatic patients for whom he had prescribed a combination of ephedrine, caffeine, and phenobarbitol. He began prescribing the combination as a weight-loss remedy, word spread around the entire country, and by 1977 the "Elsinore pill," as it became known, was being taken by tens of thousands of Danes. One pharmacy alone manufactured a million tablets a week. The timing couldn't have been better, as the use of amphetamines for weight loss, so popular in the 1960s, had plummeted after their addictive potential had been recognized. But severe skin reactions, a rare effect of phenobarbitol, were soon reported, and the Danish Institute of Health issued a warning. Then, in 1981, Axel Malchow-Moller of the University of Copenhagen published a randomized, placebo-controlled study of the "Elsinore pills" minus the phenobarbitol. He found that they still resulted in nearly nine extra pounds lost after twelve weeks compared to placebo. And, although they also produced tremors, insomnia, and feelings of exaltation, none of the side effects were what he considered "serious." Sales of the ephedrine-caffeine combination took off worldwide, not only among those seeking to lose weight but also among club-goers who wanted a buzz. In 1983, however, the FDA played party pooper by banning the combination of ephedrine and caffeine due to its growing abuse as a recreational stimulant, as well as growing concern that the one-two punch of caffeine plus ephedrine could be dangerous.

It didn't take long, however, for fans of the Elsinore pills to figure out that while the combination of caffeine and ephedrine was now illegal, pills containing caffeine plus *ephedra* (the natural herb) remained perfectly legal. The chemical ephedrine, after all, was classified as a drug, while the plant ephedra was classified as a dietary supplement. The division made no scientific sense: both the natural and synthesized versions contained the same molecules and had the same effect on the human heart and nervous system. (*"It's the molecule, stupid."*) But it made a great deal of commercial sense for companies seeking to cash in on ephedra's kick.

⊂⊃ ⊂⊃ ⊂⊃

Having been rebuffed twice by Texas district judges in his attempt to ban Formula One, the state health commissioner David Smith decided on May 12, 1994, to file a federal suit against the company, accusing it of making false claims on the label and illegally adding synthetic ephedrine. "The real issue that I need to reinforce is that this is a public health concern and threat," he said. Six months later, with over a hundred reports of stroke, psychosis, memory loss, muscle damage, nerve damage, high blood pressure, heart palpitations, or death linked to Formula One, the lawsuit had still gone nowhere when, on November 8, George W. Bush was elected governor.

At first, Bush's election changed little in the health department's attempts to clamp down on ephedra sales. It finally reached a settlement with the maker of Formula One, in which the company agreed to pay $400,000 in court costs, limit the amount of ephedra in the pills, and stop making unproved claims. Then, on March 31, 1995, the department proposed rules requiring a prescription for almost all products containing ephedrine. The public reacted with such anger and outrage, placing as many as a thousand calls per week to Culmo's office, that the department allowed the proposed rule to expire and set about planning a longer-term strategy in which it would organize a panel of medical experts to review the evidence on ephedra's safety. Part of that strategy was to bring in the feds.

Having just been thwacked upside the head by its loss in the battle over DSHEA, the FDA, unfortunately, could not ban any dietary supplement, including ephedra, without ironclad proof of dangerousness. But by October of 1995, the agency had grown sufficiently alarmed by the reports coming out of Texas that it convened an expert panel for a two-day meeting. There, Culmo described the 900 cases of adverse reactions her department had so far become aware of. Disturbingly, Culmo told the group, most of the reactions had occurred in patients who had taken the ephedra at doses recommended on the label, in striking contrast to many of the severe reactions to legitimate drugs, which are far more common among those who either intentionally or mistakenly take too much. At the end of the meeting, the panel recommended that the FDA set maximum dose limits for ephedra supplements, require warning labels, and establish manufacturing standards. But while it sought a defensible legal strategy, the agency took no immediate action.

Manufacturers, on the other hand, acted swiftly to capitalize on the remarkable profits that the makers of Formula One were earning. Some, it is true, refused to plunge in; Gerry Kessler, for instance, felt that ephedra was just not safe, and his ethical qualms no doubt cost his company millions in potential lost profits. Many others, however, were not troubled by an inconvenient conscience. Indeed, it is difficult to imagine a more apt commentary on the true nature of the ephedra business than this: two of the companies that would prove most successful were founded by felons who had been involved with methamphetamine, the illegal stimulant with a primary ingredient that is, of all things, ephedrine. Robert Occhifinto, for instance, had served eighteen months in federal prison after supplying ephedra to a methamphetamine dealer. Before that, he had been convicted of importing hashish. When he got out of prison, Occhifinto's New Jersey company, NVE Pharmaceuticals, began marketing Stacker, Black Beauty, and Yellow Jacket, all containing ephedra and caffeine. Both "black beauty" and "yellow jacket" were also the street names for speed, but Occhifinto insisted that was a coincidence. He named Black Beauty, he insisted, after the Disney movie, to connote the strength of the horse.

Michael Ellis and Michael Blevins, founders of Metabolife International Inc., had a similar story. Back on November 1, 1988, agents of the Drug Enforcement Administration had raided Ellis's California home and discovered a secret methamphetamine laboratory. In exchange for a sentence of probation, Ellis agreed to become an undercover DEA informant. Blevins, a high school buddy who had made the meth with him, was sentenced to five years in prison. Ellis drove Blevins to the prison and promised to build a legitimate business that Blevins could join when released. On January 23, 1995, less than three months after DSHEA was signed into law, Ellis formed Metabolife to sell an ephedra formula he called Metabolife 365. Within months, his old pal Blevins was allowed to transfer out of prison to a halfway house in San Diego. He wrote to the judge that a job awaited him at the new company. "With hard work and dedication," he wrote, "we are going to build something we can all be proud of." With Ellis as president, Blevins became vice president, and they decided to follow a multilevel marketing model similar to Formula One's, selling the product to distributors and the public directly from their San Diego office.

The first year, they sold 4,752 bottles and filed a corporate tax return showing gross sales of $115,024. Between 1996 and 1999, sales increased fast enough to make Metabolife one of the fastest-growing companies in the United States. In 1998, it sold 9 million bottles, generating $186,895,354 in sales, according to its tax return. In 1999, the company declared sales over $350 million. That same year, the company said it was selling 225,000 of its pills each hour. It had so much cash on hand that, according to a letter obtained by the Associated Press, "Ellis offered to pay the Russian government $15 million to put Metabolife's logo on an International Space State rocket. He suggested cosmonauts make Metabolife part of their in-space diet." Raphiella Adamson, director of retail operations for Metabolife in 1998 and 1999, said in an affidavit that the corporation was taking in about $1 million per day from the "will call" counter at its headquarters. Half of the money—up to $500,000 per day—was in cash, she said.

Both the FDA and the Texas Department of Health, meanwhile, continued to spin their wheels. In August of 1996, the FDA convened its Food Advisory Committee to review the mounting case reports. After hearing from dozens of scientists, industry representatives, and victims and their families, more than half of the twenty-six panel members concluded that, based on the available data, no safe level of ephedrine alkaloids could be identified. Most of the other members of the panel felt that a fairly low level—between one and eight milligrams per serving— would be "reasonably safe." Even so, aside from its traditional medical use as a nasal decongestant, no member could identify any proven benefit for ephedrine alkaloids that would justify any risk at all. That same month, at the urging of the Texas Medical Association, the state health department proposed rules to limit ephedra sales to prescription only. Once again the growing legions of independent distributors of ephedra products rose up in protest. Once again the proposed rules were allowed to expire.

Then, in September of 1997, Governor Bush appointed a new health commissioner, William "Reyn" Archer, MD, son of the powerful U.S. congressman Bill Archer. He appeared at first to be as determined as Smith had been to crack down on ephedra, and in May of 1998 the department issued, for a third time, proposed rules to restrict sales of ephedra to prescription only. It was then that the death threats started coming in.

"We know exactly why people like you get blown up," said one caller to the health department. "You'll never live to see this happen."

Cynthia Culmo, still the director of Drugs and Medical Devices, was told by a middle-aged female caller, "You have a daughter. Your address is public. You're going to regret this."

The department tried to shield her and other officials, screening their phone calls as best as possible. But the number of calls had reached as many as a thousand per day, and Culmo considered herself a public servant whose duty it was to hear from the public. An idealist without a shred of political interest, she also wasn't a typical bureaucrat, in that she wasn't afraid to make waves if she felt her cause was just.

"I believe you have to do the right thing, even when the right thing is difficult," Culmo later said, "which is one of the reasons I couldn't back off, even with the threats. My parents instilled a lot of it. I heard this a lot growing up, and I still believe it, that you have to tell the truth and the truth will set you free. I went into government very naive. I was clueless."

That is not to say she wasn't afraid. "We were very worried. There were many conversations with my husband. But he never told me to get out. He knew I felt committed to this, that I felt there was an obligation to the public. You can't let them manipulate you or control you. We would sort of joke about it. But my husband said, 'If one of you ends up dead, I don't care how natural it looks, someone's got to investigate it, because I don't think it's going to be natural causes.' "

For all her determination, she and others in her department decided it would be best if they did not attend the public hearing scheduled for June 3, 1998, lest their presence should incite a riot. Phil Howry did attend the meeting, however, and spoke out in memory of his wife, Julie. In the hallway outside the meeting room after his testimony, Commissioner Archer approached him. The two actually knew each other, because Howry's daughter was working that summer as an intern in the Washington office of Archer's father, the U.S. congressman.

"Reyn, you know this is not right," Howry said to him. "You've got to shut these people down."

"Phil, there's certain ways you can fight these products," Archer replied. "Let the FDA do it, let the federal government do it. The Texas Department of Health is powerless to fight business like this. They'll sue us if we try to ban it."

"Come on, Reyn," answered Howry. "You telling me the State of Texas is afraid of a lawsuit?"

Immediately following the meeting, Metabolife began buying influence commensurate with its enormous hoard of cash. As its first key lobbyist, Metabolife hired Jeff Wentworth, an influential state senator in Texas, where it is perfectly legal for legislators to be paid to lobby state agencies. Wentworth arranged a July 2 meeting between Metabolife's president, Michael Ellis, and Commissioner Archer. Around the same time, the company hired a leading San Antonio law firm, Loeffler, Jonas & Tuggey, LLP, and the partner James Jonas III met with Governor Bush's health-care advisor, Ron Lindsey. A month later, on August 11, Archer held a closed-door meeting with officials from Metabolife and seven other ephedra manufacturers. Culmo was excluded, as were any independent doctors or consumer advocates. According to an investigation by *Time* magazine's Michael Weisskopf, Archer agreed to accept industry recommendations that the maximum dose limit be set at 25 milligrams per serving, significantly higher than what the FDA's advisory committee had considered to be the safe upper limit two years earlier. But what would be the exact language of the new regulations? An aide to Archer wrote in her notes of the meeting, "Industry will draft rules."

At Culmo's urging, Archer backpedaled, announcing in mid-September that the maximum serving would be 10 milligrams. Then, according to Weisskopf's account in *Time*: "On Oct. 2, Ellis, Wentworth and Jonas contributed a total of $10,000 to Bush's re-election campaign, followed three days later by $5,000 from another Metabolife official, Michael Blevins. According to Ellis' spokesman, Jonas sought the money as co-chairman of a fund raiser for Bush. Archer held a meeting with the task force Oct. 20 and once more backed off the stricter limits. On the same day, Tom Loeffler, a former Texas Congressman hired as a Washington lobbyist for Metabolife, contributed $25,000 to the Bush gubernatorial campaign." In November, Archer decided to scrap the proposed rules altogether.

Meanwhile, at the federal level, the FDA was having no better luck getting traction with its efforts to regulate ephedra. On June 4, 1997, the FDA announced its intention to restrict supplements containing ephedrine alkaloids to no more than 8 milligrams per dose. Congress then asked the General Accounting Office to examine the scientific basis for the proposal. The GAO concluded that the reports of injury and death the FDA had received were still too flimsy a basis on which to take action. Even though hundreds of animal and human studies conducted over decades had shown that ephedrine alkaloids could speed the heart enough to cause heart attack or stroke in otherwise healthy individuals, no theoretical risk, however severe, was sufficient under DSHEA for the FDA to act. Actual injuries—bodies in the street, as it were—had to be piling up, and they had to be conclusively linked to the supplement. And so despite having received by 1999 some 1,173 reports of adverse reactions, the FDA formally withdrew its modest proposal to limit the maximum doses of ephedra tablets, and went back to watching the body count rise.

Back in Texas, the department of health proposed a rule in January of 1999 requiring a simple warning on the labels of all ephedra products, listing the possible side effects. It was the department's fourth and, by far, its most modest proposal to regulate ephedra, and this time the rule was actually allowed to go into effect. The department then tried for something stronger: a ban on sales of all ephedra products to minors, and a requirement that the labels include the FDA's consumer hotline number for reporting adverse reactions. Amazingly, this too appeared to pass muster and was slated to go into effect on September 1, 2001. By then, of course, George W. Bush had left Austin and taken up residence in the White House, and presumably should have had nothing to do with the passage of a Texas state law. But on August 1, Bush's secretary of Health and Human Services, Tommy G. Thompson, was approached by Jeff Wentworth, the state senator who was still on Metabolife's payroll. In a conversation lasting just a few minutes, Wentworth conveyed Metabolife's concern that the FDA was unprepared to handle the calls that might be generated by having its consumer hotline number listed on the labels of ephedra (a concern the FDA did not share). One of Thompson's aides then called Texas's commissioner of Health and Human Services, Don A. Gilbert. On August 28, Charles E. Bell, executive deputy commissioner of the health department, sent an e-mail to the department staff, saying, "[it] seems to be in the best interest of TDH [the Texas Department of Health] to take the advice of Secretary Thompson's office and delay either our implementation date or our enforcement of the rules that would take effect September 1st, 2001, for 60 days."

Sales of Metabolife 365 had by then reached a cumulative total of $1 billion. Having spent more than $4 million of that on lobbying fees to the firm of Loeffler, Jonas & Tuggey, Metabolife seemed to be getting its money's worth. The same could be said in California, where after the company spent $493,000 in "soft money" contributions in 2000, Governor Gray Davis vetoed legislation restricting ephedra use on September 29 of that year. On the federal level too Metabolife donated $683,000 to campaigns during the 2000 election, making it that year's seventh-largest donor among pharmaceutical companies.

The company did not confine its spending, however, to such traditional lobbying efforts. During a deposition for a court case involving another ephedra manufacturer, Wallace Winter, MD, PhD, a pharmacologist and toxicologist who served as the FDA's Pacific Region medical officer in San Francisco during the 1990s, made a sensational admission (which, it should be noted, he refused to stand by when it came time for the trial). He stated during the deposition that he met Ellis on a single occasion sometime between 1996 and 1997, when he was planning to retire from the FDA and had heard that the company was looking for scientists. During the meeting, Ellis offered him a large sum of money. "I think at the time," Dr. Winter said, "he said to me he would give me ten thousand dollars if, while I was still working for the FDA, I would say something about ephedra or something."

The lawyer conducting the deposition asked him, "And do you recall that Mike Ellis wanted you to say statements critical of the FDA's policy toward ephedra?"

"I don't recall specifically," Dr. Winter said, "but I think that would be the general context, yeah."

Dr. Winter turned down the offer, he said, "because it was inappropriate." But upon retiring, he did become an expert witness testifying to the safety of ephedra in five cases involving four companies: AST Sports Science, E'ola, NexProtein, and Metabolife.

⌐ ⌐ ⌐

The FDA's coziness with the industry it regulated deepened in August of 2001 with President Bush's appointment of Dan Troy as the agency's chief legal counsel. Troy—the older brother of Tevi Troy, then a special assistant to President Bush and a deputy cabinet secretary—had spent much of the 1990s fighting the FDA, often successfully, as one of the country's best-known lawyers for drug, supplement, and tobacco companies. After graduating from Columbia Law School in 1983, he had served two years as a law clerk to Robert Bork, the ultraconservative judge who was rejected by the Senate as a possible Supreme Court justice.

Troy's appointment came at a particularly difficult time for the agency. After David Kessler had stepped down as commissioner in February of 1997, Clinton had next appointed Jane E. Henney, MD, considered by many to be as tough, capable, and principled as her predecessor. But with Henney's resignation days before Bush took office in January of 2001, in order to let the new president choose his own appointee, the agency went for twenty-two months without a confirmed commissioner. Into this policy void came Troy. Having previously represented Pfizer Inc. in a dispute with the FDA, he now took the extraordinary step of filing a brief throwing the agency's support behind Pfizer in a lawsuit it was facing over the suicide of a patient who had been taking the Pfizer antidepressant Zoloft. A fox, it seemed, was in charge of the henhouse.

On the issue of ephedra, Troy repeatedly insisted that the agency lacked the legal authority to ban it, according to those both within and outside the FDA. Even when it became known that Metabolife was quietly settling lawsuits with victims, Troy refused a request by one of the agency's top officials to seek records from the lawsuits indicating just how many adverse event reports it had received from customers. Such information would have proven explosive, because in a 1998 letter, Michael Ellis had told the FDA that Metabolife had "never received one notice from a consumer that any serious adverse health event has occurred because of the ingestion of Metabolife 365." But Troy would not allow the agency to pursue evidence that Ellis had lied. Not until August of 2002, when Metabolife voluntarily gave up records of 14,684 adverse reactions reported by its customers (after the IRS came across the records in a raid on Ellis's ranch as part of a tax-evasion investigation) did it finally become known that eighteen heart attacks, twenty-six strokes, forty-three seizures, and five deaths had been linked to Metabolife.

By the beginning of 2003, a cynical view had taken hold among consumer advocates: that state legislators were so beholden to Metabolife and other free-spending ephedra manufacturers and the FDA was so dominated by Troy's pro-business thinking that nothing would be done until a celebrity died and grabbed the public's attention. And then it happened. On February 17, 2003, Steve Bechler, a pitcher for the Baltimore Orioles, collapsed and died of heatstroke after taking Xenadrine. The twenty-three-year-old was at spring training camp in Florida. He weighed 249 pounds and, in an effort to lose weight, hadn't eaten much solid food in two days. The Broward County medical examiner concluded that the Xenadrine and the high humidity and 81-degree temperature, combined with a history of borderline high blood pressure and other minor health problems, had all played a role in his death.

Industry officials and their advocates argued that ephedra had nothing to do with Bechler's unfortunate demise. But with intense media coverage of the celebrity death, political pressure on the Bush administration grew intense. Eleven days after Bechler's death, the FDA announced that it would immediately ban unsubstantiated claims about ephedra's supposed ability to boost sports performance, and that it was seeking rapid public comment on whether to require stern new safety warning labels. By then, between 12 and 17 million people were estimated to be taking some 3 billion doses of ephedra supplements each year, and the FDA had received more than 2,000 reports of adverse events—fifteen times more than it has received for the next most commonly reported herbal supplement. On May 26, Illinois became the first state to ban ephedra. But even as the U.S. House Subcommittee on Oversight and Investigations drew up plans for a hearing later that summer, a young man in Oklahoma continued taking his Stackers to lose a few pounds.

⸻

Born on March 4, 1981, Todd James Lee had grown up in rural Oklahoma, fourteen miles from Muskogee. In fifth grade, he had written an essay at school saying that his dream in life was to follow the footsteps of his stepfather, Karl, into the U.S. Air Force. By the time he turned twenty, living on the outskirts of Oklahoma City with his mother, working at a call center for Williams-Sonoma, his dream had yet to come true. But his winning personality still managed to make a strong impression wherever he went. His supervisor, Wendy Musgrove, didn't know anybody who didn't like him. His attitude was different from those of most of the call center's employees. He didn't get bogged down in the tedium or negativity. He didn't talk bad about anybody, didn't gossip about anybody. Instead, he would sometimes walk around the call center, rubbing people on the back.

Kristie Runion, eighteen years old when she first met him at the call center, looked up to Todd. She'd never once heard him lie or say something negative. "He was pure and kindhearted and intelligent," she said. "There was no ego with him. He had a really good philosophy on life." As much as she admired him, though, Kristie was pleased to observe a change in Todd the longer he worked at Williams-Sonoma. "When he came here, he was quiet, shy, very inward—the most quiet person I've ever met in my whole life. When he came to Oklahoma City from the country, he really got to grow. A lot of people, if you grow up in the country, you stay in the country." Gently alluding to family problems he'd faced, she said, "The fact that he came out okay is amazing. And he was better than okay. He was an angel. He was just my best friend." She also became Todd's girlfriend.

His younger sister, Shayna, likewise thought of Todd as her best friend, even after she went to live with Karl in the suburbs of Dallas. "I could talk to him about anything," Shayna recalled. "Stuff with our family—me and him would stick together. He was a real good listener. He always bragged about me, because he thought I was real mature for my age."

Even his mother, Camille, considered Todd her best friend. "He was so deep," said Camille. "One of my friends said he was an old soul; she could talk to him about her problems. We talked every day. He was my life."

After turning twenty-one in 2002, Todd decided it was time to make his dream come true. As Kristie saw it, the military was Todd's ticket to a better life. "Not that he didn't love his country," she said, "but Todd was basically joining the Air Force because he could get a good education, he could see the world, and he could make himself a better person, a worldly man."

He had just one obstacle: his weight. Nobody had ever thought of Todd as fat, but he was more than ten pounds over the 186-pound limit the air force set for a man of his height, five-nine. Even after a few days of fasting, he remained a few pounds over. Due to his low body fat percentage of 16 percent, however, he was allowed in, and on June 4, 2002, he proudly became Airman Basic Todd Lee.

After completing basic training at Lackland Air Force Base in San Antonio, he took courses in electronics and communications, receiving in April of 2003 a certificate for outstanding academic excellence, with a score of 95 percent. Meanwhile, his weight crept back up to about 205 pounds, and he was enrolled in what was informally known as the Air Force's "fat boy" program. Until he reached 186 pounds, he would not be allowed to become an Airman First Class and get his second stripe. He began dieting, working out, and taking Stacker 2, a weight-loss supplement containing ephedra. The pounds melted off.

He was sent later in April to serve in the Thirty-second Combat Communications Squadron at Tinker Air Force Base, located fifteen minutes from where his mother lived in Oklahoma City. When Kristie saw him upon his return, she was surprised at how trim he looked. One night, while they cuddled together on a couch, she noticed that his heart was beating fast.

"I'm taking Stackers," he explained. "They're awesome. They give you energy."

"I'm going to have to try one of those," Kristie replied.

The next weekend, she did try one of Todd's Stacker pills. Her heart began beating rapidly and she felt dizzy.

"Do you need to go to the doctor?" Todd asked her. "These things can kind of spin you out."

She didn't feel sick enough for a doctor, but she did find herself wondering about the pill's safety. Still, Todd said he'd bought them at a health food store, so she figured they had to be okay.

On Friday, June 6, two days after his first anniversary of joining the Air Force, still without his second stripe, Todd began the day by working out, and then volunteered to be on the flight line welcoming fellow airmen returning from Iraq. He wore his best dress uniform, standing at attention in the 80-degree heat. Later that afternoon, his mother arrived at the base, as planned, so that she and Todd could drive together to pick up Shayna halfway between Oklahoma City and Dallas, at a gas station where Karl would meet them.

"Todd, your head's not fat anymore!" Shayna said when she first saw him at the Love gas station in Ardmore, Oklahoma. She was amazed at how much weight he had lost. With her was a friend, Ambre, who was joining them for the weekend. They thanked Karl for dropping the girls off, and then began the hundred-mile trip back to Oklahoma City.

Shayna was surprised to see Todd take the passenger seat; he always liked to drive. He was so quiet that she thought something was wrong.

"No, I'm just tired," he told her. He put on his sunglasses and drifted off to sleep as they headed north.

The sun was setting as they neared Todd's base on Interstate 240, where he would have to be behind the wheel in order to get in. He started stirring, and told Camille to put the Tinker Air Force Base pass onto the dashboard. Then she heard him utter a loud sound and she looked over. His hands were clenched up to his chest.

"Todd, are you okay?" Camille asked him. "Todd?"

A tear was rolling down his left cheek from beneath his sunglasses.

"Todd!" Camille called, but heard only gurgling. Shayna leaned forward and placed her hand against Todd's chest. She felt nothing.

"Mom, his heart isn't beating."

Camille shrieked, gunned the engine and took the next exit, at Sunny-lane Road. At the end of the ramp she flew through the stop sign, past oncoming traffic and into the parking lot of a Total gas station, where she screeched to a halt up against the curb of the station's convenience store.

"Call 911!" she screamed inside the store. "My son isn't breathing!"

A crowd of people instantly formed around the car. A guy named Dave who worked inside ran out and said they needed to take Todd out of the car and place him on the pavement. Camille saw Todd's head bump hard on the concrete pavement as they laid him down.

Dave immediately began performing CPR. Someone handed Camille a telephone. The 911 operator on the line asked her what was happening. Just then, Todd vomited. Camille told the operator, who said they should stop performing CPR. Camille told Dave, and he did stop, but then Todd's face turned blue, so Dave started again. Shayna got down on her knees and started praying.

After what seemed like forty-five minutes (it was actually closer to fif-teen), the paramedics arrived. They pulled out a defibrillator, gave Todd's heart a couple of shocks, and then took him to nearby Hillcrest Hospital, with Camille, Shayna, and Ambre following close behind. Inside, a nurse told them to sit down in the waiting room. It wasn't more than ten min-utes before two doctors came out, asking questions about what had hap-pened.

"Is Todd okay?" Camille asked.

"No," said one of the doctors, "he passed away at—"

Camille didn't hear the words. "No, no, no!" she cried out, breaking into uncontrollable sobs. Shayna sat down, in shock, and Ambre hyperventilated so badly that she was given a cubicle inside the emergency room.

Kristie, visiting her sister, had gone to bed early that night, not knowing that her sister had taken the phone off the hook so they could get a good night's sleep. She'd expected to hear from Todd, and in the morning, she plugged the phone back in and checked her messages. Dozens of messages had been left for her, telling her that something had happened to Todd. Figuring he'd been in some kind of car accident, she called Camille's house.

"Todd's dead," Camille sobbed. "He had some kind of a heart attack."

Kristie thought, *"A heart attack?* How the hell could he have a heart attack?" Her brain searched for a possible solution. And then she blurted out the words: "Camille, he was taking those Stackers."

⌒ ⌒ ⌒

Less than two months after Todd's death in the summer of 2003, the House Subcommittee on Oversight and Investigations held a hearing to look into the ephedra industry. Robert Occhifinto, president of the company that made Stackers, told his bizarre story about how he had named Black Beauty, another of his ephedra products, after the Disney movie. (An incredulous Representative James C. Greenwood, Republican of Pennsylvania and chair of the subcommittee, replied, "Your testimony under oath is that you decided to use a Walt Disney character for a name for your products, that you had no notion that 'black beauty' had been used as a street drug, and you did not pick Dumbo, you did not pick Pinocchio, you did not pick Goofy, you picked Black Beauty and it was just an amazing coincidence?" To which Occhifinto answered, basically, yes.) Michael Ellis was called to testify too, but he exercised his constitutional right to remain silent while the Justice Department sought an indictment against him for making false statements to the FDA.

Despite Ellis's silence, the hearing proved to be an enlightening deconstruction of the evidence for and against ephedra's safety. One study that drew a great deal of debate was an independent analysis by the Rand Corporation (a respected research organization) of fifty-two previous ephedra studies and of all the injury reports that the FDA had received by then. As Russell Schreck, then the president and CEO of Metabolife, said in his opening remarks at the hearing: "The Rand study noted [that] no serious adverse effects were reported in the fifty-two clinical trials."

Diana DeGette, Democrat of Colorado, said she was "confused" by Schreck's comment and quoted directly from the Rand report: "Overall, people who received ephedra or ephedrine had between 2.2 and 3.6 times higher odds of suffering harmful side effects, including psychiatric symptoms, jitteriness, palpitations, nausea, and vomiting than did people taking a placebo. From the 284 reports of serious adverse events we identified two deaths, three heart attacks, nine strokes, three seizures, and five psychiatric cases as sentinel events with prior ephedra consumption. . . . In aggregate, the [reports suggest] a link between products containing either ephedra and ephedrine and catastrophic events such as sudden death, heart attack, stroke, seizure, and serious psychiatric symptoms. Regarding safety we conclude from the clinical trials that ephedrine and ephedra are associated with two or three times the odds of experiencing psychiatric symptoms, autonomic symptoms, upper gastrointestinal symptoms, and palpitations." She then asked Schreck, "Do you agree with the Rand report findings?"

"I do not agree with those," Schreck replied.

The subcommittee then turned to questioning the author of the other big study often touted by manufacturers as proving that ephedra was safe. Carol Boozer, PhD, was a nutritionist who had received her doctorate from Harvard and served on the faculty of the Institute of Human Nutrition at Columbia University. Her study had been published in the *International Journal of Obesity and Metabolic Disorder.*

Greg Walden, Democrat of Oregon, asked Dr. Boozer, "Did the findings of your six-month study show that ephedra is safe?"

"I have refrained from using the word 'safe' in defining the results of the study for this reason: I think that it is a word that can be generalized. And I have said in the papers that I do not think our results can be generalized beyond the types of people we studied."

"So nobody should ever use your study to say their product is safe, is that accurate?"

"I would not recommend that they do that. I do not use that word."

"Sometimes it is held up as the gold standard, the best scientific research out there. But yours would not be a study you would stand behind to say that this drug is safe?"

"I am not saying that it is unsafe either."

Representative Greenwood then took up the questioning of Dr. Boozer. Just five days earlier, in anticipation of the hearing, he had released an analysis of her study commissioned by the FDA and conducted by three independent experts. The analysis had found that some of the patients in the study had been mistakenly given the active ephedra-and-caffeine pills instead of the inactive placebo pills they were supposed to get; it therefore shouldn't have been surprising that the "placebo" group appeared to have the same kinds of symptoms as the ephedra-and-caffeine group. The experts concluded that the study was "severely compromised" and "impossible to rely on."

Greenwood asked Dr. Boozer if she personally would recommend to overweight patients that they take ephedra.

"No," she said. "I have worked in a medical setting for many years as a nonphysician, and I am very conscious of the difference between my ability to give medical advice and that of the physician. So I would refer someone [to a physician]."

"But you would not recommend this product, would you?"

"I limit my advice to diet and exercise."

"But I am asking you a very serious question. This is a very important policy issue. Is the reason you would not recommend this because you're just not qualified and perhaps if you had a medical degree you would know when to recommend, or is the reason you do not recommend it because you think it's not a good idea for people to use this to solve their weight problems?"

Finally cornered, Dr. Boozer answered: "I have some of the same concerns that have been expressed earlier about the widespread use of these compounds. And while I feel that within the constraints of our study that people were not at risk, I still would have hesitation in advising people who are outside the constraints to use this, because it has not been widely studied."

⊂⊃ ⊂⊃ ⊂⊃

By the end of 2003, according to sources close to the agency, Secretary Thompson made it clear to the FDA commissioner, Mark McClellan, that it was time to make the ephedra problem go away. Although Thompson's office had previously pressured the Texas Department of Health to scuttle its restrictions on ephedra, the political pressure had now grown too great. On December 30, McClellan announced that ephedra was "adulterated" under the meaning of DSHEA, meaning that it was either a "significant or unreasonable" risk. (Nine years earlier, Gerry Kessler had fought to make the standard "significant *and* unreasonable" but had had to compromise to get DSHEA passed.) According to insiders, proving it was a "significant" risk had been nearly impossible due to the haphazard nature of the injury reports that came in. But establishing that it was an "unreasonable" risk turned out to be far easier, since almost any risk at all would be too great if the product had only a slight, short-term benefit for weight loss—and no study had shown that it could do anything more than that. As a result, McClellan announced, the FDA would enact a national ban on ephedra, to take effect on Monday, March 12, 2004. In the meantime, he said, "Consumers should stop buying and using ephedra products right away, and FDA will make sure consumers are protected by removing these products from the market as soon as the rule becomes effective."

But stores and Web sites rushed to move as much product as they could. Four days before the ban went into effect, Mike Giordano, sales manager at the World of Fitness gym in Bloomfield, New Jersey, called the ban "ridiculous." In a refrigerated display case in front of the counter, beverages containing ephedra were still being sold. "I've been taking it nearly every day for six years," Giordano said. "Next they're going to have to outlaw cars because of some fool who doesn't want to drive safe. I don't see it as public safety. I see it as individual rights being taken away."

Two doors down stood Bloomfield Health Food Center, where the owners, Ken and Sam Kapoor, father and son, were hoping to sell out their last remaining supply of products containing ephedra by Sunday. There on the shelf were all the onetime favorites: Stacker 2, Ripped Fuel, Xenadrine, YellowSubs, TrimSpa, Thermo-Tek, and Up Your Gas.

"It was one of our better-selling products," said Sam, referring collectively to all the ephedra-containing products. The replacements had not been selling nearly as well among weight lifters and dieters, he added.

By then, companies like Metabolife and TrimSpa were rushing to get new ephedra-free products to market. TrimSpa switched to an ingredient nobody had ever heard of (an African cactus called hoodia gordonii) in its new formula X32, and hired the famously overweight Anna Nicole Smith as its chief spokesperson, claiming that her sudden slim-down was due entirely to TrimSpa. At the same time, its advertisements appeared to follow the letter of DSHEA to almost comical effect. In commercials and on the Internet, its glowing testimonials by Anna Nicole and others were countered by the notice: "These results are not typical. X32 may not work for everyone. Average weight loss achieved after 8 weeks using X32 with a reduced-calorie diet and exercise was between .6 to .8 pounds per week based on the interim results of an ongoing clinical trial." But for all the caution, by March of 2005 the company faced three class-action lawsuits charging that the only component of hoodia gordonii ever shown to work as an appetite suppressant (an extract called P57) was not contained in TrimSpa. A search that month of the vast database maintained by the National Library of Medicine turned up only one weight-loss study that even mentioned hoodia gordonii, and it focused on the extract P57. The test subjects were rats, not humans. Yet TrimSpa was selling well enough to spawn dozens of copycat hoodia products.

As for Xenadrine, its new ephedra-free version was promoted as "the next generation in advanced thermogenic technology." The ad went on, "This amazing, patent-pending formula produces an entirely new level of effectiveness never before seen in the diet supplement industry. In fact, it is the first product ever to be powered by an ultra-potent blend of natural, clinically proven metabolic compounds that work synergistically to produce unprecedented fat-burning results—without containing ephedrine!" Like many of the other ephedra replacements, the new Xenadrine contained bitter orange peel, better known as an ingredient in orange marmalade. Even in minuscule amounts, bitter orange contains a chemical cousin of ephedrine called synephrine. In concentrated doses, it produces an adrenaline-like kick to the heart and nervous system similar to ephedra's. A few days before the ephedra ban went into effect, the FDA revealed that it had received reports of seven deaths and eighty-five adverse reactions associated with bitter orange. By then, the *Annals of Phar-*

macotherapy had reported on the case of a fifty-five-year-old woman who showed up at an emergency room in Atlanta with chest pain and a dully aching shoulder. Tests showed she had suffered a heart attack. She had never smoked, and had no prior history of heart disease. She had, however, been taking Edita's Skinny Pill, containing 300 milligrams of bitter orange, for the past year. The doctors who wrote the report concluded that the woman's heart attack was "possibly" associated with bitter orange, and warned that supplements containing bitter orange "may present as a risk for cardiovascular toxicity."

Meanwhile, in the three and a half months between the announcement of the ephedra ban on December 30 and its scheduled implementation three and a half months later, an additional four ephedra-related deaths were reported to the FDA, bringing the total to 164. By then, the agency had received 2,570 reports of adverse events associated with ephedra, not counting the 14,000-plus that it had obtained from Metabolife.

But manufacturers were not prepared to let their cash cow go without a fight, and moved to block the ban by filing a federal lawsuit in—where else?—Utah. A second federal suit was filed in New Jersey. At ten-thirty in the morning on Monday, April 12—the day the ban was to go into effect—Robert Occhifinto, maker of the Stackers that Todd Lee took before dying, sat in the fourth row of Room 2 in the federal courthouse in Newark. Wearing a blue sport shirt that nicely showed off his muscles, he said nothing while his attorneys sought a temporary restraining order to hold up the ban.

After wrangling for more than an hour on legal minutiae, the U.S. district judge Joel Pisano posed a simple question to Walter P. Timpone, the lead attorney representing Occhifinto's company: "Is this case generated by a legitimate concern for the public's access to a short-term weight loss product, or by a concern about the economic interest of your client?"

Mr. Timpone argued forcefully that the public's interest would best be served by allowing consumers to exercise their right to choose whether they wished to continue taking ephedra. "The government is coming and saying you cannot," he said, and then turned to a personal example. "I'm a sun lover. It lowers my blood pressure and makes me feel good. I know it's dangerous, but I'm going to sit down in the sun and take that chance, at least until the FDA bans the sun. I have the right to be wrong."

But Judge Pisano ruled that the public's right to be protected from serious harm outweighed its interest in being free to buy such a product. To issue the restraining order, he would have had to find that the manufacturers' case had a strong likelihood of ultimately prevailing, that the manufacturers would suffer irreparable harm, and that the public interest would be served. On all questions, the judge came down against the manufacturers.

"Virtually every fact in this case is disputed," Judge Pisano stated. With the FDA's own records in the case totaling some 133,000 pages, and its regulation banning ephedra taking up 147 pages in the Federal Register, he said it was impossible for him to decide then which side was likely to prevail. "The resolution of the findings in this case is going to require a full evidentiary hearing and a full review of the administrative record," Judge Pisano added.

Senator Richard Durbin, Democrat of Illinois, said at the time that while he applauded the FDA's ban, he didn't believe it could be enforced. "They have a handful of people monitoring a multibillion dollar industry," he said. "Until we change the basic law, the FDA will never be able to enforce it."

But Jeffrey Shuren, the FDA's assistant commissioner for policy, said he disagreed with Durbin's view. "Right now we think we have the people we need to get the job done," Shuren said. "This is really going to be a test case."

But the test ended a year later, on April 13, 2005, when the U.S. district judge Tena Campbell ruled in the Utah case that the FDA had not sufficiently established the danger of a 10-milligram ephedra dose under the rules of DSHEA. The FDA filed an appeal on June 13, noting that it now knew of nineteen *thousand* serious adverse reactions to ephedra products. While the appeal was considered, ephedra crept back on the market. One company, for instance, began sending e-mails to millions of Americans promoting an ephedra product called Eca Fuel. "Finally," the company's e-mails stated, "the forbidden fat-burning herb banned for being 'too effective'—ephedra—is available to the public again." Officially, the FDA's view was that ephedra remained strictly illegal (except for the 10-milligram dose sold by Nutraceutical Corporation, the Utah firm that had challenged the law). Yet incredibly, the agency neither publicized nor enforced its view, and so the selling continued.

Finally, on August 17, 2006, a three-judge panel of the Tenth Circuit Court of Appeals ruled in favor of the FDA, and even Eca Fuel disappeared from the market. But ephedra was not dead yet. Nutraceutical Corporation filed an appeal to the entire court (not just the three-judge panel) on September 28. Whichever side loses is expected to appeal to the U.S. Supreme Court, meaning that one of the deadliest herbs ever sold could ultimately go back on the market.

As a practical matter, however, the marketing magic is gone. Too many people have heard about the dangers of ephedra, and too many personal injury lawsuits have been filed—including some 400 against Metabolife alone. For Michael Ellis, the firm's president, the turning point came in 2005, which was for him, as Queen Elizabeth said of the year Prince Charles and Diana divorced, an "annus horribilis." In February, he was indicted on charges of being a felon in possession of firearms, which had been found at his California ranch by federal agents searching for evidence of tax evasion. In July, although Metabolife was still selling an ephedra-free version of its product, the company filed for Chapter 11 bankruptcy protection. In October, the company pleaded guilty to underpaying one third of a million dollars to the Internal Revenue Service after failing to report more than $1 million in cash income during 1997 and 1998. "It just boils down to greed," said the IRS agent Kenneth Hines. "Greed motivates criminal enterprises and criminal individuals more than anything in the world." Ellis's buddy and vice president at Metabolife, Michael Blevins, pleaded guilty in October on charges that he too had been in possession of firearms despite his prior felony conviction. As part of the plea, Blevins agreed to provide substantial assistance in the government's cases against Ellis, which included charges that Ellis lied to the FDA when he said the company had received no reports of adverse reactions. On November 7, he agreed to sell Metabolife's remaining products for $12 million to IdeaSphere, the company that owns TwinLab, Nature's Herbs, and Alvita Teas, and whose vice chairman is the motivational speaker Tony Robbins. The remains of Ellis's and Blevins's company, now known as MII Liquidation Inc., announced on May 31, 2006, that it had settled the first 21 of the 400 lawsuits against it for $4.7 million.

Occhifinto's company, NVE, also filed for bankruptcy protection in 2005, despite projected sales of $40 million that year for ephedra-free

Stacker 2, down from $70 million the year before. A Houston attorney handling some of the 117 personal injury lawsuits filed against the company said that just two of them could reach $30 million in damages, including the case of a thirty-nine-year-old woman who suffered a stroke after taking Stacker 2 and is now a paraplegic. "We have some tragic injuries to some very young people," said the attorney, Ed Blizzard.

For all the well-earned troubles of the ephedra peddlers, however, virtually every one of the government officials who fought them also suffered. After rising quickly to her position as director of Drugs and Medical Devices at the Texas Department of Health, Cynthia Culmo never got another promotion after she began trying to regulate ephedra; at the end of 2003 she left government service to work for the private industry. More severe consequences came to two senior officials in the FDA who took a strong stand on ephedra that was at odds with the manufacturer-friendly attitude of Dan Troy. Despite stellar performance reviews, both found themselves demoted and consigned to organizational Siberia. Both were also subpoenaed by Congressman Dan Burton for any records indicating whether they had spoken with lawyers representing ephedra victims to illegally help them in their lawsuits against manufacturers. They had spoken with such lawyers, but only to receive reports of adverse events from them, which was part of their job duties. Neither is willing to speak on record now for fear of further retribution.

The real losers, however, were the American people. For the second time in twenty years—first with L-tryptophan, and then with ephedra—supplements had demonstrated remarkable potency in warding off one thing only: the type of political fallout that drugs have suffered after every major tragedy of adverse reactions. The history of drug regulation in the twentieth century may well have been built on tombstones, according to Michael Harris, but the history for supplements since the 1970s has been one of steady deregulation, the industry's health seemingly immune to the death and suffering propagated by its products. Indeed, at the precise time that some 19,000 people were suffering severe reactions to ephedra alone and at least 164 died, the supplement industry overall continued to grow unchecked. In no year since DSHEA passed, in fact, have industry sales gone down, or even been flat. By 1999, just five years after DSHEA, supplement sales reached $16.4 billion, up 63 percent overall from 1994, according to *Nutrition Business Journal.* Even in 2003, the year Steve Bechler's death made the dangers of supplements front-page news, industry sales grew by 5.7 percent, an enviable rate for any mature industry. In 2004, sales grew again by 2.6 percent, hitting $20.3 billion. Between 2005 and 2008, *Nutrition Business Journal* projects, supplement sales will continue to grow by 3 to 5 percent per year.

Many attribute the growth to the continuing power of DSHEA. "If FDA can't take a supplement as dangerous as ephedra off the market, then Congress needs to change the law to allow it to do so," said Senator Ted Kennedy after the agency's ban on ephedra had been lifted. Bruce Silverglade, the director of legal affairs of the Center for Science in the Public Interest, said, "This decision leaves no doubt that DSHEA prevents the FDA from taking unsafe products off the market. Congress should swiftly amend DSHEA to clarify and strengthen the FDA's authority to protect the public from dangerous products and mandate that the National Academy of Sciences conducts a comprehensive safety and efficacy review of dietary supplements." But so long as Orrin Hatch has anything to do with it, the prospects for any changes in federal laws regulating supplements look dim indeed. "Nobody has shown me the need to change [the law]," Hatch said. "It gives the FDA enough power to solve these problems if they do it the right way."

In fairness, it should be pointed out that not everybody suffered in the end from the ephedra boom. The biggest companies have gone bankrupt, thousands of users have been injured or killed, and the handful of government regulators who tried to do anything about it have found their careers stalled, but at least two people have gone merrily on their way. In late November of 2004, Dan Troy stepped down from his position at the FDA and, just over a month later, joined one of the largest and most prominent law firms in the country, Sidley Austin Brown & Wood LLP, where he immediately returned to representing food, drug, and supplement manufacturers in their fights with the agency. (Although lobbying the FDA on behalf of such companies would be against the law so soon after leaving office, giving legal counsel to them is, if nothing else, perfectly legal.) Another man whose career has soared since playing a role in the ephedra tragedy is the Texas attorney Jonathan L. Snare. On December 14, 2004, the U.S. secretary of labor, Elaine L. Chao, appointed Snare to be the deputy assistant secretary for the Occupational Safety and Health Administration. Some observers sniped that his main experience until then was purely political, having served, among other things, as general counsel to both the Republican Party of Texas and the Texas Senate Redistricting Committee, positions in which he worked closely with Representative Tom DeLay and the then-governor George W. Bush. But it was not true that Snare had no experience in public health. After all, he had also lobbied Texas officials on behalf of Metabolife.

PART 2

ALTERNATIVE UNIVERSE

CHAPTER 6

WHAT'S REALLY IN THAT BOTTLE?

The largest herbal extraction facility in North America abuts Interstate 80 in Hackensack, New Jersey, in an industrial neighborhood of old warehouses and abandoned factories. Founded in 1959 as Madis Botanicals, the company had achieved sales of $6.2 million by 1995 before falling into bankruptcy that year, when it was bought out by a team of investors. Reborn as Pure World, the company has since grown more than 600 percent, with revenues reaching $37.1 million in 2004. First boosted by the boom in kava, ephedra, and St. John's wort, Pure World is now riding a bull market in black cohosh and red clover for the symptoms of menopause. But beyond its balance sheet, a journey through Pure World's hulking 138,000-square-foot manufacturing, laboratory, and warehouse facility unravels the mystery of how all those leaves, roots, and berries pictured on the labels of herbal remedies get squeezed into pills, capsules, and gelcaps—and how, in the process, much of what made them natural in the first place gets squeezed out. After all, for all the industry's talk of 3,000-year-old traditions, none of the processes used at Pure World were applied to turn herbs into pills prior to the Adelle Davis era. Indeed, hardly any herbal remedies existed in pill form before the late 1970s—the very idea was a contradiction in terms—until industrial engineers like those at Pure World invented them.

Pure World extracts more than a hundred of the most popular herbal ingredients for products sold by major manufacturers (but not such oddities as the raw kidney, pancreas, and brain sold in some multi-ingredient products). In the warehouse, ginseng from China, guarana from Brazil, yohimbe bark from Africa, fenugreek seed from India, valerian root from Poland, and kava from the Pacific island of Vanuatu sit in burlap bags, canisters, and cardboard boxes as big as men. "There's not much quality control in the growing process," concedes Julius Myer, the company's assistant vice president, who happens to have a strong Long Island accent. "It's not a perfect world." That's why, he says, the company sets firm quality standards in its contracts with suppliers, and returns shipments when those standards are not met (unlike many smaller processors, which tend to accept anything that makes it through customs and the occasional inspection by the FDA). Walking through the unheated warehouse toward something with a powerful minty smell, he points out a giant heap of brown leaves, about a thousand pounds' worth of St. John's wort, sitting in a box. "The first step," he says, "is to cut it into a smaller size." A steel contraption bigger than a garbage truck takes the loose leaves in on one side and cranks out particles the size of cigarette tobacco on the other.

Next door, in the manufacturing plant, the real transformation begins in a contraption as big as a suburban house: the percolator. The extraction process is just like brewing a pot of coffee, only instead of water, alcohol is used to extract what Myer calls "the goodies" from, in this case, 8,800 pounds of passion flower. (What exactly are they extracting? Basically whatever comes out in the extraction process. Although some manufacturers then control for certain natural constituents, others prefer to use the whole extract, whatever it may be.) A nutty smell as if from a bakery pervades the huge, noisy cement-floored room, where the workers wear hairnets and the kind of inexpensive air masks used by painters. When it's finished percolating, the resulting slurry goes first into a giant rotating evaporator and then into a spray dryer, where it is blasted with hot air and flutters to the bottom like confetti. Then it heads through a roller-compactor to be made into a sheet, and finally through a mill to achieve the desired particle size.

Now it's testing time in the laboratory. Samples are taken and put through high-performance liquid chromatography, liquid crystal mass spectrometry, or nuclear magnetic resonance devices to detect contaminants and assess the potency of key molecular constituents. But all these devices cost hundreds of thousands of dollars, and while Pure World bases its reputation on a commitment to quality, many other manufacturers can't be bothered. "Buying anything from the United States or Europe, if they're not quality-oriented, it's dangerous," says Qun Yi Zheng, PhD, the president of Pure World. Born in Hunan province in China, he came to the United States in 1985 and obtained his doctorate in organic chemistry at the University of Colorado. Can a consumer expect higher quality from the supplements sold by major manufacturers? Dr. Zheng smiles. "Not necessarily. I know the companies, so I know which ones to trust. I see how they do things. A lot of people are not following the rules."

But then, at least for now, there really are no rules for manufacturers, because the FDA has yet to enact any manufacturing standards for supplements. Dr. Zheng would love to see standards enacted, because that would help them to "compete on a level playing field." In the meanwhile, the greatest danger posed by dietary supplements may lie not in the ingredients listed on their labels, but in those that are not.

○ ⊂⊃ ○

Beverly Hames's unwanted education in impure supplements began at the top of a ladder, where she climbed one crisp morning in October of 1992 to clean the leaves out of her gutters. Beverly was used to working on the house; she'd repainted it herself after divorcing in 1989. But this particular morning, perhaps because she was rushing to get to her job as senior office assistant for the Multnomah County Parole and Probation Department in Portland, Oregon, she reached a little too far and felt it: something gave way in her lower back. Soon, jolts of excruciating pain were coursing up her spine, but she went to work anyway.

When the pain didn't pass after a couple of days, seeing an herbalist was the last thing on her mind; she did not have a New Age bone in her body. Beverly, at forty-eight, had a tough, no-nonsense style well suited to her work with female offenders. Deeply conservative, yet tender enough to take in stray dogs, she had grown up never missing a day of school, and for years had won awards at work for having taken no sick days. From her father, who'd owned his own store, gas station, and RV park, she'd learned that to get ahead in life, you needed to work your butt off, sunup to sundown. So she made an after-work appointment with an orthopedist. She had to wait several weeks to see him, however, and when she did, she found him rude and unprofessional. He diagnosed her as having a ruptured lumbar disc at the L4 and L5 segments of the lower back, and recommended that she undergo spinal surgery to repair it. But Beverly, who had heard horror stories of botched back surgeries, had such a bad impression of him that she was frightened at the idea of him operating on her. She thought, "I wouldn't bring my dog in here to have surgery by you," and left.

A few days later, still in severe pain, she spoke with a coworker. "Maybe you'd like to go see this acupuncturist I go to," the woman suggested. Skeptical about nontraditional treatments, Beverly was nonetheless eager to avoid surgery and willing to give a gentler alternative a first shot. After work on December 9, the coworker drove Beverly from their office in downtown Portland fifteen minutes south to the nearby suburb of Beaverton, where the naturopath Mitchell Stargrove practiced.

Then in his midthirties, with an unlined face and chestnut brown wavy hair and mustache, Stargrove had the gentle, soft-spoken manner of a historian. Raised in Minnesota as Mitchell Bebel, he'd attended Oberlin College before moving to Portland. On the wall of his examination room were framed certificates from the Oregon College of Oriental Medicine (where he taught the history of medicine), the National College of Naturopathic Medicine (where he lectured), the National Certification Commission for Acupuncture and Oriental Medicine, and the State of Oregon Board of Naturopathic Examiners. Above the desk in his office was a collection of old, worn books, some dating back to the 1880s, which he used on a daily basis in choosing and preparing his homeopathic remedies. He practiced with his fellow naturopath Lori Beth Stargrove; although not married, they lived together with their three young children. Stargrove was a name they'd made up for themselves. They also worked with a chiropractor, an acupuncturist, and a counselor by the name of Gaea Laughingbird.

Sitting in his examination room, Beverly was tearful, angry, and frustrated with the unrelenting pain. She also said she was feeling depressed and stressed out by her job. With lights lowered and soft music playing in the background, Stargrove treated Beverly with acupuncture. Then he took out a bottle of a Chinese medicine that he said contained snake bile, told her to open her mouth, and placed a few of the tiny pellets on her tongue. In traditional Chinese medicine, he explained, snake bile is used for what is called "thick phlegm." He gave it sometimes to his own children, to treat their asthmatic flare-ups. Then he prescribed hypericum, also known as St. John's wort, for her depression; Specific Lumbaglin, an imported Chinese patent medicine used for lower back pain; homeopathic preparations of arnica and magnesium phosphate; PSI, a compound of herbs, vitamins, and minerals; and another Chinese patent medicine, Jin Bu Huan, used in both adults and children for pain and lack of sleep. When Beverly asked about the safety of the products, he assured her they were all safe because they were natural. "Homeopathic remedies do not have any toxicity," he once stated, "due to the dilution factor." But, he cautioned, she would not get immediate relief from her pain; it would take time.

Beverly saw him again on December 11, 15, 19, and 26. Each time he performed acupuncture on her, and kept her on all the prescriptions except the arnica. (Although homeopathic remedies are regulated as dietary supplements, and thus do not require a prescription, Stargrove wrote out the remedies and doses much as a physician would, so that they could be properly filled by an herbalist.) On the December 19 visit, Beverly told him that her pain was worsening with exertion, but that the St. John's wort seemed to be helping. That day he prescribed her another supplement, Ligaplex II, a combination product designed to strengthen ligaments and tendons. By December 26, however, she had gotten worse, with severe pain and spasms. On January 9, 1993, he prescribed liquid amber, a Chinese remedy for back pain. Two days later he prescribed salvia. On January 23, he prescribed a homeopathic remedy called lachesis 200, containing the venom of the bushmaster snake, also known as the lachesis muta or surukuku. On February 6, he prescribed eucommia bark, a traditional Chinese treatment taken from the hardy rubber tree. On February 26, he added clematis to the treatment plan. Sometimes she filled her herbal and homeopathic prescriptions at an adjoining pharmacy, in which Stargrove was a 33 percent owner; other times she went to stores he recommended. By late March, having received more than ten different prescriptions, Beverly's most acute pain seemed to be lessening, and she stopped seeing Stargrove.

Then, on the morning of March 30, while driving to work, she decided to avoid a traffic light by detouring through a strip mall's parking lot. A woman driving ahead of her came to a stop, and Beverly stopped behind her. Then, without warning, the woman backed up into Beverly's car, giving her a bad jolt. By the time they had finished filling out the police reports, Beverly's back pain was worse than ever.

Stargrove began treating her again, but decided to also refer her to a chiropractor, Robin Grimm-Schaefer, who worked nearer to Beverly's home and was more of an expert in the use of Chinese herbs. He continued prescribing Chinese medicines himself, however, maintaining the Jin Bu Huan, while adding another patent medicine, Chin Koo Tieh Shang Wan, as well as a box of Chinese herbs for sciatica, the exact contents of which he wasn't certain. He also added the homeopathic remedies rhus tox, made from poison oak, and bryonia alba, made from a climbing vine also known as snakeweed or devil's turnip. Between the two practitioners, Beverly received additional prescriptions for Chinese medicines containing asarum, clerodendron, cyperus, stephania, the tail of a gecko, and dried earthworm. In all, Beverly received more than twenty different prescriptions from Stargrove and Grimm-Schaefer, most containing multiple ingredients. She saw Stargrove seventeen more times through midsummer of 1993, and saw Grimm-Schaefer thirty-eight times through January of 1994.

But the pain didn't let up, and in December of 1993, Beverly began seeing a second orthopedic surgeon, Paul M. Puziss, MD. She liked him, and trusted him when he suggested she might be able to get relief from a physical therapist, John Bonica. Over the next six months, under the care of Bonica and Dr. Puziss, Beverly's back finally began to feel better. But then a new set of problems popped up, seemingly unrelated to the first. Stomach acid was refluxing into her esophagus; she didn't want to eat or drink; her head ached, and her energy level was bottoming out. When Dr. Puziss mentioned to her during a routine exam in July 1994 that her hair didn't look as perfectly coiffed as she usually kept it, Beverly broke into tears and confessed that she felt absolutely horrible.

"There's something going on with you," Dr. Puziss said. Fearing she might have some type of cancer, he referred her to an oncologist, Dr. Ralph Weinstein, who suspected leukemia. But her blood test came back negative, so Dr. Weinstein had her blood drawn a second time.

The next day, when she returned to Dr. Weinstein for a follow-up visit, he told her, "I need you to talk with my colleague Dr. Parker at the Northwest Renal Clinic."

She left Dr. Weinstein's office and walked the two blocks to the Northwest Renal Clinic. Seated in Dr. Parker's office, looking out at the beautiful western hills and the Fremont Bridge, she asked him what was going on.

"Do you have any idea what's wrong with you?" Dr. Parker asked her. He was younger than she was, tall and bespectacled.

"No," Beverly said. "I'm just sick. My head's been killing me. I feel like someone's been playing basketball with my head for three weeks. I've only been eating low-fat foods lately. Maybe I screwed myself up like that?"

"No," Dr. Parker said. "You're in kidney failure." Beverly looked back at him, speechless. "You're very sick."

"How can I be in kidney failure?" she asked. She didn't have diabetes, one of the leading causes of kidney failure, and had no family history of kidney disease. "How did this happen? How could this happen?"

"You need to be in the hospital," Dr. Parker told her.

"I can't afford a hospital bill," she said, even though she had medical insurance through her job. "Can't I just go home and stay in bed?"

Dr. Parker reluctantly agreed to let her go home, and she spent the weekend in bed, sleeping. On Monday, however, he had her visit St. Vincent's Hospital for the first of three intravenous injections of prednisone, in hopes of reversing the kidney failure. That did not work, and on July 27 she entered the hospital for a kidney biopsy. She had to be kept fully awake for the painful procedure, to hold her breath or breathe when told to by the doctor. She was shaking so hard afterward that the doctor gave her Valium, and she also needed a blood transfusion. Yet for all that, the biopsy revealed nothing to explain her kidney failure—no heredity factors, no ibuprofen overdose, no signs of pesticides or other known nephrotoxins. As she grew progressively sicker, sliding inexorably toward kidney dialysis, fearing that she would die, one question kept repeating in her head: How had this happened to her?

◯ ◯ ◯

Unknown to Beverly, her case bore a striking similarity to twelve other cases of kidney disease linked to Chinese herbs that had first been described in a prominent medical journal on February 13, 1993—months before she had been prescribed one of the same herbs, stephania, highlighted in the report. According to the article in the *Lancet*, two Belgian women had shown up at the nephrology clinic of the University of Brussels in early 1992 with unexplained kidney failure. Though unexplained cases remain a stubborn fact of life (there's even a fancy medical word for them: idiopathic disease), a sharp-eyed doctor, Jean-Louis Vanherweghem, noted an odd coincidence in the women's background: both had followed a weight-loss regimen at the same medical clinic. Curious, Dr. Vanherweghem decided to interview all of the seven other women in Brussels under the age of fifty who had gone into kidney failure between 1991 and 1992. Sure enough, all seven of them had gone to the same weight-loss clinic, an association that no other doctor had noticed. Then he decided to survey twenty-five other women, seemingly healthy and randomly selected, who had attended the weight-loss clinic in the same period. Three of them, it turned out, had impaired kidney function. However, the clinic had specialized in weight loss for fifteen years without any problems. What could be causing the recent disease?

In May of 1990, Dr. Vanherweghem discovered, the clinic had added to its standard therapy two Chinese herbs: stephania and magnolia. But no previous cases of kidney failure due to ingestion of either stephania or magnolia had ever been reported. The only similar type of case, known as Balkan nephropathy, had been possibly linked to aristolochia, but Dr. Vanherweghem could find no trace of aristolochia in the samples of weight-loss formula it tested. Even so, he concluded that something about the herbs almost certainly prompted the kidney failure, and stated in his *Lancet* report that the link "add[ed] support to the arguments against uncontrolled therapy with herbal preparations."

Following publication of the study, a distributor of Chinese herbs in Portland wrote a paper for the American Botanical Council titled "Stephania and Magnolia Bark: Targets of a Misdirected Investigation." The distributor, Subhuti Dharmananda, PhD, was director of the Institute for Traditional Medicine. Casting the *Lancet* study in terms of a turf battle between Eastern- and Western-style practitioners, he asserted that Dr. Vanherweghem was simply seeking to "enter the fray about herb regulation in Europe." Dharmananda saw only "flimsy circumstantial evidence" to support the claim that herbs had anything to do with the patients' kidney failure. In fact, he wrote, "No safety problems have been noted in the U.S. where stephania and magnolia bark (sometimes used together) have been utilized since at least 1976 and continue to be used extensively."

In January of 1994, Dr. Vanherweghem published an addendum to his original paper in *Lancet*. By then, 70 cases of what he called Chinese herb nephropathy, including "30 of whom had terminal renal failure," had been linked to use of the same clinic's weight-loss formula. Using improved methods to analyze herb powders sold in Belgian pharmacies as stephania, he did indeed find traces of aristolochic acid in eleven of twelve samples. He concluded that aristolochia had been substituted in place of stephania at markets in China, where the herbs originated. "This report underscores, once again, the absolute necessity of the introduction of measures to control the correct identification of herbal preparations," he wrote.

In response, Dharmananda wrote an addendum to his paper for the American Botanical Council. Calling Dr. Vanherweghem's conclusion that aristolochia had caused the kidney disease a "strained hypothesis," he referred to a recently published report on toxicity and side effects of some Chinese herbs: "Aristolochia species are not listed among the nephrotoxic herbs. If one clinic in Belgium can produce 70 cases of renal failure, including 30 fatal cases, in a period of about two years using minuscule amounts of aristolochia, one would expect that the Chinese literature would be filled with cautions about the toxicity of these herbs (which all contain aristolochic acid), since they are extensively used at much higher doses."

Although he did nothing at that time to directly warn the buyers and prescribers of the herbs he sold, and had publicly cast doubt on the Belgium study, privately Dharmananda felt concerned enough that he called his contact at Taising Trading, the Hong Kong company from which he bought his Chinese herbs. He asked his contact, a guy named Frank, to double-check that the stephania he'd been ordering was not being substituted with aristolochia, as had happened in the Belgium cases. Frank assured him that no such substitution was taking place, and that the company had a Chinese medical doctor who confirmed that the stephania they ordered was the stephania they got. Still privately concerned, however, in 1995 Dharmananda contacted a Chinese pharmacologist he knew and asked him to personally go to the marketplaces in China, buy some stephania, make an extract, and test it for aristolochic acid. The pharmacologist, Dr. Kazhi, did so, and found no trace of aristolochia. At that point, Dharmananda, whose company annually grossed some $1.4 million selling herbs, did nothing more to check on the safety of the 500 to 900 bottles of stephania tablets that he sold each year, even though he did not actually know where Taising obtained its stephania. This much he did know, however: neither Taising nor the California company that turned its raw herb into tablets did any testing of the stephania or any of the other herbs they sold; and neither did Dharmananda himself ever test any of the herbs he sold. He also knew that the purity of the stephania and other herbs he bought from Taising were protected by nothing more, during shipment from China and storage in warehouses, than plain cardboard boxes or burlap bags.

A couple years earlier, Dharmananda had decided to expand beyond merely importing and distributing Chinese herbs and had opened a clinic, the Immune Enhancement Program, for treating people with AIDS, cancer, multiple sclerosis, diabetes, rheumatoid arthritis, hepatitis C, and pain syndromes. He wrote hundreds of articles describing the use of Chinese herbs to treat everything from Lyme disease, brain tumors, liver cancer, Alzheimer's disease, hemorrhoids, and hepatitis, and even wrote one entitled "Chinese Herbs to Promote Breast Development." The articles, although sober, well-researched, and often voicing support for Western medicines, also include many statements that, at the very least, skirted the edges of DSHEA's prohibition against the sellers of dietary supplements making claims that their products heal or cure diseases. For instance, his article on brain tumors flatly stated: "Outcomes can be improved by utilizing Chinese herbal medicine in addition to standard therapies, or, in cases of diffuse or large cancers that are inoperable, in place of them." In a paper on HIV, dated October of 1997, he listed seven ingredients in an herbal formula called Baicalcumin and then asserted, "Together, these ingredients can reduce the inflammation that occurs in persons with HIV infection, such as intestinal and skin disorders, and it may reduce the rate of HIV replication." In his paper on leukemia, he wrote: "There is reasonable evidence from China that leukemia patients can get symptomatic relief and may have prolonged life span (perhaps 50% longer than that normally expected with standard chemotherapy) by the use of herbs and improved nutrition." In an appendix on treatment strategies for acute leukemia, he quoted two recipes, one for "Toad Skin Wine" with 1.8 kilograms of toad, "viscera discarded," and another, An Lu San, containing centipede, scorpion, silkworm, and something called eupolyphaga, combined in equal amounts and ground to a powder. And what was eupolyphaga? A kind of cockroach.

Given the huffy article Dharmananda had written about Dr. Vanherweghem's *Lancet* study, it was a sad twist of fate when it turned out to be Dharmananda's Institute for Traditional Medicine that supplied, under its Seven Forests brand, the tablets labeled "stephania" that Beverly Hames had taken for months.

⌐⌐ ⌐⌐ ⌐⌐

Thinking she was going to die, Beverly bought herself a forest green 1994 Mustang convertible GT with a white roof and white leather interior. She figured if she only had six months to live, she'd spend her remaining time on earth with the top down and the stereo blasting. And the car would be her casket.

She began attending a support group for people in kidney failure. The psychologist who led it told her it was time to downsize her life. "You've got to minimize," he said. "You can't keep doing yard work and chopping wood." At the time she had a huge yard and heated her home with firewood, which she enjoyed, and her mortgage was nearly paid off. But she decided the psychologist was right, and so she sold her home and moved to half of a two-family house nearer to the city.

But of course she couldn't afford to stop working, despite growing increasingly tired from the progressive failure of her kidneys. Finally, three days after Thanksgiving 1994, unable to put it off any longer, Beverly was hospitalized to have a shunt inserted into her abdomen for dialysis, leaving a double tube sticking out of her like a nozzle on a tire. From then on, she would have to spend forty-five minutes, four times each day, waiting while one bag of fluid slowly drained into her through the shunt, while a second bag slowly filled with the waste products that her kidneys could no longer remove.

Then began the waiting for a transplant. She carried a beeper with her at all times, in case a kidney became available. In the late summer of 1995, one did become available, and her doctors tried to beep her. But she happened to be driving with her then-boyfriend on the wrong side of a mountain, which interfered with the signal. When she found out that she'd missed her chance, she was devastated.

But on January 18, 1996, she got a second chance. Beverly and a coworker were attending a meeting in northwest Portland when it began snowing hard. Departing early, they returned to the office, which had already been closed due to the weather. Inside, they heard the front office phone ringing. It was Beverly's boyfriend, calling to tell her that Oregon Health and Science University (OHSU) had been trying to get through. "They've got a kidney for you. You've got to get out there."

"I've got the Mustang and I can't get out of the parking lot," she told him.

Luckily, her boyfriend's son had a four-wheel-drive Toyota. He picked her up and took her to her home, where she grabbed her overnight bag, and they made it to the hospital. Beginning before midnight and ending early in the morning of January 19, surgeons placed a new kidney in her abdomen, leaving the old ones in, as is often done.

Once released from the hospital, Beverly had to begin taking prednisone and Prograf, an expensive anti-rejection drug. Her weight ballooned, hair began growing all over her body, and her face became round and moon shaped. And every other day for the first year after the transplant, she had to go to the hospital to have her blood drawn.

It was during one of those early post-transplant visits that she met for the first time with William M. Bennett, MD, head of the division of nephrology at OHSU. She told him what she had been telling everyone else who would listen for the past eighteen months: "I don't understand why I got kidney failure, why this happened to me."

With a trim graying beard, glasses, and thinning hair, Dr. Bennett began asking her the usual questions. "Were you taking any new medicines or drugs?"

"I never took any drugs in my life," she answered. Like most patients asked about "drugs," she didn't consider herbs to fall in that category.

But, thinking of the *Lancet* study, Dr. Bennett pressed on. "Any herbs?"

It was the first time in more than eighteen months of medical care for her kidney failure that anyone had thought to ask Beverly that question. At the time, physicians and pharmacists virtually never thought to ask their patients about the use of supplements; few health professionals understood how prevalent they had become, or how dangerous they could be. Even now, as many have added questions about supplement use to their standard intake forms, they have found that patients often refuse to talk openly about the subject.

"Just getting them to tell you that they're taking it is difficult," explains Sarah A. Hein, a pharmacist and drug safety specialist at Tampa General Hospital in Florida. "And if you tell them they can't take it in the hospital, a lot of them get angry. They tell me, 'This is what I take and I want to take it now!' "

Catherine Ulbricht, a senior pharmacist at Massachusetts General Hospital, says that it's difficult for hospitals to even know how many of their patients are taking supplements. "One of the biggest problems is that patients don't tell us," she says. "It may be we don't ask or we aren't comfortable discussing them because we're not trained. Or patients may think we're not going to accept an alternative therapy."

A survey published in the *British Journal of Cancer* indicated just how few patients tell their doctors about their use of supplements. The survey of 318 outpatients receiving cancer treatment at London's Royal Marsden Hospital found that 164 of them, or 51.6 percent, used some type of "alternative" medicine, yet fewer than half had discussed their supplement use with a health-care professional involved in their care.

In response to Dr. Bennett's question, Beverly replied, "Well, I did take these herbal preparations for my back, but that was months before I got sick."

He asked her what kinds of herbs she'd taken. When she mentioned stephania, his ears pricked up. He told her about the report in *Lancet*. "If you have any of the herbs left, it would be helpful if you could bring them in."

Two days later, she brought in a dozen bottles of the various herbs she'd been prescribed by Stargrove and Grimm-Schaefer, most of them distributed by Dharmananda's Institute for Traditional Medicine. Dr. Bennett sent samples of each herb first to a colleague of Dr. Vanherweghem's in Belgium, and then to the FDA.

Karen A. Wolnik, director of the Inorganic Laboratory Branch of the FDA's Forensic Chemistry Center in Cincinnati, had each of the samples ground and an extract made. The extracts were analyzed for the presence of aristolochic acid by high-performance liquid chromatography. The Seven Forests gecko was negative for aristolochic acid, as were the Seven Forests eucommia, cyperus, and salvia. But the Seven Forests asarum, stephania, and clerodendron were each positive for aristolochic acid, as were the Jin Bu Huan and Chin Koo Tieh Shang Wan made by other companies. And the arnica, one of the homeopathic remedies that Stargrove insisted had no toxicity, was also positive for aristolochic acid.

○ ⊂⊃ ⊂⊃

Kidney failure turned out to be just one of aristolochia's side effects. In 1994, one of the Belgian patients was diagnosed with bladder cancer. By 1999, 40 percent of the kidney biopsies of the Belgian patients were found to have multiple small tumors. Doctors then recommended to all the Chinese herb nephropathy patients whose kidneys no longer functioned to have the entire organs surgically removed as a precautionary measure. By then, they had a total of 105 patients with some degree of nephropathy caused by aristolochia, and 43 with end-stage renal failure. Of the thirty-nine patients who agreed to undergo surgery, eighteen of their kidneys were found to be cancerous, and nineteen of the twenty-one remaining had precancerous cells, according to a report by the Belgian doctors in the *New England Journal of Medicine*. Combined with animal studies showing that aristolochia could induce cancer, the case seemed clear that the herb was not only nephrotoxic but also a potent carcinogen.

In an editorial accompanying the *NEJM* report, David Kessler, by then having left the FDA to become dean of the Yale School of Medicine, engaged in a bit of I-told-you-so. "Congress has shown little interest in protecting consumers from the hazards of dietary supplements, let alone from the fraudulent claims that are made, since its members apparently believe that few of these products place people in real danger," he wrote. "Nor does the public understand how potentially dangerous these products can be. Examples like that described by [the Belgian doctors] should persuade Congress to change the law to ensure the safety and efficacy of dietary supplements before more people are harmed." In the meanwhile, since aristolochia had now been shown to be so dangerous, Kessler wrote, "It is likely that the agency will take some action in the very near future."

The herb was quickly banned in seven European countries, as well as in Egypt, Japan, Canada, and Venezuela. Eventually, hundreds of medical articles were published by researchers across the world, attesting to the herb's dangers. Even Dharmananda was finally convinced by the evidence, writing in a new article published by his institute: "It is appropriate to discontinue use of all herb materials containing aristolochic acid."

And then the FDA did act, within the scope of powers that Senator Hatch and his colleagues in Congress had left it to deal with dietary supplements. On May 16, 2000, the agency wrote a letter to manufacturers and distributors, "urging" them—that is, asking them—to stop selling supplements containing aristolochia. On April 9, 2001, the once-proud agency that had been created nearly a century before to protect Americans from unsafe medicines wrote manufacturers a second time, asking them again to please (pretty please) stop selling the dangerous herb. By then, seven more cases had been reported in France, and two cases, including Beverly's, had been reported in the United States. The second case involved Donna Andrade-Wheaton of Cranston, Rhode Island, whose acupuncturist recommended she take herbs, including aristolochia. In September of 2002, still in her late thirties, she had to undergo a kidney transplant.

To this day, only those two U.S. cases of kidney failure due to aristolochia have been described in the medical literature or the news media. Many others have occurred, however. According to Richard Ko, a pharmacist with the California Department of Health: "There are three others that I'm aware of, at least. At least two were for weight control, and one was for arthritic pain. One was in San Diego, two in the San Francisco Bay area. All suffered kidney failure."

According to Arthur P. Grollman, MD, a professor of pharmacology and medicine at the State University of New York at Stony Brook: "I've been called on at least ten or twelve cases. I get calls from public health departments. I've had calls from Texas and at least three or four other states. There's no way to know what the true number is."

(Knowing the true number of cases of liver failure caused by herbs is also difficult. More than a hundred cases have been reported in the medical literature in recent years, including thirty due to kava, sixteen to chaparral, ten to germander, five to comfrey, and five to pennyroyal. But the national surveillance system tracking liver failure cases does not list herbs as a possible cause, so the full extent of the problem is impossible to know. William Martens Lee, MD, a distinguished professor in liver diseases at the University of Texas-Southwestern Medical Center in Dallas, and chief investigator of the Acute Liver Failure Study Group, estimates that about forty herb-linked cases occur each year.)

How could aristolochia have been so widely used in China and the rest of the world for millennia without apparent ill effect until now? The herb, after all, is one of the oldest known. Theophrastus, who in the third century BC succeeded Socrates as head of the Lyceum, knew of its uses. Pedanius Dioscorides, the first-century Greek physician who traveled with the armies of Nero, wrote of it, and the plant's heart-shaped leaves and winding stems are still perfectly recognizable in a sixth-century illuminated manuscript of his *Materia medica*. It is described in the *Pen ts'ao kang mu*, completed in 1578 by the Chinese physician Li Shih-chin. Other civilizations of the world have also used aristolochia, and many still do, including India, Egypt, and the native peoples of both North and South America. Its primary uses can be inferred from its folk names: birthwort (to induce labor) and snakeroot (to treat the bites of snakes and other reptiles). For centuries, it was given to nearly all European women during birth. It has also been widely used around the globe for treating stomachache, headache, and joint pain; as a wound healer, fever remedy, and malaria treatment; and as an aid to induce menstruation and abortion. Yet for all its millennia of uses, almost nowhere in the abundant literature of Eastern and Western herbology was there ever a mention of toxicity or danger.

"The reason, of course, is quite simple," says Dr. Grollman. "It's painless, and the damage happens much later, so you don't put together the fact that you took this medicine and four years later, you have kidney failure. That's what makes it different from most other nephrotoxic agents.

This is a delayed symptom. It's been part of Indian medicine for thousands of years. It's been part of South American medicine, Chinese medicine, European medicine. All these great civilizations have used it. And not one reported its toxicity until the Belgians did. There are certain things tradition can't tell you."

Since aristolochia's toxicity was recognized in the West, he adds, "hundreds and hundreds of people in China have been documented with aristolochic acid poisoning. They have whole clinics just for aristolochic acid poisoning in Beijing. The pattern is exactly the same as in the West. They take it for arthritis, etcetera, then one day their feet swell up and someone says, 'You have advanced renal failure.' "

Xiaomei Li, MD, director of the renal division of Peking University First Hospital in Beijing, published an editorial in the June 2004 issue of the journal *Nephrology*. After describing the large number of cases that have occurred there, she wrote, "The best way to prevent aristolochic acid nephropathy is to ban the use of herbs that contain aristolochic acid from the pharmaceutical market. This principle has...been introduced in some Eastern countries and regions such as Japan, Korea, and the mainland of China and Taiwan. These actions will no doubt reduce the incidence of aristolochic acid nephropathy."

○ ⊂⊃ ⊂○

Warnings by health authorities about contaminants in traditional remedies from China, India, Mexico, and other foreign countries have gone ignored for years now. On July 20, 1999, Jerry Oliveras, the lab director of Anresco Laboratories, a company that tests foods, drugs, and supplements for safety, testified before an FDA panel on dietary supplements. "Botanicals coming out of the People's Republic of China," he said, "have everything from no real detectable levels of heavy metal to just about every heavy metal you want to think about. We have products coming into this country that are predominantly cinnabar. Not just cinnabar, which is a mercury salt, but also cinnabar heavily contaminated with soluble lead salt. They are sold over the counter. Go down to Chinatown, get some little red pills and take them, and go about your happy way while you're slowly poisoning yourself to death. We sometimes get samples in our laboratory that are fifty-three different herbal products as a composite, and we're [asked] to analyze those in one single test and say, yes, the heavy metals are too high, or no, there's no detectable pesticide. It's a farce. We know it's a farce. They know it's a farce, but because they don't want to spend the money, they're not going to test each of those ingredients separately. They're only going to test them as a single composite so they can get a report that says, 'no detected pesticide residues, must be organic, must be good for you.' There are also companies that are very concerned about what they're doing, but they are the exceptions."

In September of 2000, doctors writing in the journal *Pediatrics* described the case of a five-year-old Indian boy living in Los Angeles who had been born developmentally delayed due to a temporary loss of oxygen during childbirth. Referred for persistent anemia, he could stand only with assistance and could not walk. The mother, who was well educated and spoke excellent English, initially denied any exposure to lead or use of any folk medications. But after further questioning, she admitted giving her son a Tibetan herbal vitamin, in the form of tablets, three times per day for the past four years of his life. A traditional medicine healer had told the parents that the tablets were pure herbs prepared according to ancient Tibetan traditions by a physician close to the Dalai Lama. They were said to be free from any harmful or toxic substances and to promote brain growth and improve his mental capabilities. The doctors, based at the city's Children's Hospital, tested the tablets and found them to be very high in lead and arsenic. The boy too was found to have a remarkably high level of lead in his blood. Although it was difficult to know how much of his developmental delay was caused by his birth trauma and how much by the lead poisoning, three months after undergoing treatment to remove the lead he was able to walk with minimal support and was more communicative. Within six months of his stopping the herbal vitamin and undergoing therapy, his mother and grandmother felt that he had made significant progress in social interactions characterized by more awareness and joy of others, and responsiveness to directions.

On November 5, 2003, the New York City health commissioner Thomas R. Frieden warned residents to stop using the popular folk remedy litargirio from the Dominican Republic because it contained high lead levels. Litargirio has been widely used for years by Dominican immigrants in the United States for a variety of ailments, but earlier that year in Rhode Island, children who used the product were diagnosed with lead poisoning, and samples of it were found to be made of 79 percent lead. "There is absolutely no health benefit from using it, only danger," Dr. Frieden said. "If you're using it, stop right away, and go to a doctor to get a blood test for lead." The FDA investigated the product and found that it had "no proven health benefits and, because of its high lead content, poses health risks when used in contact with the skin or ingested. These risks are particularly serious for children." While the agency almost certainly would have placed a ban on all litargirio products in the years prior to DSHEA, the law prevented any such blanket bans without the kind of lengthy effort and extensive evidence it had brought to hear against ephedra. And so rather than ban the poisonous product, it issued a warning in English and Spanish.

On July 9, 2004, the Centers for Disease Control and Prevention published in its *Morbidity and Mortality Weekly Report* a review of twelve cases in five states of adults who had suffered lead poisoning from taking remedies made in keeping with the Ayurvedic tradition of medicine practiced in India and other Southeast Asian countries. (In the United States, Deepak Chopra is a leading proponent of Ayurvedic treatments, as popularized in his bestsellers *Quantum Healing* and *Ageless Body, Timeless Mind*.) In New Hampshire, a thirty-seven-year-old woman with rheumatoid arthritis showed up at an emergency room after suffering a stomachache, nausea, and vomiting for six days; she had been taking Ayurvedic medicines high in lead. In California, a thirty-one-year-old woman visited an emergency room with stomachache, nausea, and vomiting after having suffered a spontaneous abortion two weeks earlier; she had been taking nine different Ayurvedic medicines prescribed by an Indian practitioner for two months. Ten other cases were reported in Texas and New York involving five other women and four men who had been taking the medicines for conditions ranging from infertility to diabetes.

On December 15, 2004, doctors at the Division for Research and Education in Complementary and Integrative Medical Therapies at Harvard Medical School published the results of a survey they had made of products from all thirty stores located within twenty miles of Boston City Hall that sold Ayurvedic herbal remedies. Concerned by reports of brain damage, paralysis, deafness, and other effects of lead poisoning caused by such remedies, they bought a total of seventy Ayurvedic products from the stores and tested them for lead. They found that fourteen of the seventy, or 20 percent, had dangerously high levels. "Testing of Ayurvedic herbal medicine products for toxic heavy metals should be mandatory," they concluded.*

The day after the Boston study was published in the *Journal of the American Medical Association*, the FDA issued a nationwide alert after discovering residue of the pesticides procymidone and quintozene in ginseng imported by FCC Products, Inc., of Livingston, New Jersey.

Such warnings, however, are notoriously ineffective, as evidenced by a 2003 report in the *New England Journal of Medicine*. Two years after the FDA had issued its alert about aristolochic acid, Lois Swirsky Gold, PhD, of the University of California at Berkeley, reported on her online check of the herb's availability. She found nineteen products definitely containing aristolochic acid, and ninety-five more suspected to contain it, available for sale on approximately one hundred Web sites.

One should not assume that only foreign-made supplements from Third World countries pose a risk of contamination. In 2004, Consumer-Lab.com analyzed dozens of children's multivitamins and reported that Li'l Critters Gummi Vites, a popular children's brand sold in Costco and Wal-Mart, contained 2.5 micrograms of lead per serving. Rather than recall the product or notify the public of the problem, the manufacturer mounted a publicity campaign questioning the lab's results.

○ ○ ○

That the ingredients in supplements might be adulterated with heavy metals or other contaminants is bad enough; that they would be secretly larded with pharmaceuticals—the very thing consumers taking them are trying to avoid—is downright bizarre. Yet the practice is so common that

---

*One can only hope that U.S. stores will not soon be stocking Ayurvedic products sold under the brand name Goratna, or "jewels of the cow." Reportedly selling briskly in New Delhi, India, they include sanjivani ark, a potion made of cow urine for treating cancer, and cow dung toothpaste. The product may be bullshit, but the story is true. Purushottam Toshniwal, the general secretary of the cooperative that manufactures the products, was quoted by the Associated Press as saying: "Even in the United States, they now recognize the worth of cow urine."

when Lawrence R. Schiller, MD, clinical professor of medicine at the University of Texas Southwestern Medical Center in Dallas, recently told the Drug Enforcement Administration that he had discovered Valium in a Chinese herbal remedy used by a patient to treat chronic diarrhea, the DEA was not surprised. "They said it happens all the time and suggested that I report it to the Texas attorney general's office," Schiller said. "I did and nothing happened."

In March of 1998 a supplement called Sleeping Buddha, marketed as an herbal alternative to prescription sedatives, was found to contain a prescription-strength dose of the sedative estazolam. In February of 2000, five Chinese herbal supplements marketed to treat diabetes were found to contain the prescription diabetes drugs glyburide and phenformin, the latter of which had been outlawed two decades earlier in the United States. In April of 2002, Utah-based E'OLA International agreed to stop selling AMP II Pro Drops after the FDA found they contained synthesized ephedrine, which can be sold only as a drug. A year later, in April of 2003, Ultra Health Laboratories and Bionate International recalled Vinerol, marketed to increase sexual desire and performance, after Viagra was found in it. That same month, the FDA warned Global Vision Products that it could not legally continue to sell its baldness remedy Avacor, widely advertised on radio, because it contained minoxidil, the active ingredient in Rogaine. That June, Viga for Women was found to contain Viagra, and NVE was found to be manufacturing five different products, all supposedly natural enhancers of sexual performance, when in fact they all contained tadalafil, the active ingredient in Cialis. That September, twelve cases of liver injury, including one death and one transplant, were reported in Japan due to an "herbal" Chinese weight-loss supplement containing the weight-loss drug fenfluramine. The next month, New Zealand health authorities recalled four Chinese supplements containing Viagra and Cialis. On November 2, 2004, the FDA warned consumers not to buy or use Actra-Rx, a supplement marketed for erectile dysfunction, after it was found to contain Viagra. Less than a month later, on November 30, the Beverly Hills manufacturer of Male Power Plus was shocked—*shocked!*—to find it contained Cialis, and promptly issued a voluntary recall. Just six days later, Thomas and Linda Hardy, former owners of a Southern California store called the Herbalist, agreed to pay $167,000 in fines and reimbursements for mixing the likes of Tylenol, Motrin, Benadryl, and Unisom into their "100 percent herbal" remedies.

But undoubtedly the most notorious case of drug-adulterated herbals involved PC-SPES, marketed to promote "prostate health." Its creator, Sophie Chen, PhD, a chemist who had immigrated from Taiwan, held an unpaid position as an adjunct professor at New York Medical College. After patenting PC-SPES and setting up a California company, BotanicLab, to sell it, she scored the ultimate scientific coup for it: publication of a study by independent scientists in the *New England Journal of Medicine*. Published in September of 1998, the small study reviewed the response of just eight men to the supplement. In all eight, their blood level of prostate-specific antigen (a protein produced by the prostate that rises in cases of prostate cancer) dropped. In six of the eight men, the level of testosterone in their blood also dropped significantly—a positive finding, since testosterone can spur the growth of prostate cancer. However, the researchers also found that PC-SPES had potent effects similar to estrogen, the female hormone. Not surprisingly, all eight of the men developed breast tenderness and loss of interest in sex. But another finding was more puzzling: one of the men developed a dangerous clot in a vein. "Use of this unregulated mixture of herbs may confound the results of standard or experimental therapies and may produce clinically significant adverse effects," the researchers concluded.

Still, the hoopla generated by the prestigious publication and the promising results led to an invitation from Congressman Dan Burton, Republican of Indiana, for Chen to appear before Congress. On September 23, 1999, his Committee on Government Reform held a hearing on whether the U.S. government was doing enough in the fight against prostate cancer. In his opening statement, Burton asked: "Are we looking enough into the natural approaches to healing? Are we moving forward in getting real answers about the nutritional aspects of cancer prevention, including organic and plant-based diets and the role of dietary supplements? Are we looking at the role of pain management issues, including complementary approaches like meditation, guided imagery, acupuncture, aromatherapy, and music therapy?"

Called to testify, Chen began, "I appear before you today as a medical researcher. The good news I can say today is there are botanicals that can be beneficial for cancer treatment and prevention. The bad news is we do not have enough clinical studies and there is still a long way to go." She described PC-SPES as a "standardized botanical formulation composed of seven purified Chinese herbs and one American herbal extract." With "many different prestigious laboratories and hospitals across the United States" studying it, she estimated that over a thousand men were taking it. At the University of California, San Francisco, Dr. Eric Small had found that twenty-seven of sixty-one men with advanced prostate cancer "responded 100 percent," she said, and the other thirty-four men "responded with 57 percent." The only side effects seen so far, she said, were decreased libido and "some breast tenderness."

"Is the NIH funding any studies on your invention, your scientific research?" Burton asked.

"No, Mr. Chairman. As a matter of fact, I wrote an application for NIH funding and it was rejected."

That soon changed, and NIH eventually awarded $2.1 million to study PC-SPES. But by the time of Burton's hearing, reports of dangerous complications due to the supplement were already emerging. Some men were developing enlarged breasts, and some developed an effect most unwelcome: a shrunken penis. On September 14, 1998, sixty-four-year-old John Meyer of Sonoita, Arizona, died of a blood clot—the same kind of problem seen in the original *New England Journal of Medicine* study—that had lodged in his heart and lungs. He had recently begun taking PC-SPES for nothing more than a harmless enlargement of his prostate, because he had preferred a natural treatment over standard medical care—even though PC-SPES cost as much as $500 per month.

Doctors and patients alike began to wonder if something other than herbs were responsible not only for the good effects, but also for the bad—both of which were reminiscent of those of diethylstilbestrol, or DES, an artificial estrogen banned in 1971. Finally, a Connecticut man's wife became so suspicious when the supplement, which had been producing good results for him, suddenly stopped working that she decided to have it tested. She obtained a sample of the older batch that had been effective, and sent it along with a sample of the new, ineffective batch to a laboratory. Sure enough, DES was found in the old batch, but not in the new.

Then, instead of clot formation, PC-SPES was suddenly being linked to the opposite problem: bleeding disorders. In a study published in October of 2001, two Seattle doctors reported on a traveling businessman who had nearly died after he spontaneously began to bleed from every orifice. Even as other labs were confirming the presence of DES in some samples, the state's health department now found warfarin, a blood thinner. Subsequent tests of samples going back to 1996 found low levels of DES from the beginning, with the warfarin apparently added later on to counteract the first drug's clotting effects.

Eventually, drugs were found in all eight products that Chen's company sold. Because the case was circumstantial, however, she and two other executives of the company got off with pleading no contest to state misdemeanor charges. The company pleaded no contest to a felony, paid $500,000 in penalties, and agreed to never sell supplements in California again. At least twenty-five lawsuits have been filed against Botanic-Lab alleging serious injuries or death. Chen, whose company is believed to have grossed some $50 million before being shut down in 2002, retains her faculty title (although she is not paid and no longer teaches) at New York Medical College.

⊂⊃ ⊂⊃ ⊂⊃

Not only do dietary supplements commonly include adulterants or pharmaceuticals that are not listed on the label, but they also often contain far less or far more of the ingredients they do list. "I'd say you have a three out of four chance of a supplement having what it claims on the label—nothing more and nothing less," says Tod Cooperman, MD, president of ConsumerLab.com. "It's not a good record, particularly because these are products people rely on for their health." What about supplements produced by the big chains and name-brand companies, which often claim on their label that they follow the good manufacturing practices, or GMPs, promulgated by trade groups? "We routinely find problems with products that claim to follow GMPs," says Dr. Cooperman. "You've got to take what they say with a grain of salt."

He should know. Since 2003, Dr. Cooperman's laboratory has tested hundreds of dietary supplements to check for potency and purity. In

2004, it tested forty-four multivitamin products and announced that eleven had failed their tests due to, among other problems, having too much of some of their listed ingredients. When it tested forty-nine brands of glucosamine and chondroitin in November of 2003, it gave four a failing grade, including one that included only 18 percent of the promised 500 milligrams of chondroitin, and two veterinary brands for pets that contained no chondroitin at all. When it tested eleven brands of CoQ10 in late 2003, it found one that contained none. In March of 2004 the laboratory tested eleven brands of echinacea; five failed. One was contaminated with lead and four were low in phenols, the plant chemicals used to measure the potency of echinacea. One contained less than 5 percent of the expected level of phenols.

Incredibly, no government agency is presently responsible for testing dietary supplements to assure their purity and potency. One hundred years after Congress passed the Pure Food and Drug Act of 1906, supplement manufacturers continue to enjoy a free pass to operate outside the bedrock principle that all drugs should be, at the very least, pure and of reliable potency. Although DSHEA authorized the FDA to establish rules for so-called good manufacturing standards for dietary supplements, the agency has seen its proposed standards shot down time and again by the industry. In 2004, then–Commissioner Lester Crawford promised to issue the long-awaited regulations by year's end. But by the time of his hasty resignation in September of 2005, his promise remained unfulfilled. A month after his departure, the FDA finally submitted the regulations to the Office of Management and Budget for review. On April 24, 2006, the agency published an announcement in the Federal Register saying that it expected "final action" on the proposed rules by December of that year. But according to George Whitmore, a spokesperson for the agency, the December date "was established for planning purposes only. It has no bearing on the final disposition of the proposed rule, and does not constitute any sort of deadline. The proposed rule remains under OMB review. While the proposed rule is under review, and pending final disposition of the proposal, FDA has no ability to predict final action." Assuming the rules ever do take effect, they will be modeled on the relatively lax standards governing foods, not the far tighter standards for manufacturing drugs, because DSHEA deemed supplements to be foods, not drugs. Even then, they will almost certainly be challenged in court by manufacturers seeking an injunction against their enforcement, as occurred following the FDA's attempt to ban ephedra.

○ ⊂⊃ ⊂

Contaminants in dietary supplements have injured not only many users' health but the careers of athletes competing in the Olympics. In January of 2003, the U.S. swimmer Kicker Vencill tested positive for steroids, but he denied taking any. The only pills he had taken were a vitamin supplement, Super Complete. He sent a sample of the pills to a testing lab, which found them contaminated with a steroid precursor, 19-norandrosterone (sold as a dietary supplement in the United States until a 2004 law reclassified it a controlled substance). The U.S. Anti-Doping Agency reduced his suspension from four years to two, but he still was unable to compete in the 2004 Athens Olympics. "I paid for it," Vencill told the Associated Press. "I paid for it dearly." He sued the maker of Super Complete, Ultimate Nutrition of Farmington, Connecticut, and in May of 2005 a California jury found the company liable and ordered it to pay $578,635 in compensation.

Similar cases occurred during and preceding the 2000 Olympics in Sydney, including the loss of the Norwegian wrestler Fritz Aanes's bronze medal after he tested positive for steroids. He complained that he had been taking only a supposedly natural dietary supplement made in Utah; when tested, it turned out to be contaminated with the steroid nandrolone. Three other Olympic hopefuls had the same unhappy experience in Sydney, finally leading the International Olympic Committee to blast the U.S. supplement industry at a press conference in December of 2000. Prince Alexandre de Merode, chairman of the IOC's medical commission, went so far as to blame Orrin Hatch's involvement in the passage of DSHEA for the lack of purity in U.S. supplements. "He [Hatch] is directly implicated in this affair," said the prince. The former Olympic speedskater Johann Olav Koss of Norway, a member of the IOC athletes' commission, also expressed dismay with the Utah supplement industry. Hatch then fired back, "I am tired of this childish finger-pointing. The last time I checked, neither the prince nor the athlete were experts in food and drug law." He insisted that under DSHEA, supplements had to be properly labeled. But Dick Pound, chairman of the World Anti-Doping Agency (WADA), told the Associated Press: "Labeling is not at all reliable."

The same thing happened two months before the 2002 winter Olympics in Salt Lake City, when the U.S. bobsledder Pavle Jovanovic tested positive for another banned steroid, 19-norandrostenedione, resulting in a two-year ban from the sport. He claimed to have taken only a supplement called Nitro-Tech, and decided to sue both the manufacturer and the GNC stores where he bought it. The manufacturer countersued, and while awaiting a trial expected to begin in April of 2006, Jovanovic told the *New York Times* that he would no longer take any supplement—not even a vitamin.

After the IOC randomly tested 240 supplements and found one fifth of them to be contaminated with banned substances, it decided to join with WADA to create an education campaign for all would-be Olympic athletes, said Gary I. Wadler, MD, an expert on drug use in sports who has frequently testified before Congress and currently serves on WADA's Prohibited List and Methods Committee. "We told athletes not to take supplements because they had no assurance of purity," said Dr. Wadler. But in November of 2005, the U.S. Olympic Committee decided that such advice just wasn't working after a survey found 90 percent of their athletes were taking them. As a result, the USOC announced that it had contracted for the first time with a company to manufacture a supplement, with every batch to be tested at the company's expense at a laboratory run by the University of California at Los Angeles, the only such laboratory approved by WADA for testing of banned substances. The company was not, however, based in Utah, or anywhere else in the United States. The ninety-six-year-old food company, Ajinomoto, is based in Japan.

⊂⊃ ⊂⊃ ⊂⊃

Following the recognition that the unlabeled aristolochia in her supplements could cause kidney cancer, Beverly Hames underwent a second surgery in 2000 to have what was left of her original kidneys removed. By then she had settled for an undisclosed sum from a lawsuit against Stargrove, his company, Dharmananda's company, and others involved in the case. Living with her Maltese, Sally Anne, in a modest middle-class home, she continues to pay a monthly mortgage, lives frugally, and remains at high risk, due to the aristolochia, of developing cancer elsewhere in her body.

"It's been a nightmare," she says. "I'll never live out my true life. It's like someone murdering you slowly. Don't use the word 'natural' on me ever again. That's how they get away with selling this garbage, by calling it 'natural.' It just needs to stop. They're killing people."

CHAPTER 7
ONE A DAY

Cooper Burkey had stopped eating his vegetables. The smart, big-hearted, gleeful four-year-old boy had rarely suffered so much as a cold, but his parents, a New York real estate agent, Wayne Burkey, and Marcy Lynn, a filmmaker, were big believers in the benefits of whole foods—unprocessed and untouched by modern manufacturing methods. So rather than give him an ordinary Flintstones vitamin, their pediatrician recommended they give him the Perfect Food Super Green Formula, made by a fast-growing Florida supplement company called Garden of Life. The greenish brown caplets, measuring nearly seven-eighths of an inch long, were labeled as containing concentrated beets, carrots, broccoli, cucumber, tomato, kale, parsley, asparagus, brussels sprouts, bell pepper, garlic, ginger, onion, garbanzo beans, kidney beans, lentils, flax seeds, sunflower seeds, pumpkin seeds, sesame seeds, barley grass, oat grass, wheat grass, alfalfa grass, and fifteen other natural ingredients. An adult serving of five caplets was labeled as containing 2,500 IU of vitamin A as carotene, 60 milligrams of vitamin C, 100 milligrams of calcium, and 3 milligrams of iron. Children were recommended to take one fourth to one half of the adult dose, or up to two and a half caplets.

At 12:55 p.m. on Friday, February 16, 2006, Cooper's mother, Marcy, gave him one of the caplets to swallow. But the large caplet caught in his throat. He began to choke and then turned blue. Unable to help him, Marcy immediately dialed 911. When emergency responders arrived at the apartment in downtown Manhattan, they found the little boy unconscious and not breathing. Despite frantic efforts, they were unable to revive him. The boy lay limp as he was taken outside, placed in an ambulance, and driven to New York University Downtown Hospital. At 2:20 p.m., he was pronounced dead.

Though at first glance Cooper's tragic death may seem like a freak accident, adverse reactions to vitamins and minerals are not nearly as rare as one might think, according to an alarming set of national statistics that has gone unreported, and apparently unnoticed, by any news outlet in the United States, buried as they are each September in the pages of the *American Journal of Emergency Medicine*. But anyone willing to tabulate twenty-two years' worth of reports would find that between 1983 and 2004, poison control centers around the country received a mind-boggling 1.3 million reports of adverse reactions to vitamins and minerals, of which 175,268 required treatment in a hospital and 139 resulted in death. In the decade following the passage of DSHEA in 1994, during a time when yearly reports of all other types of poisonings grew by just 24 percent, incidents related to vitamins and minerals jumped by 62 percent, reaching a record 95,540 in 2004.

To some, it may not be surprising that a little-known herb like bloodroot can burn off a person's nose, or that an exotic Chinese herb like artistolochia can cause kidney failure. But in the United States today, vitamins and minerals are regulated under DSHEA precisely as herbs are, manufactured under the same near-total lack of standards, and permitted to make the same unproved claims about their powers to "support heart health" or "maintain a healthy immune system." Nevertheless, they are looked on by the majority of consumers as not only safe but essential to health. And they are the very bedrock of the dietary supplement industry, accounting for an estimated $7 billion, or about one third, of the industry's $21.2 billion total sales in 2005. More than half of U.S. preschoolers are now given a multivitamin by their parents every day. According to the National Maternal-Infant Health Survey, in which the mothers of 8,285 preschool children were interviewed in 1991, 54.4 percent said they gave their children a daily vitamin or mineral supplement. Adults too take vitamins in enormous numbers. The most recent and thorough survey of adult usage, the National Health and Nutrition Examination Surveys (NHANES) conducted during 1999 and 2000 among 4,862 adults, found that 35 percent of Americans regularly took a multivitamin. After his annual physical in July of 2005, even President George W. Bush was reported to be taking one. Could Adelle Davis have asked for anything more?

Such high use shouldn't be surprising, given the consistency of the public message voiced by leading advocates, manufacturers, and trade organizations who repeat the seductive term "nutritional insurance" so often that it has been assumed into our collective cultural consciousness as gospel. Jeffrey Blumberg, PhD, professor of nutrition at Tufts University in Boston, stated in a recent article that remains on the sites of WebMD and Fox News: "Most people need a multivitamin as 'insurance.' Everybody needs to eat more healthfully. While you're trying to get there, take supplements." Chris Rosenbloom, PhD, a spokeswoman for the American Dietetic Association and associate dean of health and human services at Georgia State University in Atlanta, was quoted on the Web site of a Blue Cross insurer as saying: "A well-formulated vitamin and mineral pill for seniors is the best bet. It's an insurance policy." A 2004 article on the Web site of the Harvard School of Public Health was headlined "Dietary Insurance: A Daily Multivitamin" and concluded by calling multivitamins "about the least expensive insurance you can buy." An article in the spring 2005 issue of the free newsletter distributed by CVS used the same "nutritional insurance" line, as does an article on the Web site of Centrum, maker of one of the most popular multivitamins on the market.

While we take it for granted that such advice is supported by major medical groups and government agencies, it is not. In fact, no major medical group or government agency actually recommends the routine use of multivitamins for otherwise healthy children or adults, with only a few particular exceptions. While single, targeted vitamins or minerals are recommended for particular ages or ailments, the idea that everyone needs the "nutritional insurance" of a daily multivitamin has no basis in science or any official guidelines. Indeed, according to the American Academy of Pediatrics, for children between the ages of five and twelve, "supplements are rarely needed." The American Medical Association's only official policy on vitamins is that women of childbearing age take a folic acid supplement to prevent birth defects, and that newborns receive a onetime dose of vitamin K within one hour of birth to prevent a rare bleeding disorder. The U.S. surgeon general Richard H. Carmona, in designating 2005 as the "Year of the Healthy Child," had only one vitamin recommendation: that every woman of childbearing age take a folic acid supplement. Even the American Dietetic Association states in a position paper, "There is little scientific evidence of benefit to the average person" from a low-dose multivitamin or multivitamin-mineral supplement. Most recently, a panel of thirteen experts convened by NIH on May 17 and 18, 2006, to resolve some of the confusion over multivitamins concluded, "The state of evidence is insufficient to recommend either for or against the use of multivitamin/multimineral [supplements] by the American public."

"Most of the vitamin supplements consumed in the United States are unnecessary," agrees Benjamin Caballero, MD, PhD, director of the Center for Human Nutrition at Johns Hopkins University in Baltimore and a member of the Food and Nutrition Board at the National Academy of Sciences. "But don't rely only on my opinion. Look at the 2005 Dietary Guidelines for Americans. They don't recommend any vitamin supplement for the healthy population consuming a variety of foods."

The guidelines, jointly prepared by the Department of Health and Human Services and the Department of Agriculture, represent the federal government's best effort to give science-based advice on nutrition and physical activity. While the guidelines recommend B_{12} for adults over fifty and folic acid for women of childbearing age who may become pregnant, nowhere do they recommend a multivitamin for anyone. "Nutrient needs should be met primarily through consuming foods," the guidelines state. "Foods provide an array of nutrients (as well as phytochemicals, antioxidants, etc.) and other compounds that may have beneficial effects on health. Supplements may be useful when they fill a specific identified nutrient gap that cannot or is not otherwise being met by the individual's intake of food. Nutrient supplements cannot replace a healthful diet. Individuals who are already consuming the recommended amount of a nutrient in food will not achieve any additional health benefit if they also take the nutrient as a supplement. In fact, in some cases, supplements and fortified foods may cause intakes to exceed the safe levels of nutrients."

Another nationally prominent nutritionist who advises against the use of multivitamins is Robert M. Russell, MD, director and senior scientist of the Jean Mayer USDA Human Nutrition Research Center on Aging at Tufts University in Boston. "I don't take them myself," he says. "Instead of paying attention to their diet and a mixed variety of foods that they should be eating, people think they're getting everything they need from a multivitamin, which is not the case. If you're just depending on a multivitamin, you're missing out on many, many, many benefits that come from eating a variety of foods."

But where Adelle Davis left off in 1974, self-interested manufacturers and retailers, as well as an outspoken coterie of opinionated nutritionists, have picked up, selling many vitamins on the basis of an irresistible scientific conjecture that came into vogue shortly after Davis's passing: that they prevent disease by acting as "antioxidants" to protect the body from the ravages of "free radicals." The theory had just one inconvenient problem: it would turn out not to be true. But by the time scientists would figure that out, the healing powers of vitamins would already be an article of faith among tens of millions.

⊂⊃ ⊂⊃ ⊂⊃

The first time the words *vitamin* and *antioxidant* appeared together in the *New York Times* was in 1946, in a business story about a new way to efficiently extract vitamins from vegetable, animal, and fish oils. It didn't appear in the *Times* again until a quarter century later, in 1972, in an article about the use of vitamin E as an underarm deodorant. Over the next ten years, it appeared eight more times, including in an Estée Lauder advertisement for skin cream containing vitamin E. The following decade saw a doubling of such pieces, with twenty published through March of 1992. The next two years alone brought thirty-three pieces—mostly health news articles, but also some advertisements for beauty products and vitamins that picked up on the growing frenzy. Only then were the results published in the *New England Journal of Medicine* from a study designed to bring scientific certainty to the question of whether antioxidant vitamins actually prevent disease. Unfortunately, the answer was not what the public had been led to expect all those years.

Faith in vitamins, of course, long predated the antioxidant craze, and from the earliest days of the twentieth century had been based on bits and pieces of provocative scientific research championed by iconoclasts like Adelle Davis. Vitamin E, for instance, had long been touted as a kind of natural Viagra for sexual potency; even its chemical name, alpha tocopherol, is Greek for "oil of fertility." And vitamin C enjoyed widespread popularity for preventing and treating colds, thanks largely due to Linus Pauling, PhD. Pauling remains the only person ever to win two unshared Nobel Prizes (one for chemistry and another for peace), and his impeccable credentials lent his utterances enormous weight. In his 1970 book *Vitamin C and the Common Cold,* he claimed that 1,000 milligrams of vitamin C per day would cut people's risk of catching a cold by 45 percent. Yet as time went on, studies failed again and again to support such claims.

The antioxidant story was different. Its theoretical underpinnings were sound, and the evidence from a variety of preliminary studies looked undeniably promising. Scientists had known since 1900, after all, that a "free radical" could be formed in organic compounds when a spare electron in one molecule glommed on to another molecule in order to nab itself a fellow electron—like birds in the springtime, electrons like to pair up—thereby forming a chain reaction as the odd-man-out electron in each molecule reached out to steal an electron from its neighbor. Such an effect could be beneficial: Plexiglas, polyethylene, and latex are all made from organic free radicals, their very plasticity caused by the gooey mingling of their electrons. But in living things, the free radicals that form as a natural by-product of oxygen metabolism were found capable of latching on to and harming cells essential to health. Antioxidants, however—otherwise known as "free radical scavengers"—stopped the oxidation process by latching onto and deactivating the free radicals, thereby preventing them from doing harm. It was well established by the late 1960s that the body had its own army of natural antioxidant substances, including the enzyme glutathione peroxidase and a class of proteins called superoxide dismutase. But then, beginning in the 1980s, researchers began to find that vitamins A, C, and E, as well as carotene, selenium, and some of the B vitamins, also had antioxidant properties. For instance, academic researchers in California and Texas published studies showing that vitamin E could prevent LDL cholesterol, the so-called bad cholesterol, from becoming oxidized, thereby (the researchers theorized) preventing the LDL from doing harm. Two biochemists at the

University of California, Berkeley, Lester Packer and Bruce Ames, became especially well known for their research, and their views, on the importance of antioxidants.

By the late 1980s, the once obscure theory of antioxidants and free radical scavengers became the talk of health clubs and cocktail parties, the stuff of headlines and best-selling books, as studies of large numbers of men and women began finding that those who took vitamins had lower rates of heart disease and cancer. The studies were not conclusive, however, because the people involved had not been randomly assigned to take either the vitamins or placebos. And without randomly assigning the people, one could never be sure whether the vitamin poppers were healthier for other reasons—such as that they ate healthier foods and jogged more often. Still, the early studies' results were certainly tantalizing. As papers by prominent researchers began finding rates of heart disease or cancer as much as 50 percent lower among those who happened to be taking vitamins compared to those who were not, the press pounced. A headline from the *Washington Post* stated in 1989: "Free-Radical Fighters: Vitamins A and E and Carotene May Reduce Cancer Risk." That same year, the *New York Times* ran a story headlined "New Research Bolsters Long-Held Beliefs That Vitamin E Can Provide an Array of Benefits." Another piece in the *Times,* from 1990, began, "If preliminary findings presented at the annual meeting of the American Heart Association two weeks ago hold up, carotene may be the next nutrient in the public spotlight." The following year, the *Post* titled a story "Researchers Are Taking a Fresh Look at Vitamin C." Although the scientists quoted in the articles often urged caution in interpreting the results, the impact on vitamin sales was unmistakable. According to a *Wall Street Journal* article on February 13, 1993, vitamin E sales in the three prior months were up 31 percent compared to those of the same period a year earlier, with sales of carotene and vitamin A up 19 percent and vitamin C up 13 percent. Manufacturers were rushing "all-antioxidant" vitamin formulas to market (many of which remain on the market to this day); a company named Free Radical Sciences was said to be developing antioxidant drugs against cancer; and tests were being sold to measure the level of antioxidants in people's blood.

And then the first randomized, placebo-controlled study of antioxidants—vitamin E and beta carotene—was published in the *New England*

Journal of Medicine on April 14, 1994. Carried out by the National Cancer Institute in partnership with Finland's National Public Health Institute, the study involved 29,000 Finnish men, all long-term smokers over the age of fifty. Smokers had been picked specially because of their increased risk of getting cancer and heart disease sooner. They were each given either vitamin E, beta carotene, a pill that combined both, or one that contained neither. The shocking results: those taking the vitamins saw no benefit over those getting the placebo. Instead, the men taking beta carotene were actually slightly more likely to die of lung cancer or heart disease. Experts expressed surprise, but held out hope that other studies already under way would find the expected benefits.

Less than two years later, two more randomized studies of beta carotene appeared. The Physicians' Health Study followed 22,071 doctors for twelve years and found no difference in health outcomes for those given beta carotene rather than the placebo. The Carotene and Retinol Efficacy Trial involved 18,314 people at high risk for lung cancer because they had worked with asbestos, giving them either beta carotene, vitamin A, both, or a placebo. The study was ended twenty-one months ahead of schedule, on January 10, 1996, when the researchers realized that the death rate from lung cancer was actually 28 percent higher among people taking the vitamins than those taking the placebo, and the death rate from heart disease was 17 percent higher. The findings were considered so important that they were announced at a press conference by the National Cancer Institute, which had funded both studies, before being published in medical journals. "With clearly no benefit and even a hint of possible harm, I see no reason that an individual should take carotene," said the NCI's director, Dr. Richard Klausner.

Similarly disappointing results appeared in studies of other antioxidants, leading the Institute of Medicine, an arm of the National Academy of Sciences, to issue a report in April of 2000 saying that there was no convincing evidence of benefit in taking any of the antioxidants at the high doses that had long been recommended. And the news kept getting worse. In October of 2004, the British medical journal *Lancet* reviewed fourteen randomized trials involving 170,525 people who took either a so-called antioxidant cocktail of vitamins A, C, and E and carotene or a placebo, to see whether gastrointestinal cancers could be prevented. It concluded: "We could not find evidence that antioxidant supplements can prevent gastrointestinal cancers; on the contrary, they seem to increase overall mortality." In the seven best-designed studies, they noted, death rates increased an average of 6 percent in those who took the vitamins.

Three months later came the first of two studies that, by any reasonable standard, should have put the final nails in the coffin for vitamin E's reputation as a beneficial antioxidant. Examining the evidence from nineteen previously randomized trials involving a combined total of 135,967 adults, the study, published in the *Annals of Internal Medicine* in January of 2005, found a slightly increased risk of death associated with vitamin E. Dr. Caballero told the *New York Times:* "This reaffirms what many have already said. The evidence for supplementing with any vitamin, and particularly vitamin E, is just not there. This idea that people have that even if it does not have any effect, at least it will not hurt, may not be that simple." Then, on March 16, 2005, the *Journal of the American Medical Association* published a study involving 9,541 people at 174 medical centers in Europe and North America. After an average of seven years, it found that patients taking 400 International Units of vitamin E had derived no benefit from it in terms of preventing heart disease or cancer, and were in fact 13 percent more likely to develop heart failure than those who took placebo, and 21 percent more likely to be hospitalized for heart failure.

It seemed the time had come for the great antioxidant theory of vitamins as free radical fighters to be put out to rust alongside the battered remains of countless other theories that initially sounded great and looked promising but ultimately proved not to mesh with reality. But the Council for Responsible Nutrition, the country's leading trade group for dietary supplement manufacturers, was having none of it. In full-page advertisements in the *New York Times,* the *Los Angeles Times,* and *USA Today* published soon after the *Annals* study, the group stated that its goal was to "reassure the public of the safety and benefits of vitamin E." At the same time, the newsman Larry King kept right on pitching vitamin E supplements in his paid commercials for Ester-E. Such propaganda appeared to be paying off. In the decade since the antioxidant bubble popped among scientists, the public has remained deaf to the bad news.

In July of 2005, a large national survey found that 12 percent of U.S. adults, or 24 million people, were still consuming high doses (400 International Units or more) of vitamin E supplements each day.

⊂⊃ ⊂⊃ ⊂⊃

Other theories of vitamins' benefits proved equally disappointing. No good studies exist to support the use of vitamin E to improve the appearance of the skin or to prevent colds. Many good studies do, however, show that vitamin C does *not* prevent colds. Indeed, few theories in the history of medicine have undergone more scientific scrutiny than Linus Pauling's claims about vitamin C. The National Institute of Allergy and Infectious Diseases' current position is as follows: "Many people are convinced that taking large quantities of vitamin C will prevent colds or relieve symptoms. To test this theory, several large-scale, controlled studies involving children and adults have been conducted. To date, no conclusive data has shown that large doses of vitamin C prevent colds. The vitamin may reduce the severity or duration of symptoms, but there is no clear evidence. Taking vitamin C over long periods of time in large amounts may be harmful. Too much vitamin C can cause severe diarrhea, a particular danger for elderly people and small children."

If not vitamin C, can the "nutritional insurance" of a daily multivitamin protect against a cold? Researchers from the Netherlands sought to answer the question in a carefully designed study published in the *Journal of the American Medical Association* in August of 2002. They gave 652 people aged sixty or older either a multivitamin, 200 milligrams of vitamin E, both, or a placebo. Those given a multivitamin did no better on any measure of colds than those given a placebo, whether on the number of colds per year, their severity or duration, the number of symptoms, or the need for bed rest or medication—and those given vitamin E actually did worse. A 1992 study in *Lancet* by Ranjit K. Chandra, MD, a prominent immunologist at Newfoundland Memorial Hospital in Canada, did report a significant drop in illnesses due to infectious diseases. However, the same Dr. Chandra also reported in 2001 in the journal *Nutrition* that multivitamins improved immediate and long-term memory, abstract thinking, problem-solving, and attention in older adults. In February of 2005, the journal took the almost unheard-of step of retracting that study, revealing that Dr. Chandra had refused to answer charges that his data had been invented. "A group of scientists and investigators found some of the claims made [were] implausible [and] not reproducible, [and] that the basis on which the data was analyzed was not appropriate and could not yield the results claimed," the editor of the journal told the Canadian Broadcasting Corporation. What's more, the retraction stated, "Chandra failed to declare that he holds a patent on the tested supplement formula and has a financial stake in it because the supplement was licensed to Javaan Corporation, a company founded by his daughter, that sells the supplement." In the retraction, similarly serious questions were raised about the validity of the *Lancet* study. Dr. Chandra now lives in India, where he serves as president of Javaan Corporation.

And what of the supposed benefits of the B vitamins? Americans spent $237 million on B vitamins in 2003, according to *Nutrition Business Journal,* an increase of 7 percent over the year before. The eight water-soluble B vitamins are often packaged together and sold as "energy boosters," because they help the body convert carbohydrates into sugar. Yet the evidence of benefit is limited to a few special cases, while the potential for harm is widespread. Vitamin B_3, better known as niacin, has been shown at high doses to lower cholesterol and prevent the progression of heart disease. But because it can raise diabetics' blood-sugar level, cause facial flushing and liver damage, and prevent the proper absorption of medications, it should be used only under a doctor's supervision. Vitamin B_6 is widely promoted to treat everything from depression and migraines to carpal tunnel syndrome, PMS, and high levels of homocysteine (a risk factor for cardiovascular disease). But it's never been proven to relieve any of these conditions, and in fact doses less than 500 milligrams per day—widely sold in single-dose capsules, even though the Institute of Medicine has set the upper tolerable limit at 100 milligrams—can cause neuropathy, a kind of nerve damage marked by tingling and numbness in the arms and legs. B_9, better known as folic acid (when synthesized), has been added to all enriched breads, cereals, flours, cornmeals, pasta, rice, and other grain products in the United States since 1996, based on strong evidence showing that it would greatly lower the risk of the birth defect spina bifida. But hopes that it would also lower rates of heart disease have yet to be borne out, and a 2004 study found tentative signs of a slightly increased risk of death, and of breast cancer, in women years after they took it during pregnancy. As for B_{12}, because all adults over fifty have a reduced ability to absorb it, the 2005 Dietary Guidelines for Americans recommends that they either eat foods fortified with it or take supplements. But because folic acid can worsen a B_{12} deficiency, leading to anemia and even brain damage, taking both folic acid and B_{12} together can be dangerous.

Perhaps the most surprising disappointment among the many unproved claims for vitamin and mineral supplements are those made for calcium. By far the most popular mineral supplement in the United States, calcium is regularly used by 8.7 percent of U.S. adults, who spent just over $1 billion on it in 2003, a sharp rise of 19 percent over the year before, according to *Nutrition Business Journal*. A wealth of studies back the view that calcium in the diet, particularly when vitamin D intake is adequate, builds strong bones during adolescence and early adulthood. But does taking calcium in a supplement rather than in food actually make a difference in preventing the problem that postmenopausal women take calcium to prevent: hip fractures? It would seem like a slam dunk, but the Women's Health Initiative (WHI)—the same study of 36,828 postmenopausal women that proved that hormone replacement therapy increases the risk of stroke, breast cancer, and dementia, and that a low-fat diet prevents neither heart disease, cancer, nor obesity—reached similarly disappointing findings about calcium supplements. In a study published in the *New England Journal of Medicine* on February 16, 2006, the leaders of the WHI reported that after seven years, calcium with vitamin D supplements resulted in a small improvement in hip density, but "did not significantly reduce hip fracture, and increased the risk of kidney stones." The same group reported in another study in the same issue that the supplement also did not prevent colorectal cancer. In an accompanying editorial, the Harvard physician Joel S. Finkelstein, MD, wrote: "We must conclude that calcium with vitamin D supplementation is not an effective means of preventing fractures in this population. Many people may be disappointed with these results." But, he added, "With the widespread marketing of calcium and vitamin D, many women believe that they are completely protected against the development of osteoporosis if they are taking these supplements. This study should help correct this important misconception and allow more women to receive optimal therapy for bone health."

○ ▭ ▭

If people simply feel better taking vitamins or mineral supplements, or if they believe, despite the lack of scientific evidence, that they're doing themselves and their kids some good with them, where's the harm? The case of Cooper Burkey and the 1.3 million Americans who have experienced adverse reactions since 1983 would seem enough of an answer, but in truth the effects of taking them—in pills that almost always contain concentrations far beyond what could ever be obtained from foods, or, for that matter, has ever been consumed in the history of the human race—may prove far more widespread and harmful than has previously been imagined. In July of 2004, the journal *Pediatrics* published a frightening analysis of data from 8,285 preschool children obtained from the National Maternal-Infant Health Survey. It found that African-American children who had been given a simple multivitamin supplement in the first six months of their life had a 27 percent increased risk of asthma, and that exclusively formula-fed children of all races who received vitamins in their first six months had a 63 percent increased risk of developing food allergies. In addition, all those who had received vitamin supplementation by the age of three had a 63 percent increased risk of food allergies if they had been breast-fed, or a 39 percent increase if they had been exclusively formula-fed. The lead author of the study, Joshua D. Milner, MD, a clinical fellow at the National Institute of Allergy and Infectious Diseases, said he did the study after reading basic research suggesting that vitamins can alter the immune system. Because it was only a survey, the results may have been skewed by demographic variables. Still, he and his fellow researchers agreed that the findings warrant further study. As to whether the immune-altering effects of multivitamins could be playing any role in the rising rate of autism is, at this point, unknown and virtually unstudied.

More certain, however, is the harm that vitamin A can do. Even the amount in an ordinary multivitamin, researchers now believe, can weaken adults' bones. The strongest evidence to date comes from the Nurses Health Study, which examined the relationship between hip fractures and vitamin A in more than 72,337 postmenopausal women. Those who took at least 2,000 micrograms of retinol (a primary component of vitamin A), whether through food or supplements, were 89 percent more likely to have suffered a hip fracture than those who took less than 500 micrograms. The study, published in the *Journal of the American Medical Association* in January of 2002, concluded: "Long-term intake of a diet high in retinol may promote the development of osteoporotic hip fractures in women. The amounts of retinol in fortified foods and vitamin supplements may need to be reassessed." The FDA has set the Daily Value of vitamin A intake at 5,000 international units, or 1,500 micrograms of retinol, and most multivitamins contain at least that much. But according to Meir Stampfer, MD, chair of the Harvard School of Public Health's Department of Epidemiology: "Between supplements, fortified breakfast cereals and milk, it's easy to get up to 10,000 or more international units per day, and that's a level where you start to see clinical harm in terms of increased susceptibility to fractures and other adverse health effects."

Without question, the most dangerous supplement in the home of any family with a toddler is iron, because of the tragic consequences that can result when a child gets into a container of iron-containing supplements and consumes a toxic dose. On the Friday following Valentine's Day of 1993, the Centers for Disease Control and Prevention published an alarming article on the subject in its *Morbidity and Mortality Weekly Report*. "Iron is the most common cause of pediatric poisoning deaths reported to poison control centers in the United States," the CDC reported. In just the six previous months, five children between the ages of eleven and eighteen months had died in the Los Angeles area alone after taking supplements containing iron, the CDC revealed. The first involved a sixteen-month-old boy who got into a loosely capped container of his mother's prenatal iron tablets and ate between thirty and thirty-five of them. The tablets were disc-shaped, colored red or green, with a glossy sugar coating—just like M&M's. Because the boy did not show the usual initial symptoms of iron overdose (vomiting and diarrhea), his parents did not seek prompt medical attention. By the time he had lapsed into a coma, doctors were unable to revive him. That was in June of 1992. Three months later, in September, an eighteen-month-old boy swallowed a similar number of prenatal iron tablets with the same M&M's appearance, and he too died. A twelve-month-old died the same way in November. The next month, a two-year-old boy fed his eleven-month-old sister somewhere between thirty and thirty-five of the tablets that he'd found in a box on the floor, and she died. The spate of deaths led the Los Angeles Department of Health Services to issue a media alert on January 20 about the dangers of iron overdose, but on January 28, a fifth death there involving a thirteen-month-old girl was reported.

Looking back to 1991, the CDC noted in its report, "5,144 ingestions of iron supplements were reported to poison control centers in the United States; 11 were fatal. Children aged less than 6 years accounted for 3,578 (69.6%) ingestions of iron and 9 of the deaths. In addition, 18,457 ingestions of iron in the form of multivitamin or combination preparations were reported; 16,021 (87%) occurred among children aged less than 6 years. During 1991, consumption of multivitamin preparations in the form of prenatal vitamins with iron caused two additional deaths among children aged 17 and 18 months."

The CDC went on to note that more than 120 different iron-containing preparations were then available. "Although in three cases the iron supplement was a prescription item," the report stated, "the 60 mg per tablet dosage is also available in over-the-counter preparations. Ingestion of as few as five or six tablets of a high-potency preparation could be fatal for a 22-lb child." The CDC was especially concerned because until the mid-1980s, only about 1,200 children had overdosed on iron each year—less than one fourth the number in 1991—usually resulting in "only" a couple of deaths. Clearly, the increased use of iron supplements, whether alone or with multivitamins, was having an unintended and tragic side effect.

In response to the CDC's report, some in the supplement industry argued that such cases are unavoidable accidents having nothing to do with the inherent safety or dangerousness of vitamins or minerals. Such an argument ("accidents will happen") can be highly convincing; indeed, it served the automobile industry exceedingly well for decades, allowing it to sidestep responsibility for the deaths that inevitably resulted from car crashes and to avoid making such essential safety features as seat belts and side-view mirrors standard on all cars. But the FDA didn't buy such a fatalistic view. In 1997, it issued regulations requiring that any supplement containing iron have a warning label, and that those with more than 30 milligrams of iron be sold in unit-dose packaging—blister packs—to make it harder for toddlers to eat too many of them. Those two strategies helped bring down the number of deaths due to iron ingestion to five in 2002 and four in 2003. But the number of nonfatal iron poisonings has remained staggeringly high, reaching 32,995 in 2003, with four out of five involving children under the age of six. Thirty of those cases were considered life-threatening or resulted in permanent neurological damage.

Yet soon after the FDA issued its regulations, Gerry Kessler and his Nutritional Health Alliance filed a lawsuit charging that under DSHEA, the agency had no authority to issue regulations for the purpose of poison prevention. Incredible as it may seem, on January 21, 2003, the U.S. Court of Appeals agreed, voiding the unit-dose packaging requirement. Explaining his motive in filing the suit, Gerry Kessler said: "Although our company does make an iron pill in a childproof container, and I believe they should be [in childproof containers], we didn't believe the FDA had the right to [require it]. So the NHA took the FDA to court and proved that it didn't have the right. They were usurping a power that didn't belong to them. In fact, they were right to do it. We just didn't believe the FDA *had* the right to do it." As things stand now, then, manufacturers are free to put as much iron into a tablet as they see fit, and are under no obligation to use special packaging to prevent toddlers from getting into their containers.

○ ▭ ⬭

If concerns about the safety of vitamins and minerals are hastily dismissed by most adults in the United States, they are taken far more seriously in some European countries. On August 11, 2004, the Danish Veterinary and Food Administration announced that it had refused an application from Kellogg's to fortify Corn Flakes, Rice Krispies, Special K, and fifteen other products with iron, calcium, folic acid, and vitamin B_6. A statement in Danish by Paolo Drotsby, deputy chief of the administration's nutrition division, was translated into English as saying that the products would "have toxic effects in the doses Kellogg's uses." The European press ran headlines about "toxic cereal," and spokesmen for Kellogg's expressed shock. Chris Wermann, director of corporate affairs for Kellogg's in Europe, told the *Guardian:* "Most of us are a bit incredulous. It is quite clear from nutritionists that diets around the globe are deficient in vitamins and minerals. We are quite worried about the Danish authorities challenging this. We don't believe there is any danger at all. There is every reason for people to have these."

But Danish health authorities believed otherwise. Salka E. Rasmussen, PhD, a senior researcher at the Danish Institute for Food and Veterinary Research, was one of four scientists who concluded, after reviewing the safe upper limits for vitamins and minerals that had previously been established by the European Community Scientific Committee on Food, that the amounts that Kellogg's wanted to add would bring some citizens, particularly children, over the safe upper limits.

"It's all a question of doses," said Dr. Rasmussen in a telephone interview from her home in Copenhagen, where she lives with her husband and two young children (with a third on the way). "If you take too much calcium, you get calcium in your kidneys and can develop kidney stones. If you take iron, you can very easily get levels in your blood that are too high. You can get heart problems and can die of it. During evolution, humans developed to absorb very efficiently the limited amounts of vitamins and minerals we got from our foods. We have a very good absorption of iron, because there were such low amounts in our food. It was hard to get meat. Now many males have a problem with too high iron levels in the body. This iron overload increases their risk for heart disease and heart problems. That's really a problem."

Asked whether she was concerned that some children, due to poor diets, might not get enough of their necessary vitamins, she replied, "That's an entirely different problem. If you're concerned that somebody gets too little of certain vitamins, then you should have mandatory fortification of the necessary nutrient, like with iodine in salt or folic acid in bread. In that way, you can make sure nobody gets too low an amount if it's really necessary." And what of the children who eat peculiar diets, refusing to eat anything but, say, macaroni and cheese or cornflakes? "But just adding vitamins to the cereal won't give children everything they need to grow," she pointed out. "There's more to foods than vitamins and minerals. You need the fiber. You need all the compounds, known and unknown, that are in foods. That has always been the authority's viewpoint in Denmark. Vitamins and minerals are just not the solution. That is pretty much proved now in many studies. A lot of studies supplementing people with vitamins and minerals have not shown a decrease in mortality. Many times they see an *increase* in mortality. Especially for children who eat an unhealthy diet, the solution is not to add vitamins to the macaroni and cheese or the breakfast cereal. It's to feed them a better diet."

Health officials in other European countries, including the United Kingdom and Sweden, are now studying whether children in their countries are likewise getting overly high doses of vitamins, she said.

◯ ◯ ◯

Almost drowned out amid the white noise of unsubstantiated claims comes, sotto voce, the case for vitamin D, which just may be the only vitamin that the average American needs *more* of. In February of 2005, the *Journal of the National Cancer Institute* published two studies showing that increased exposure to sunlight is linked to increased survival in melanoma patients, as well as a lowered risk of developing lymphoma. According to an editorial accompanying the studies, the effect was likely due to vitamin D, which the skin makes in response to sunlight. "It's long been known that Vitamin D is a critically important agent in bone health," the editorial stated. "More recently it has become increasingly obvious that Vitamin D has important regulatory functions in the cell, in terms of cell division."

According to Michael F. Holick, PhD, MD, professor of medicine, physiology, and biophysics at Boston University and one of D's biggest advocates, deficiency of the vitamin is "an unrecognized epidemic in the United States. At the end of winter, thirty-two percent of Bostonians are deficient in vitamin D due to lack of sunlight exposure. In Maine, of girls between the ages of nine to eleven, forty-eight percent are D deficient at the end of winter." Among the studies he quotes is a 2004 study in the journal *Neurology*, which found that vitamin D might decrease women's risk of developing multiple sclerosis. And a December 2005 study in the journal *CHEST* found that the more vitamin D people have circulating in their blood, the better their lungs function.

According to the Institute of Medicine, 200 international units of vitamin D daily is adequate for men and women alike from birth through fifty, an amount easily obtained by two cups of milk or two ounces of cheese, while 400 international units are necessary from age fifty-one to seventy, and 600 international units daily thereafter. But the government's 2005 Dietary Guidelines for Americans recommends 1,000 international units for the elderly as well as for African-Americans (because their dark skin synthesizes less vitamin D in response to sunlight) and the housebound. Other researchers have suggested such levels for others. For instance, a paper in the February 2006 issue of the *American Journal of Public Health* concluded that taking 1,000 international units of vitamin D per day could lower an individual's risk of colon cancer, breast cancer, and ovarian cancer by 50 percent. But at this point, such assertions are no better proved than were the antioxidant claims of the early 1990s. And taking much more than 1,000 international units could be dangerous; the Institute of Medicine has found that the safe upper limit for vitamin D is 2,000 international units per day, except for infants in the first year of life, for whom 1,000 international units per day is the limit.

Thus we must face an increasingly certain conclusion, unpopular though it may be, that vitamin and mineral supplements, with the possible exception of vitamin D, are not only unnecessary for most people, but in many cases harmful. This is far more disturbing news than the revelation that a drug like Vioxx does more harm than good. Drugs, after all, are not marketed and promoted as essential to everybody's health; to the contrary, they are always sold with a lengthy list of possible side effects. Yet so thoroughly do we believe in vitamins and minerals—so carefully have we been manipulated to believe—that many mothers would consider themselves negligent *not* to give them to their children, even if in an unchewable caplet nearly an inch long. But as the growing evidence shows, our trust in vitamins and minerals has been misplaced. The very bedrock of the dietary supplement industry turns out to be a swamp where the facts go to die.

CHAPTER 8
WOMEN AND CHILDREN FIRST

Established in 1957, the Long Island Regional Poison and Drug Information Center is one of the largest in the country, serving some 3.6 million residents of the New York City suburbs. Located in the leafy town of Mineola, its staff includes a pharmacist, Elaine Kang-Yum, who found herself receiving so many calls about dietary supplements that she established the Herb Watch Program, the first launched by any poison center in the country. The need for it became tragically apparent one day in 1999, when a call came in from the emergency room at Jamaica Hospital in nearby Queens. A mother had walked into a local health food store earlier that day seeking a remedy for her eighteen-month-old son's fever. The clerk had told her that a teaspoonful of eucalyptus oil would be a good treatment, even though any physician or pharmacist would know that eucalyptus oil, when ingested, is poisonous. But the mother bought the eucalyptus oil, went home with her sick son, and gave him the recommended teaspoonful. Within minutes, the toddler began to choke and went into a convulsion. The mother dialed 911, the boy was taken by ambulance to the hospital, and now the emergency room doctor wanted some advice on how to treat him.

The standard treatment would have been to pump the stomach to remove as much of the eucalyptus oil as possible and to give activated charcoal, a powder mixed with water and taken by mouth, to absorb what remained. But by the time the boy arrived at the hospital, the damage had already been done. Like other essential oils, including the most popular—Vicks VapoRub, which includes a combination of them—eucalyptus oil is intended for external use only, as it can cause vomiting, breathing difficulty, depression of the central nervous system, seizures, and coma when taken by mouth, in even tiny amounts. With the rise in popularity of "natural" essential oils, however, the number of such cases reported each year to poison centers around the country had jumped from 2,661 in 1990 to 4,099 in 1999, the year the Long Island center received the call about the toddler. (Five years later, the number would hit 7,310.)

Soon after arriving at Jamaica Hospital, the little boy suffered another seizure and was then transferred to the much larger North Shore University Hospital. Again he suffered another seizure and was given Valium to stop the seizing. But his condition only worsened. His breathing became so labored that doctors had to insert a breathing tube and place him on assisted ventilation. He survived, but ultimately suffered significant and permanent brain damage.

In the history of the dietary supplement industry, when did ordinary mothers begin to trust more in the safety of untested herbs for their children than in drugs regulated by the FDA? When did the tipping point occur? For Judy Robinson, a pediatric nurse practitioner with a PhD in nursing, it was certainly not while she served eight years as a school nurse during the early to mid-1990s, when questions about herbal remedies came rarely if ever. But between 1998 and 2003, when she served as executive director of the National Association of School Nurses, things changed. "We began to see a significant increase in the number of parents wanting to use herbals," she says. "In some cases, the nurses were being told that the parent expected their child to be given an herbal remedy during the school day. The nurses were concerned, because they didn't have a doctor's orders to give those herbs, they didn't know the amount of active ingredients in them, and they didn't know what else was being given at home. Many parents didn't understand that if something happened to the child based on an herb that wasn't tested by the FDA, if they had some kind of liver, kidney, or any kind of side effect, the school could be liable. And there were confrontations sometimes when the nurse said she couldn't give it."

Today dietary supplements are targeted at children everywhere. Chamomile Calm, made by Botanical Laboratories, Inc., is said to be "wonderful for soothing the over-energized, anxious, or exhausted child." Herbs for Kids Respiratory & Throat Support is "designed to ease a dry, irritable cough." HealthAid Children's Echinacea Drops formula "provides the purest echinacea herbal support during exposure to colds and flu." And Nordic Naturals sells strawberry-flavored capsules called DHA Junior (the "n" in "Junior" is backward on the label, a la Toys "R" Us), described as "a delicious way for children two years & up to supplement their diet with the essential fatty acid DHA to support development of the brain and visual system."

As the market has grown, so have the claims. In the past decade, the Federal Trade Commission has taken action fourteen times against supplement manufacturers whose products target children, including products that claim to help children lose weight or treat their attention deficit and hyperactivity. Some of the products, according to the FTC, contained stimulants, hormones, or herbs known to be toxic. "False claims exploit parents' fears about giving their children prescription drugs," says the FTC's Howard Beales. "But these alternative therapies may actually do the children more harm than good." The latest action came in April of 2006, when the FTC settled charges against Dynamic Health of Florida, the maker of Pedia Loss, for falsely claiming that it could "cause weight loss in overweight or obese children ages six and over." The only ingredient listed on the label having any history as a diet aid was hydroxycitrate, an extract from the garcinia plant that was shown in a 1998 study in the *Journal of the American Medical Association* to be no better than a placebo in achieving weight loss.

Says Hilary Perr, MD, a pediatric gastroenterologist and director of the Evolving Foods and Children's Health Program at California Pacific Medical Center in San Francisco, "My office is filled every day with people who don't provide their kids with a basic, adequate diet and think that a granola bar or a dietary supplement will fix it. I put [such parents] in a realm of a growing population of people who are educated and who have resources and access to medical care but who are overwhelmed by the complexity of the world and misinformed about proper nutrition."

Critically ill children are especially likely to be given dietary supplements by their parents. A 2001 study by the Fred Hutchinson Cancer Research Center in Seattle found that 54 percent of pediatric cancer patients in western Washington State were given herbal remedies by their parents to treat the cancer or cope with side effects from standard medical treatments, and that 59 percent were given high-dose vitamins. "While the data are conflicting about harm or benefit regarding use of these products among children undergoing cancer treatment, some caution may be advisable," stated the study's author, Marian L. Neuhouser, PhD. She noted that antioxidants such as vitamins C and E can reduce the effectiveness of chemotherapy, and that herbs such as yew needle and the herbal tea essiac have been linked to heart and kidney impairment, particularly when taken with certain cancer drugs.

Tales of sick children gravely injured by the very supplements their parents thought to be safe and natural date back to the Adelle Davis era. Susan and Donald Pitzer of Pompano Beach, Florida, were close followers of Davis's *Let's Have Healthy Children,* and when their newborn twin sons, Ryan and Darren, suffered from colic in April of 1978, they tried a cure she recommended: potassium chloride. After buying some at a health food store, Susan added it to a bottle of her breast milk. Ryan drank down his bottle eagerly, but Darren refused. A few hours later, Ryan vomited and turned pale—not a particularly unusual thing for a three-month-old baby to do. Next morning, he was colicky again, so Susan gave him some more. Ryan coughed, threw up, and stopped breathing. Susan tried to give him mouth-to-mouth resuscitation while Donald called an ambulance. Doctors at Cypress Creek Hospital revived him briefly, and then transferred him to Jackson Memorial Hospital in Miami. At 3:30 in the morning of April 4, Ryan died. As the subsequent lawsuit would later show, Davis had once again badly misinterpreted the study on which she had based her advice. And it was not the last time "Mother Nature" would reach out from the grave to harm a child: in 2005, Australian physicians reported the hospitalization of an anemic eleven-month-old whose parents had followed the advice in *Let's Have Healthy Children* by feeding their baby a diet of barley water, corn syrup, and goat's milk.

To Dr. Perr in San Francisco, such cases have become almost routine. She tells of a sixteen-year-old boy who came into her office recently due to persistent nausea and stomach pain. "What I learned was that he was taking eighteen preparations in a day. Two out of the eighteen were prescription drugs, the rest were all supplements—thymus extract, ribonucleic acid, different types of algae. I discovered that many of the preparations contained vitamin A, and in combination, he was inadvertently being poisoned by it." Another child she treated was born with biliary atresia, in which the ducts that drain bile from the liver wither away, causing bile to back up and damage the liver. "The treatment is liver transplant, and it works," says Dr. Perr. "But until the child is ready for transplant, our job is to help them be as nutritionally complete and develop as normally as possible. This one family was also seeing a naturopath, who prescribed a supplement. I asked the family to bring it in so I could see what it was. The label wasn't very informative, so I called the company. It was crushed sheep adrenal glands. The liver is the body's filter and detoxifier, and here they were putting their child's liver under stress. This was an upper-class, educated, cosmopolitan, sophisticated family with all the resources you could ever hope for, living under the popular misconception, held by so many people, that if something is simply called natural it couldn't possibly cause harm or interfere with healing."

Another example of what can happen when parents give their children supplements walked into the office of Tor A. Shwayder, MD, a pediatric dermatologist at Detroit's Henry Ford Hospital, in November of 2003. Accompanied by his mother, the sixteen-year-old boy—tall, muscular, and good-looking—said he had been taking a daily teaspoon of colloidal silver for two years to prevent colds; the whole family had. There was only one problem: his skin had turned silvery gray.

Made of microscopic silver particles suspended in a liquid, colloidal silver has been aggressively marketed since the mid-1990s as an antibiotic treatment for AIDS, cancer, tuberculosis, malaria, lupus, syphilis, scarlet fever, shingles, herpes, pneumonia, typhoid, tetanus—even, most recently, as a cure for bird flu. Originally sold in nose drops before the development of legitimate antibiotics, it was discredited in the 1950s as ineffective and found to have a truly macabre side effect. After months or years of ingesting colloidal silver, a patient was likely to find his or her skin turning slate gray, a result of the microscopic silver particles becoming embedded in the skin and every internal organ. The condition, called argyria, was found to be permanent and irreversible.

Such was the case with the young man who walked into Dr. Shwayder's office. "He looked like Papa Smurf," Dr. Shwayder recalled, referring to the blue cartoon character. "He was very gray, especially in the sun-exposed areas. So I did a punch biopsy behind the ear, which showed many, many silver granules deposited in the dermis." He also took a blood sample. The normal level of silver in the blood is 0 to 14 nanograms per milliliter; the boy's was 209. Dr. Shwayder called the local poison control center to see what could be done for the boy. Nothing, came the answer. "Not only is it permanent," Dr. Shwayder said, "but silver is a noble medal. That's why it's used in coins; it doesn't change with time. Silver dug up from ancient Agean ruins still looks fine five thousand years later. So he's stuck with it. And silver is a photo-reactive compound. It will get darker when the sunlight hits it."

The boy's family, he said, were working-class folks from farm country north of Detroit. "They didn't seem nutty," Dr. Shwayder said. "But they seemed the type that could be easily swayed by a drugstore display. They kept saying 'We feel better; we haven't got any colds; it really works.' No one expressed any anger to me. That seemed odd. They kept justifying their use of it. I had to almost twist their arms to get them to stop." In fact, he had to point out to the mother that she was "getting gray at the corner of her jaws too."

⬭ ⬭ ⬭

For most teenagers, the problem is not so much the supplements given to them by their parents but the kind they take on their own—the kind once sold at a bland stucco-and-cinderblock storefront in the shadow of Pikes Peak, at the corner of West Colorado Avenue and Fourth Street in Colorado Springs. On February 13, 2004—Friday the thirteenth, as it happened—two high school students entered the store, Cell Page Communications, but not to buy a cell phone. It was nearly five p.m. when they walked past the cashier and into a side room on the left devoted to a separate retail operation called Mind Excursions. There, displayed under a glass counter as at a vitamin shop, were products with names like Trance,

Schmooz, Krypto, Meltdown, Snuffadelic, Trip2Night, Liquid Speed, Cloud 9, Ragga Dagga, Wizard Smoke, Orange Speedball, and a sixteen-ounce bottle of pale green fluid called Green Hornet. The two boys, Billy and John, both recently turned eighteen, had heard the owner of the store, Kevin Schnitker, interviewed on a local radio station, KILO, where he was called the "herb man." They had come to buy some of the safe, natural, legal supplements that he sold there and online for getting high.

They paid forty-five dollars for the Green Hornet, went outside to their three waiting friends—Sam, Andrew, and Jeremiah, none of whom was yet eighteen—and then drove a mile and a half to a nearby Travelodge. If they were going to get high, they wanted to do it someplace where they wouldn't be bothered. By five-thirty p.m., having told their parents various stories, the boys were sitting in Room 228 taking two ounces each of the sweet green liquid—twice the dose recommended on the label. Ten minutes later, their judgment already seriously impaired by mild hallucinations, the boys each drank another ounce or two.

Billy opened the motel room door, thinking he'd take a walk. Down the corridor he saw creatures from the game "Doom" running toward him, spitting fire, and he could actually feel the heat of it. He closed the door, walked to the bed, and saw spiders the size of coffee mugs crawl onto his leg.

"The spiders are on me!" he shouted. When he kicked them off, he felt the weight of their bodies. He heard wood cracking above him and looked up. People were crawling out of the ceiling. On the floor, he saw pigs running around with forks in their butts. "Get over here," he called to the pigs, and ran around the room, chasing them.

John, who had been sitting at the wooden table in the corner of the room, stood up and said, "I'm tripping." He turned to walk away from the table, then fell backwards, striking his head on the table's edge. Crumpled on the floor, his body jerked spasmodically in a convulsion.

Billy snapped out of his hallucinations long enough to realize that his friend was in trouble. He picked up the phone to call 911 but couldn't remember how to dial it. Moments later, he too fell to the floor, his face beet red, and began to convulse.

Jeremiah, the big football player and the least affected of the group, managed to call 911. When the ambulance arrived, Billy grew so combative with the attendants that they had to tie him down to the pallet.

Moments after arriving at Memorial Hospital, Billy's dark brown eyes rolled up into his head and he had another seizure. His blood pressure was rising and his heart was racing, but still Dr. Mark James, director of pediatric emergency medicine, didn't know what was in the Green Hornet, because its label listed no ingredients. (A laboratory analysis would later show that it contained, in addition to numerous herbs, high levels of the over-the-counter cold remedies diphenhydramine and dextromethorphan.) With Billy's life in jeopardy, Dr. James called Rocky Mountain Poison Control. The doctor there, Dr. Dean Olsen, had a tentative list of twenty ingredients in Green Hornet and suggested that the best approach would be to simply give the kids intravenous fluids. By Sunday morning, all the boys were out of the hospital and on their way to a complete recovery. Kevin Schnitker, the owner of the store that sold them the Green Hornet, suffered no lasting consequences, either. The FDA sent him its standard warning letter for sellers of supplements that are marketed as street drug alternatives. Schnitker stopped selling the herbs from his store and shifted to offering them exclusively on his Web site, changing the name from mindexcursions.com to smokelegalbuds .com. The site, like many others, continues to operate.

Other teens experimenting with street drugs sold under the guise of dietary supplements have not been so lucky. GHB, once touted as an alternative to L-tryptophan until its mind-altering and life-threatening qualities led it to be outlawed, was linked to more than 45 deaths and 5,500 emergency room overdoses between 1990 and 2000, according to the U.S. Drug Enforcement Agency. More recently, on January 23, 2006, Brett Chidester, a seventeen-year-old straight-A student in Wilmington, Delaware, committed suicide after having frightening hallucinations under the influence of salvia, another herb sold on the Internet. (Illegal only in Louisiana and Missouri, it is now the subject of a bill that would similarly outlaw it in Delaware.) But the most widely used mind-altering herb that remains legal in nearly all states is kava, made from the crushed root of a South Pacific pepper plant. Canada, Germany, Singapore, South Africa, and Switzerland all banned kava after more than twenty-five cases of severe liver disease were associated with it, including four that required a liver transplant. On March 25, 2002, after a healthy young U.S. woman required a liver transplant after ingesting kava, the FDA sent out a warning against taking it. *Consumer Reports* has it listed among the

"Dirty Dozen" most dangerous supplements, and DUI arrests—for driving under the influence of kava—have led to convictions in California and Utah. So far no state has specifically outlawed it, although in 2005 Louisiana outlawed the use of any plant for mind-altering purposes. And so kava, which is also sometimes taken as an antidepressant and sleep aid, remains a standard component of multi-ingredient products sold in convenience stores and gas stations, and was used by 2.4 million people in the United States in 2002, according to the National Health Interview Survey. Incredibly, nonalcoholic kava bars have recently opened in Florida, Oregon, and Hawaii, including Boca Raton's Nakava, "the world's first kava bar chain," where "you don't have to be 21 to enter," where the kava drinks' potency is rated from 1 ("chill") to 4 ("you're in the spirit world"), and where the drinks' ability to induce "numbness" is likewise rated up to 4 ("you're at the dentist"). But hope for an unexpectedly important medical benefit from kava flared briefly on February 15, 2006, when news was published that researchers from the University of Aberdeen in Scotland and the Laboratoire de Biologie Moleculaire du Cancer in Luxembourg had found laboratory evidence of a protective effect against ovarian cancer and leukemia. The research, however, was not published in a medical journal. Rather, it was simply announced at a press conference at which the president of the Fiji Kava Council, Ratu Josateki Nawalowalo, said, "It's exciting news and it's a blessing and as we've always said, we have been sitting on a potential multibillion-dollar industry for the Pacific Islands, and this news has been received gladly by the island countries."

○ ○ ○

Mind-altering substances are hardly the only dietary supplements endangering the health of teenagers, yet an insidiously symbiotic relationship seems to exist between this age group's use of herbs and their risk of using illegal drugs. A study published in the March 23, 2006, issue of the *Journal of Adolescent Health* found that teens who have ever used herbs of any kind are six times more likely to use cocaine and nearly fifteen times more likely to have used anabolic steroids than are teens who have never used herbs. "Children who are open to experimenting with herbal products may be more open to trying illicit drugs," concluded the study's author, Susan Yussman, MD, assistant professor of pediatrics at the University of Rochester Medical Center.

Far more widely used by teens than any herb, however, are the performance-enhancing supplements taken by high school athletes. The most popular is creatine, used by about 17 percent of male high school athletes, according to recent surveys in both Iowa and Wisconsin. An amino acid made by the body, creatine is used by the muscles to derive energy. A search for "creatine" on Google pulls up an impressive 8.5 million results, the first of which, from bodybuilding.com, states, "Everyone consistently using creatine is making HUGE, AMAZING gains!" Studies have in fact shown that it can improve performance in sports that require speed and power, particularly weight lifting and sprinting. And in a medical context, creatine may have an important role to play in treating the muscle wasting caused by muscular dystrophy. A 2004 study in the journal *Neurology* found that, compared to placebo, four months of creatine significantly increased fat-free mass and handgrip strength in the dominant hand while reducing a marker of bone breakdown. But as used by young athletes, there are clear dangers. In 1998, the FDA listed thirty-two adverse events associated with creatine, including seizure, vomiting, cardiac arrhythmia, and death. A 1999 survey in the *Journal of the American Dietetic Association* of college athletes who used creatine found that 31 percent had experienced diarrhea, 25 percent experienced muscle cramps, 13 percent, unwanted weight gain, and 13 percent, dehydration. Between 2001 and 2003, U.S. poison centers received a total of 733 reports of adverse reactions to creatine, 334 of which required treatment in a hospital and 11 of which were life-threatening. Two studies have also reported impaired kidney function associated with the supplement.

Even more worrisome is dehydroepiandrosterone (DHEA), a steroid precursor that the FDA banned back in the 1980s before DSHEA permitted it to be resurrected as a dietary supplement. Senators tried to include it in a 2004 bill that outlawed other such precursors, including androstenedione, the supplement that Mark McGwire used while setting the Major League Baseball home run record. But the law ended up carving out a special exception for DHEA. Why? "Because that's sixty percent of the supplement market out in Utah," says Arthur P. Grollman, MD, the professor of pharmacology and medicine at the State University of New

York at Stonybrook who advised Senator Richard Durbin of Illinois on drafting the bill. "The only reason Utah would agree to go along with the bill is because he [Senator Hatch] thinks steroids are very bad for our young people, but he would just like DHEA kept out of it." While some studies have found potential medical uses for DHEA, other studies have shown that it may promote the formation of fatty plaque in arteries and increase the risk of suicide. It also raises men's levels of the female hormone estrogen—not a good thing for men, unless they want to develop breasts. DHEA is converted into steroids within the body, and like steroids can lead to shrunken testes, oily skin, increased aggression, and, over the long term, heart and liver failure. Moreover, because it remains regulated as a supplement, shoddy manufacturing standards have allowed some manufacturers to sell doses that differ from what is listed on the label. Such concerns show why Canada regulates DHEA as a prescription drug.

Even illegal anabolic steroids are being injected by a growing portion of student athletes determined to gain muscle mass. A 2004 survey by the University of Michigan's Institute of Social Research found that 3.4 percent of all twelfth-graders had tried steroids at least once. (The figure, however, includes girls, even though almost all the users are boys.) But such hard-core "juicing," as steroid use is popularly known, has to be viewed in context: supplements of all kinds have become absolutely commonplace in high school locker rooms. In Lodi, California, the *News-Sentinel* conducted a survey of high school football players and found that forty-one out of seventy-three, or 56 percent, had used some type of supplement. Gary I. Wadler, MD, a member of the World Anti-Doping Agency's Prohibited List and Methods Committee and lead author of the book *Drugs and the Athlete,* blames DSHEA and the marketing blitz it engendered for fostering the perception among teen athletes that they need supplements to compete. "DSHEA created the mindset that you needed a pill, a powder, or a potion to be competitive, to be healthy, and without a pill you were lacking," he says. An example of such marketing messages can be seen on bodybuilding.com: "Creatine is bodybuilding's ultimate supplement, and for good reason. For one thing, creatine can significantly increase lean muscle mass in just two weeks. It is also responsible for improving performance in high-intensity exercise, increasing energy levels, and speeding up recovery rates. It's no wonder athletes who use it have such of an edge over those who do not. Soon nearly every athlete who competes will use it (if they don't already)."

High school coaches have also come under fire lately for not only recommending supplements but also selling them to students. Michigan, Illinois, and Texas had all banned coaches from promoting supplements when Governor Arnold Schwarzenegger vetoed a similar measure in California in 2004, saying the bill was too vague in defining supplements. But the next year it was revealed that the former Mr. Universe and Mr. Olympia had taken a second job, in addition to being governor: American Media had agreed to pay him more than $8 million over five years to serve as a consultant and columnist for two of its magazines, *Flex* and *Muscle & Fitness,* both of which are chock-full of supplement advertisements. After denying that the veto had had anything to do with the deal, Schwarzenegger announced on July 15, 2005, that he was severing his ties to the magazines. Three months later, on October 7, he signed a bill requiring student athletes to sign a pledge against using supplements, banning companies from promoting them at sporting events, and requiring coaches to take a course about steroids and supplements.

Jackie Speier, the Democratic state legislator who introduced both bills and had previously fought for years to see a state ban on ephedra passed, says she has made few political friends, and many enemies, by fighting against the supplement industry. "The only people who are concerned about supplements are the people who have had adverse events, or the family members of those who have died," she says. "But protecting the health and safety of the public is our number one charge as legislators, and I don't think that allowing our children to be guinea pigs is protecting their health and safety."

○ ○ ○

The vulnerability of children and teens stems in part from the messages passed down to them by their parents, and women in particular have been the focus of intense marketing campaigns by supplement manufacturers in recent years. They are, after all, 60 percent more likely on average to use supplements than men are, according to the most recent National Health and Nutrition Examination Survey (NHANES). And with the number of menopausal baby boomers rising, in April of 1998 an

Australian company launched a $5 million advertising campaign in the United States for an herbal alternative to estrogen. Promensil, made from red clover, would make "midlife as nature intended," the ads proclaimed in magazines such as *Better Homes and Gardens* and *Martha Stewart Living.* "What time takes away, new Promensil successfully replaces: estrogens. Safe, natural plant estrogens derived from specially cultivated Australian red clover." What the ads failed to disclose was that the maker, Novogen Ltd. (owned in part by a subsidiary of the chemical giant DuPont), had sponsored two studies of Promensil's effects on women, neither of which found any benefit. But other companies were also charging into the market. Enzymatic Therapy, a supplement company out of Wisconsin, spent more than $800,000 in the first three months of 1998 to advertise Remifermin, a product containing another source of plant-based estrogens, black cohosh. And Connecticut-based Amerifit began placing commercials in March of that year on *Wheel of Fortune* and *Live with Regis and Kathie Lee* for Estroven, a supplement containing soy (another source of plant estrogens), black cohosh, and other herbs, vitamins, and minerals.

Concern about the growing numbers of supplements targeted to women led the National Institutes of Health to hold a two-day conference called "Dietary Supplement Use in Women" in January of 2002. According to a report on the meeting coauthored by Paul M. Coates, director of the Office of Dietary Supplements at NIH, "Because of the important developmental milestones (both physiological and behavioral) that occur in women in the period encompassing adolescence through menopause, it is essential that the health care community have a clearer understanding of how diet and nutrition may interact and affect developmental processes. Little is known about the interaction between the use of the broad range of dietary supplements and health outcomes in women throughout these critical periods of development. Such knowledge is essential to the evaluation of both the justification and safety of dietary supplements [use] by women."

Six months later, in July of 2002, researchers with the Women's Health Initiative reported that hormone replacement therapy, taken by millions of postmenopausal women, appeared to actually raise the risk of breast cancer, strokes, and heart attacks. Within days, the supplement industry was off and running with advertisements and promotions for red clover, black cohosh, and other natural alternatives. At that November's meeting of the North American Menopause Society, Novogen offered doctors $1,000 to attend an informational session on Promensil. By year's end, sales of black cohosh alone had soared to $59 million, up more than 500 percent over 1998, according to *Nutrition Business Journal*.

Sales have continued climbing in the new millennium, even as the evidence that such products are neither safe nor effective has grown. A 2002 review in the *Annals of Internal Medicine* noted, "Two trials have shown that red clover has no benefit for treating hot flashes." In July 2003, the *Journal of the American Medical Association* published the results of a randomized, double-blind, placebo-controlled trial of Promensil and another red clover supplement, Rimostil. "Neither supplement had a clinically important effect on hot flashes or other symptoms of menopause," the study concluded. In April of 2003, Yale researchers reported that women taking black cohosh who were undergoing chemotherapy for breast cancer experienced increased toxicity. That October, a University of Chicago doctor reported on a fifty-seven-year-old woman who developed hepatitis after taking black cohosh for three weeks. Three similar cases have been reported in Australia. In July of 2004, the *Journal of the American Medical Association* published a double-blind, randomized trial of 202 postmenopausal women given either soy protein powder to mix with their foods or an identical-looking placebo. The study found none of the effects—neither sharper minds, stronger bones, nor lower blood fats—for which soy powder had been touted as a supplement for postmenopausal women. And as with black cohosh, the safety of soy supplements is also a concern. "Taking large amounts of soy protein, as found in most soy pills or powders, could have effects on cancer risk that are not yet certain," states the American Cancer Society.

Susan Cruzan, a spokesperson for the FDA, cautions women to consider all plant-based estrogens as having the same risks of prescription versions "until research shows otherwise. We're asking manufacturers to do further studies. Until we have that information, women who use any of these products should work with their doctors to use the lowest effective dose for the shortest duration of time." Yet dietary supplement companies continue marketing such products with fervor, leading both the FDA and the FTC to send warning letters to the operators of thirty-four Web sites selling natural alternatives to hormone replacement therapy. The letters noted, "The FTC staff is not aware of any competent and reliable scientific evidence to support claims that the types of products advertised could prevent, treat, or cure cancer, heart disease, or other diseases, prevent osteoporosis, or increase bone density."

⊂⊃ ⊂⊃ ⊂⊃

Children and menopausal women are not the only vulnerable groups the supplement industry targets. Indeed, as much as the industry would have us believe that use of their products is associated with glowing health and vitality, no one takes them at higher rates than do the seriously ill. A survey published in the December 2004 *Journal of Clinical Oncology* found that of 102 patients with advanced cancer who were participating in studies of experimental chemotherapy agents at the Mayo Clinic in Rochester, Minnesota, 84—or 82 percent—were taking some kind of self-prescribed dietary supplement. Some of those supplements, the Mayo team noted, might "interact with investigational agents and affect adverse effects and/or efficacy."

Doctors and pharmacists in hospitals across the United States have been slowly learning just how difficult it is to get patients to tell them when they're taking supplements. "We find pregnant women and nursing mothers taking these things all the time, but often they don't want to tell us," says Catherine Ulbricht, PharmD, a senior attending pharmacist at Massachusetts General Hospital in Boston.

An example of the dangers facing other patients with health challenges occurred in late November of 1998, when a twenty-nine-year-old woman who had received a kidney-pancreas transplant four years earlier began taking St. John's wort to improve her mood. Assuming it was safe, she didn't tell her doctors at the University of Arkansas in Little Rock. By Christmas, a blood test showed that her level of cyclosporine, a common anti-rejection drug she was taking, had fallen to about half of its previous level. When questioned, she insisted that she was taking her cyclosporine as usual and was taking no other new drugs. By mid-January, her blood level of cyclosporine had fallen even further, measures of her kidney and pancreas function worsened, and she began feeling pain over the site of her pancreas transplant—all signs of acute transplant rejection. Only then did she finally think to tell her doctors that she was taking St. John's wort. They told her to stop taking it, raised her level of cyclosporine, and took other measures to regain the transplant's health. But nothing worked. By January of 2000, the rejection was considered permanent. By the time the Arkansas doctors published a report of her case in 2001, dozens of other cases of kidney transplant patients whose cyclosporine levels had fallen to dangerously low levels after taking St. John's wort had been reported. The herb has also been found to seriously interfere with the body's use of digoxin (used for treating heart failure), the anti-HIV drug indinavir, and certain anti-cancer drugs.

While many physicians today have come to be accepting, even supportive, of patients who take supplements in addition to their prescribed medicines, so long as they do so in consultation with their health-care providers, worries remain about those who refuse standard care altogether. Johannes Wolf, MD, professor of pediatrics at the University of Texas M. D. Anderson Cancer Center in Houston, estimates that about 5 percent of parents now refuse standard cancer care for their children in favor of alternative therapies. "If you put in a lot of time explaining and discussing it with the parents, most of them will turn around and follow scientifically evaluated treatments," Dr. Wolf says. "But not all of them. Normally they'll come back a week later, and we can turn them around. There are cases, though, where it is fatal."

Writing in Salon.com in 2002, the author Peter Kurth told of two friends, both infected with HIV, who had "dropped dead of heart attacks after embarking on healthful, 'life-enhancing' diet and exercise regimes," rather than taking their prescribed antiretroviral medications. In doing so, they had been following the kinds of recommendations made by Gary Null, the author, lecturer, and radio broadcaster who advocates alternative remedies and whose book, *AIDS: A Second Opinion* (Seven Stories Press, 2001), asserts that the disease is not caused by HIV and is actually made worse, not better, by taking antiretroviral drugs. Having seen his friends die after following such advice, Kurth calls Null's book "irresponsible" and writes, "Null's blithe disregard of the evidence seems less blinkered than criminal."

Similar concerns about the effects of ignoring standard medical care in favor of supplements were described on the afternoon of June 8, 2004, moments before Senator George V. Voinovich, Republican of Ohio, adjourned a hearing on the decade-long aftermath of DSHEA. "I am personally very concerned about this," he said, "because I had a brother who took all kinds of dietary supplements and kept urging them upon me. He died from a massive stroke two years ago. I am not saying these supplements caused his stroke, but there is reason to be concerned. I think there are a lot of Americans out there that for one reason or another think that these pills are going to be the thing that is going to keep them going, and they really are not."

Examples of tragedies occurring after people switched from standard medical therapy to natural supplements have been popping up in the news with increasing frequency. Debbie Benson, a nurse in Portland, Oregon, refused radiation or chemotherapy for her breast cancer, seeking acupuncture, homeopathy, herbs, and a special diet instead, and died fourteen months later, on July 15, 1997. Lucille Craven of Pelham, New Hampshire, refused surgery for her breast cancer, taking natural remedies instead, and died two and a half years later, just short of her fifty-fifth birthday. Sixteen-year-old Megan Wilson was brought by her mother to a naturopath for treatment of an asthma attack on July 25, 2001, and after receiving acupuncture, an injection of vitamin B_{12}, and an herbal remedy, died later that day. Charlene Dorcy, a schizophrenic, followed her husband's advice to switch from her antipsychotic drug to St. John's wort, after which she ended up shooting and killing her two young daughters on June 12, 2004. And twenty-three-year-old Jeanette Sliwinski, who suffered from severe manic depression, likewise gave up her antipsychotic medications for herbs and ended up so depressed, agitated, and suicidal that on July 13, 2005, she plowed her car into another carrying three men in Skokie, Illinois, killing them all.

◯ ◯ ◯

In September of 2001, the Senate Special Committee on Aging convened a hearing called "Swindlers, Hucksters, and Snake Oil Salesmen: The Hype and Hope of Marketing Anti-Aging Products to Seniors." According to NHANES, people aged sixty and older are 2.7 times (or 270 percent) more likely to use supplements than are those in their twenties and thirties. Howard Beales, director of the Bureau of Consumer Protection at the Federal Trade Commission, testified that "the elderly are particularly vulnerable because of the high incidence of health-related problems in [their] age group." Dennis M. Lormel, chief of the Financial Crimes section of the FBI, said that the bureau "has identified elder fraud and fraud against those suffering from serious illness as two of the most insidious of all white collar crimes being perpetrated by today's modern and high-tech con man. These schemes target those who are most concerned about reversing the effects of aging, the elderly."

One of the ailments of aging that has been well targeted by supplement manufacturers is the so-called senior moment. Ginkgo biloba, marketed to improve mental sharpness, is the third most popular herb in America today, used by 3.9 percent of adults and generating $130 million in sales in 2003. Back in 1999, Bayer began airing television commercials featuring the actress Annie Potts pitching a new formula of One-A-Day vitamins with added ginkgo. About the same time, the actor Hector Elizondo appeared in commercials for another gingko supplement, Quanterra Mental Sharpness Product. Yet in August of 2002, the *Journal of the American Medical Association* published a study involving 230 men and women aged sixty and over to see whether ginkgo performed as advertised. After six weeks, those taking the ginkgo performed no better on tests of memory, learning, attentiveness, or other signs of mental sharpness than those taking a placebo. In 2005, the *Journal of Arthroplasty* reported a case of a patient whose wound kept bleeding following a total hip replacement. When it was discovered he was taking ginkgo, which acts as an anticoagulant, he was asked to go off it and the bleeding finally ended. That same year, ConsumerLab.com reported that of thirteen ginkgo supplements it had tested, only six had passed for having the expected compounds, and that three had high levels of lead. In response, two of the companies whose ginkgo products failed the tests, Jarrow Formulas and Olympian Labs, told *Vitamin Retailer* that they had recalled their products from store shelves.

Insomnia, another perennial problem of the elderly, is the supposed reason for taking melatonin, one of the most peculiar supplements on the market today. Neither an herb, a vitamin, nor a mineral, melatonin is actually a hormone (like insulin, testosterone, and thyroid hormone). Yet rather than being sold as a drug, it is for reasons that defy logic and prudence sold as a supplement. And as such, it accounted for $67 million in sales in 2004, an increase of 7 percent from the year before, according to *Nutrition Business Journal.* In November of 2004, the U.S. Agency for Healthcare Research and Quality published a review of all the available scientific studies of melatonin's effect on sleep disorders. It concluded that melatonin does not make people sleep longer or allow them to wake up feeling more rested. It does not improve sleep quality, and offers no benefit for people battling jet lag or shift work. The only possible benefit, AHRQ found, was that in people who have trouble falling asleep, it might help them reach dreamland about ten minutes sooner. But, on average, they'll wake up that much sooner in the morning, suggesting that the supplement is simply giving a slight phase-shifting nudge to the sleep-wake cycle. Even that limited finding, however, is based on just two studies involving a total of fewer than twenty-five participants.

The agency concluded that melatonin was safe, at least when taken for no more than a few days or weeks. But in recent years, no supplement tracked by U.S. poison centers has seen a faster rise in reported reactions than melatonin has, from just 51 in 2001, of which 22 required hospitalization, to 1,705 in 2004, of which 415 required hospitalization. Reported side effects have included seizures, hallucinations, paranoia, dizziness, and decreased effectiveness of blood-thinning medications. Another possible concern is that melatonin, being a naturally occurring brain hormone, is often obtained from the pineal gland of beef cattle—cow brains, that is—and therefore poses at least a theoretical risk of transmitting mad cow disease. The synthetic version of melatonin carries no such risk, but then, one has to wonder how a synthesized brain hormone ever wound up being sold as a "dietary supplement" in the first place.

Of course, no one is forcing the elderly to ingest cow brains, or making cancer patients take strange plants and potions. How is it, then, that the most vulnerable members of our society have gotten in so deep? With no government authority or prominent medical group recommending that otherwise healthy children receive vitamins, why do so many parents give them to their kids anyway? Why do we believe?

CHAPTER 9

SHARK BAIT

6 *0 Minutes,* **the most honored news show** in television history, virtually created the market for shark cartilage overnight on February 28, 1993, when it broadcast a segment entitled "Sharks Don't Get Cancer." Mike Wallace introduced the nation to Bill Lane, a Florida businessman then in his sixties who just happened to own a shark fishing company when he came to believe, as Wallace said, that there was "something in the cartilage of a shark that stops cancer tumors from growing, growing in sharks and in humans." In an interview that Lane gave years later, he said that immediately following the show's airing, "There were thirty new [shark cartilage] products on the market in about two weeks." A market that had hardly existed before the *60 Minutes* segment aired had ballooned into a $30-million-a-year business two years later, and by the late 1990s, surveys found that more than 25 percent of some cancer patients were using the supplement.

Lane, who held a PhD in biochemistry but had spent his life as an executive in the fishing industry, had authored a book titled *Sharks Don't Get Cancer*, and when *60 Minutes* caught up with him was working as a consultant to one of the few companies trying to sell shark cartilage supplements to a skeptical public. His interest in the field had begun ten years earlier when he saw a CNN broadcast about research being conducted by the famed Judah Folkman, MD, chief of surgery at Boston Children's Hospital. Dr. Folkman had found that a bit of cartilage taken from either cows or sharks would, when surgically placed next to a tiny implanted tumor, prevent it from growing. It would take years of further research for Dr. Folkman to begin figuring out what it was in the cartilage that thwarted the growth of tumors, but just from seeing the segment on CNN, Lane was off and running. He became convinced that taking pulverized shark cartilage by mouth could prevent cancer, even though shark cartilage, like all other cartilage, is made of proteins that are broken down by digestion in the stomach—just as insulin would be broken down and become useless if taken by mouth rather than injected.

To support his theory, Lane found studies suggesting that sharks rarely developed cancer, but failed to uncover the forty reports of tumors in sharks and their close relatives on file in the National Cancer Institute's Registry of Tumors in Lower Animals. Nevertheless, he succeeded in persuading Belgian researchers to test his pulverized shark cartilage on animals. Although Lane would later insist in his book that the results were positive, the Belgian researchers decided not to seek publication in a scientific journal because, they later told *60 Minutes,* the results were not significant. Even so, Lane next got doctors in Mexico to test shark cartilage on terminal cancer patients. Then he persuaded Cuban officials to try it in a small study involving twenty-nine terminally ill cancer patients who had nothing to lose.

That's where *60 Minutes* came in. Wallace and his crew accompanied Lane and a doctor he brought along to see how the Cuban patients were doing. Lieutenant Jose Menendez, the Cuban official in charge of the study, told Wallace on air, "I am prepared to show the evidence of my data."

Asked by Wallace whether the study was showing "extraordinary results" (Wallace's words), the Cuban lieutenant interrupted the question three times to say "yes," "mm-hmm," and "yes," only to add, "We are getting results. We are trying to emphasize that we are not talking about cancer cure." In fact, of the twenty-nine patients who began the study, only three showed what Wallace called "signs of progress." When Wallace showed the results to the former chief of radiation oncology at the National Cancer Institute, he commented, "I can't say that I'm totally ex-

cited about it," but agreed that the preliminary results were worth further investigation. Even the doctor whom Lane had brought along to review the Cuban study—Dr. Charles Simone, an oncologist who had once
done research at the National Cancer Institute—cautioned Wallace that
while shark cartilage merited further research, "You can't put a green
light out for millions of patients to do this. You need—you need to work
within the structured community. That's very important."

"So you don't go to the nearest health food store and—and get shark
cartilage," Wallace said.

"I think if you do it on your own," Dr. Simone replied, "you'll get in
trouble."

But, of course, that is precisely what cancer patients did, because unlike experimental cancer drugs put through years of careful study before
going on the market, shark cartilage was already being sold by the company Lane consulted with. As other companies quickly entered the market, Lane's son, Andrew, founded Lane Labs–USA to sell a product called
BeneFin, as well as other products said to be effective against HIV and
skin cancer.

With so many cancer patients now taking shark cartilage, legitimate
researchers began conducting well-designed studies. A 1998 study of
sixty patients with a variety of advanced cancers found no benefit, and a
Danish study of seventeen breast cancer patients came to the same conclusion. Even so, NCI and the National Center for Complementary and
Alternative Medicine took the surprising step of approving two further
studies of shark cartilage. The reasons had less to do with scientific merit,
said Dr. Jeffrey White of NCI, than with "the tremendous utilization by
cancer patients." The larger of the two studies, costing more than $1 mil-
lion of taxpayer money, was to be carried out by Charles L. Loprinzi, MD,
of the Mayo Clinic. He and a team of thirteen researchers from nine in-
stitutions across the country planned to study the effects of BeneFin,
made by Lane Labs, on 600 breast and colorectal cancer patients considered otherwise incurable.

But even as its product was finally undergoing rigorous study, Lane
Labs was using marketing materials claiming that BeneFin could cure
cancer, in plain violation of DSHEA. The FDA warned the company to
tone down its marketing, and when it didn't, the FTC charged it with
making unsubstantiated claims. The company agreed to a $1 million set-

tlement, but kept on distributing brochures and newsletters that made cancer cure claims nevertheless. Finally, on Friday, July 9, 2004, after years of exhaustive investigations and court hearings, the U.S. district judge William Bassler got fed up with the company and ordered it to destroy its inventory (except for a small amount for research purposes), to never again sell BeneFin, and to refund money to anyone who had purchased BeneFin in the previous five years.

But Dr. Loprinzi's study continued, and on November 19, 2004, he reported his results at a complementary medicine meeting in New York that received almost no media coverage. Because the BeneFin powder had a recognizable smell and taste, Dr. Loprinzi reported, he had taken the trouble of making the placebo similarly fishy. Patients were asked to drink a chilled beverage containing the powder thirty minutes before a meal, three or four times each day. One month after enrolling only 83 of the planned 600 patients, half of the patients dropped out, in part because of the "very fishy smell that you could detect across the room." Concerned about the patients' responses, he decided to check the results so far to see if there was any point in continuing. It turned out there was not. On the basis of the limited number of patients, he found no difference in survival between the patients given BeneFin over those given the placebo. However, Dr. Loprinzi noted, "There was a statistically and clinically significant decrease in quality of life at one month for patients receiving the shark cartilage, compared to those taking placebo." Innocent people dying of cancer, in other words, had spent what for many was the last month of their life drinking a disgusting, fishy drink for which there had never been any good scientific evidence of a likely benefit.

Yet shark cartilage continues to be sold in drugstores and on Internet sites to this day, including on the Web site of Lane Labs. Although permanently banned from selling BeneFin, the company was permitted to sell shark cartilage under another name, so long as it made no unsubstantiated claims or compared it to BeneFin. The company has so far toed the line, boasting only of its "trusted ingredients, integrity, and clinical support." But other Web sites are under no such obligation, and so Vitaminproshop.com, for instance, sells Lane Labs' shark cartilage as "formely [sic] known as BeneFin." And old articles written by Bill Lane, in which he boasted of his appearance on *60 Minutes,* remain posted on other sites.

⊂⊃ ⊂⊃ ⊂⊃

60 Minutes is hardly the only media outlet to have misspent its credibility on supplement manufacturers. For much of the 1990s, glowing reports based on preliminary research filled even the most prestigious newspapers, magazines, and network newscasts. On January 20, 1997, the *Wall Street Journal* ran a page-one story titled, "Echinacea: Does It Cure What Ails Ya? Indians Thought So—Many People Believe It Helps Stave Off Colds and Flu; Neighbors Recommend It." That May, *Newsweek* ran a story about St. John's wort under the headline "A Natural Mood Booster." A month later, the ABC news show *20/20* ran a feature on St. John's wort introduced by co-host Hugh Downs. "Well, now a truly startling medical breakthrough—one that could affect millions of people who suffer from mild depression," Downs began. "Right now, many of them are treated with drugs like Prozac. But there may be a better way. Researchers say an amazing herb is proving to be safer, cheaper, and just as effective as prescription drugs in treating depression. Traditional medicine is slowly holding out a hand to some alternative therapies." When the segment concluded, Barbara Walters said, "This is awfully important and very good to hear about." Hugh Downs added lightheartedly, "I've written the name down. There are days." That November, *Newsweek* ran another article, entitled "Brain Boosters," highlighting the supposed ability of ginkgo biloba to improve mental sharpness. The next month, the venerable *Reader's Digest* ran a story about St. John's wort, echinacea, zinc, and other supplements under the banner "Herbs That Heal." On November 9, 1998, *Time* got into the act with a story about kava, entitled "The Root of Tranquility." Two weeks later, *Time* ran a cover story called "The Herbal Medicine Boom."

Mitchell Balbert, president of Natrol Inc., one of the country's larger supplement manufacturers, said the effects of such news coverage could not have been more dramatic. "When Barbara Walters [said], 'Oh my goodness, this is absolutely remarkable,' that was the event that turned that product," he said. "All of a sudden you had a market that emerged overnight. Our company in 1998 did $12 million in out-the-door sales of St. John's wort." Industry-wide, sales of St. John's wort took a meteoric ride from a mere $10 million nationwide in 1995 to a staggering $305 million in 1998, according to *Nutrition Business Journal*. But the effects went far beyond St. John's wort, Balbert said. "In the second half of the nineties, the industry grew due to the dramatic stories that were published in *Time* magazine, *Newsweek* magazine, *20/20*. There were sensational stories about ginkgo biloba, DHEA, melatonin, St. John's wort, echinacea. You couldn't pick up a newspaper without finding a favorable story. Because of the belief that was propagated by the favorable media, dozens and dozens of companies entered the business, and the mass market embraced the philosophy. If you read *Mass Marketing News* in those days, the VMHS [vitamin-mineral-herbal supplement] segment was the number one growth area. It really was the golden child."

The direct effect that positive news reports can have on consumers' purchases of supplements was seen in a national survey conducted in 1996 by Opinion Research Corporation for Leiner Health Products, a large supplement maker. The survey asked 1,008 adults what factor would make them decide to take an herbal supplement. A physician's recommendation was cited by 66 percent of the respondents, more than any other factor. But the next most influential source was "news coverage discussing herbal supplement benefits," cited by 26 percent of those surveyed—far more than the 15 percent who said they would be influenced by their friends' use of herbs.

Of course, news stories about preliminary research are a staple of medical journalism, and rightly so: they make for provocative reading and keep people abreast of what's happening in the research world. And virtually all the major media outlets, including *60 Minutes* and *20/20*, always made a point of peppering their reports with cautions about the lack of scientific certainty. In other words, journalists were doing nothing different in their coverage of supplements than they did in their coverage of ordinary drugs.

But that was the problem. When an emerging drug is the subject of a news report, consumers can't rush out and expose themselves to the potential dangers of taking it until large studies involving thousands of patients have been carefully reviewed by independent scientists and the FDA—a hurdle that most drugs will never clear. In the double-standard world created by DSHEA, however, positive news reports on preliminary research involving a supplement are almost guaranteed to send consumers shopping, and manufacturers advertising. "As seen on *20/20*," boasts an Internet ad for Hot Plants for Him, which supposedly "supports healthy sexual drive." Another site for a weight-loss supplement has gone so far as to take the URL of today-show-hoodia.1effects.info and boasting on its main page, "Hoodia Gordonii featured on the *Today Show* on NBC, October 24." In fact, a search for the generic terms "as seen on" and "dietary supplement" brings up 155,000 results on Google. As a result of such widespread practices, many journalists have unwittingly become the sock puppets of supplement manufacturers. Positive news reports, after all, are the industry's lifeblood, giving them the credibility they crave. By devoting airtime and page space to preliminary studies of supplements that "may" curb cancer, "may" prevent heart disease, and "may" be safe, the media has given consumers a powerful basis for believing in and buying the stuff.

◯ ▭ ◖

But news coverage is only one way that supplement marketers have been able to sway the average consumer in recent years. Another means toward this end is seen in the industry's pervasive use of misleading and downright illegal advertisements, particularly on the Internet, cable television, and talk radio. "For several years, supplement advertising has been one of our top enforcement priorities," says Richard Cleland, assistant director of the Division of Advertising Practices at the FTC. "We've probably taken more actions in this one area than in any other. We're a little frustrated when we see these ads keep popping up. There are many thousands of products out there, and we're not in a position to evaluate every single one of those claims. There have been changes in technology that have really aggravated or facilitated the problem. Virtually anyone can become a national marketer these days. Since 1999, we've sent out a thousand advisory letters to companies operating on the Internet selling products as cures for serious diseases. A lot of them had no clue there were even government regulations that applied to the products they sell."

Infomercials for a weight-loss supplement, Cleland says, can rake in as much as $100 million in sales revenue a year. Perhaps it should not be surprising, then, that between February 2004 and January 2005, the FDA and FTC took at least thirty-five separate actions against manufacturers for making illegal and deceptive claims for products like Carb Zapper, Extreme Carb Blocker, Super Starch Blocker 1000, and Ultra Carbo Blocker 2000. One of the most ubiquitous infomercials was for CortiSlim, which claimed it could cause rapid, substantial, and permanent weight loss, and that fifteen years of evidence proved that its ingredients blocked the body's release of the hormone cortisol, the cause of "every modern lifestyle disease that is associated with this fast-paced twenty-first-century lifestyle." On October 19, 2004, the FTC announced that the makers of CortiSlim had signed a stipulated interim agreement to stop making such false claims. Yet to this day, the product remains an unavoidable presence on cable television, its commercials having been only slightly tweaked to avoid the most outrageous claims that got it in trouble with the FTC.

Enzyte has been another heavy advertiser. Its early commercials described it as "the first all-natural male enhancement program that adds one to three inches to your size in just eight months or get double your money back," with "100% Safe with a 98.3% Success Rate" flashing on the screen. Its manufacturer, Berkeley Premium Nutraceuticals, was founded in a suburb of Cincinnati in 2001 by a former hockey rink advertising salesman; by 2003 it was pulling in $100 million per year, sponsoring NASCAR drivers, and forecasting sales of $260 million in the coming year. As its claims drew the scrutiny of the FTC, however, its advertisements began using a "Smiling Bob" character and switched to vaguer claims, even conceding that the product will not change the shape or size of the penis while still claiming that Enzyte could achieve "fuller, firmer, better-quality erections." In March of 2004, a class-action suit was filed against the company by a Dayton, Ohio, man who alleged that the company "continues to engage in unfair, deceptive, and fraudulent promotions and advertising by propagating a claim of 'male enhancement' that is no less fraudulent than its former, explicit claim of penis enlargement." Six months later, the Center for Science in the Public Interest filed a complaint with the FTC. "The FTC requires that advertising claims for dietary supplements, including those based on testimonials of users, 'be backed by sound, scientific evidence,'" the complaint stated. "Berkely, however, has conceded that it has no scientific studies of Enzyte substantiating any of Berkeley's claims." None of the sixteen ingredients listed on its label, including gingko, ginseng, saw palmetto, or the evocatively named "horny goat weed extract" has ever been shown to increase penis size or improve erections. In January of 2006, four of the company's former executives pleaded guilty to charges of conspiracy to defraud consumers of some $100 million of supplements they never ordered. That same month, the FTC charged the company with making false claims and improper billing. Yet Enzyte and "Smiling Bob" remain in business.

Arguably more persuasive than either advertisements or news reports, however, is the hybrid of the two, in the form of paid personal testimonials made by senior newsmen such as Larry King and Paul Harvey. While it's one thing for media figures to put their reputations, and that of their news networks, on the line for a vacuum cleaner, it is difficult to see the justification for endorsements of unproved supplements. By buying the endorsements of newsmen known and trusted by millions, the marketers cleverly co-opt the credibility of the news media itself, lending a veneer of legitimacy to their products and playing a game of "respectability by association" that has deceived even the savviest of buyers.

CNN's King, for instance, has said that coral calcium "has changed [his] life and could change yours." He has come in for particular drubbing by the Center for Science in the Public Interest for the advertisements he does for Ester-C, a brand of the vitamin that includes calcium ascorbate and other ingredients. The manufacturer claims to have performed a study showing that Ester-C is better absorbed than other vitamin C products, but has not published it in a peer-reviewed journal. Of published studies, one found the ingredients in Ester-C to be better than ordinary vitamin C at relieving scurvy in rats, but another study found no difference between the two in dogs, and a test tube study from Norway concluded: "No differences were observed when ordinary ascorbic acid and Ester-C, a commercial vitamin C product, were compared." The Center for Science in the Public Interest calls Ester-C "an overhyped brand of vitamin C that is twice as expensive as regular vitamin C." Commercials for another product pitched by King, Garlique, have been seen or heard by 98 percent of U.S. adults, according to its manufacturer. The label of Garlique claims that it "supports cardiovascular health." But a 1998 study in the *Journal of the American Medical Association* found that garlic extract has no effect on cholesterol. In October of 2000, the Agency for Healthcare Review and Quality concluded, "Garlic preparation may have small, positive, short-term effects on lipids; whether effects are sustainable beyond three months is unclear." No well-designed study has ever been published showing that garlic reduces deaths or heart attacks, and the agency found no consistent evidence for its ability to lower blood pressure or blood-sugar levels. Then again, the agency noted: "Multiple adverse effects, including smelly breath and body odor, dermatitis, bleeding, abdominal symptoms, and flatulence, have been reported." David Schardt, a senior nutritionist at CSPI, commented, "Either Larry King has a knack for picking weak products to pitch, or manufacturers seek him out to lend credibility to supplements that could use some."

Longtime ABC Radio newsman Paul Harvey, famous for his daily spots featuring the closing line "And now you know the rest of the story," has for years done advertisements for Premier Formula for Ocular Nutrition. Although Harvey doesn't say that he uses the product, his years of reading commercials for it certainly creates the impression of a personal endorsement. The manufacturer originally claimed that Premier Formula for Ocular Nutrition could restore vision lost from age-related macular degeneration and eliminate "floaters" (small specks in the field of vision). But on February 15, 2005, the maker settled charges by the FTC that these were unsubstantiated advertising claims and agreed to stop making those claims and pay the FTC $450,000. Nevertheless, Harvey has since kept right on reading the new advertisements.

To this day, no radio or cable television station has ever suffered a sanction due to airing the misleading commercials from which it profits. No newscaster has either. But perhaps a few of them should. As the FTC commissioner Pamela Jones Harbour said in a speech on February 28, 2005, before a group of direct-response marketing executives: "Media outlets should be responsible for not running false advertising. They should demand substantiation for the claims they allow to run on their air, and if they don't, the media should be called to account by consumers."

The selling of supplements gets up close and personal through multilevel marketing, or MLM, the Amway-style approach in which the company sells products to large district distributors, who turn around and sell them for a piece of the action to smaller district distributors, who do the same to even smaller distributors, and so on down the line until every-body's Aunt Tilly is selling it to her friends on the block. MLM has been a boon to supplement companies because individual distributors can make dramatic personal claims about their products to customers while talking in their living rooms or on the telephone. Best of all from the companies' point of view, the FDA and FTC are none the wiser if Aunt Tilly steps over the line to essentially practice medicine without a license by pitching the products as cures for illnesses—not that the companies (big money) would ever officially condone such practices (big money) in their official literature or training (big money).

When it comes to MLM, no supplement company has done better than Herbalife, founded in 1980 by Mark Hughes, a high school dropout who spent much of his teens in an institution for troubled youth. Badges em-blazoned with the company's "Lose weight now, ask me how" motto be-came a ubiquitous sight on the lapels of distributors in the mid-1980s. Even after Hughes's death in May 2002 due to an accidental overdose of alcohol and drugs, Herbalife has continued to grow, reporting record net sales in the third quarter of 2005 of $401 million, with a market capital-ization of $2.37 billion.

Having settled a suit brought by the state of California for making "un-true or misleading" claims, as well as suits brought by customers injured after taking its original weight-loss formula that contained ephedra, Herbalife is now promoting a new product, Niteworks. The "key benefits" of Niteworks, the company claims on its Web site, is that it "keeps blood vessels toned, flexible and youthful for improved circulation"; "helps to support healthy blood pressure levels already within the normal range"; "supports energy, circulatory and vascular health"; and "enhances blood flow, which ensures blood efficiently nourishes the heart and tissues of the entire body." Prominently displayed on the label is the signature of Louis Ignarro, PhD, who shared the 1998 Nobel Prize in medicine for re-search into nitric acid's beneficial role in relaxing blood vessels, and who is credited with developing the product. Niteworks contains the amino acid L-arginine, which Ignarro believes the body converts to nitric oxide (unproved); L-citrulline, which he believes the body recycles into argi-nine (also unproved); as well as vitamins A and C, which he believes pro-tect against the body's oxidation of nitric oxide (likewise unproved). Indeed, only one study—in mice—has shown that L-arginine and vitamins A and C benefit the heart vessels. "You can't assume it will work in people," Marcia Angell, MD, former editor of the *New England Journal of Medicine,* told Bloomberg News, a business news service. And Robert Furchgott, PhD, the pharmacologist who shared Ignarro's Nobel, told Bloomberg, "I haven't seen any properly controlled studies. It just seems to me a mouse model isn't transferable to humans. I think with the sort of money they're raking in, they could have done some human studies." Furchgott also told Bloomberg that he regrets Ignarro's association with an unproved supplement that has been linked to their shared prize. "That's sad," he said. "Sometimes I get angry. Right now, I'm just sorry." L-arginine, it should be pointed out, was found in a study in the *Journal of the American Medical Association* to have no benefit for heart attack survivors. But of course, Aunt Tilly doesn't have to mention such pesky facts when she sells Niteworks to her friends and family. As a result, business at Herbalife is booming, due in part to the $89.95 price for a thirty-day supply of Niteworks. With such bright financial prospects based on opinions rather than facts, perhaps it shouldn't be surprising that Herbalife's two top executives—Michael Johnson, CEO, and Greg Probert, president and COO—were both brought over from another company that specializes in make-believe, the Walt Disney Company.

But MLM has its limits—Aunt Tilly has only so many friends, after all—and so far more herbs and vitamins are sold in retail stores, where even the loose rules permitted by DSHEA are skirted by retailers whose clerks routinely make claims for products and give medical advice despite strict laws forbidding them from doing so. The consequence of such ill-informed recommendations were dramatized in the case, described in chapter 8, of the mother who was told by a store clerk to give her eighteen-month-old son eucalyptus oil, resulting in the child's permanent brain damage. Although large retailers like Vitamin Shoppe and GNC insist that they train their employees not to give any advice, the difficulty of enforcing such policies was addressed at the Las Vegas meeting of the National Nutritional Foods Association in July 2004. Two speakers— Rakesh Amin, a Chicago attorney, and Jay Jacobowitz, president of a retail consulting firm—attempted to untwist DSHEA's pretzel logic governing what retailers are allowed to say to their customers about the products they sell. "There's the law, and then there's the practical retail experience of interacting with your customers," Jacobowitz said.

After explaining that retailers of supplements cannot prescribe or recommend a particular product for the treatment of any disease or the relief of any symptoms, Amin asked, "How do you get around it? Trust me, these consumers are smart. You have to ask them, 'Have you seen a doctor? Has he diagnosed anything?' Let *them* say it. Sometimes you have to act dumb. 'Do *you* know what you have?' Jay would probably say he has arthritis. If not, I can tell you a way to get the word 'arthritis' out there. 'We have products that help support healthy cartilage and joint function.' Then you take them to a reference area in your store. Without saying 'arthritis,' you point to [an article about] glucosamine. It's going to say 'arthritis' there."

A retailer in the audience raised her hand. "A lot of people ask us to read the third-party literature to them," she said, referring to the books and pamphlets kept in stores' "reference" areas. "They say they didn't bring their reading glasses."

"Technically you can't do it," Amin said. But realistically, he added, "You're not going to get caught."

Despite advice from the likes of Amin and Jacobowitz on how to stay within the letter of DSHEA, most retailers don't even bother to try. Visits to fifteen supplement retailers in ten states during a two-month period in late 2004 revealed that only three of them kept within the provisions of DSHEA by not recommending particular supplements as treatments for diseases. Many did not hesitate to recommend multiple supplements to treat multiple conditions, without a thought to possible interactions or reactions. The responses from a clerk named Rafi at a GNC in Washington, D.C., were typical. Asked if he had anything to lower cholesterol, he said the best treatment was red yeast rice. According to the label, red yeast rice "helps maintain healthy LDL cholesterol levels."

When asked if garlic also promoted lower cholesterol levels, Rafi answered directly, "Garlic just maintains your cholesterol steady. Red yeast rice lowers it forty points."

Asked if he had anything to treat cancer, Rafi walked over to a shelf and pulled out a bottle of Ulta Pycnogenol, containing pycnogenol powder, grape seed extract, and bilberry fruit extract.

Anything for depression?

"SAM-e is best," Rafi said.

What about taking SAM-e and St. John's wort together?

"Yes, you'll have no problem. No problem at all."

What about something for diabetes? Rafi pointed out a stack of boxes labeled Diabetic Nutrition Plan, "for the special dietary needs of diabetics. Helps support normal glucose response. Supports eye and circulatory health."

Finally, Rafi recommended a box of Mega Men, labeled as a "maximum performance formula for men," with fifty-six active ingredients. He also recommended a box of Women's Ultra Mega, likewise containing dozens of ingredients.

"Do you need anything else?" Rafi asked five times at the checkout counter. The final price of all the purchases, after discounts, came to $216.93.

○ ○ ○

The sleek, modern appearance of the leading supplement retailers, as bright and shiny as any Gap or Target, has proved to be another effective sales tool for widening the use of supplements. The Vitamin Shoppe on Route 1 in Woodbridge, New Jersey, located just minutes from where the Garden State Parkway and the New Jersey Turnpike intersect, is typical. On a warm wet night in August of 2004, the first aisle on the right was devoted to non-ephedra versions of weight-loss aids, including Zantrex-3, which claimed on its label that it causes "546% more weight loss than America's #1 selling ephedra based diet pill." In the back, shelves were laden with king-size canisters of protein powder and other supplements aimed at athletes. Against the left wall was a reading area with newsletters and books, including a few by Stephen Holt, MD, a Bill Clinton lookalike who gave up gastroenterology to sell supplements. And up front, near the cash register, was a nearly life-size stand-up cardboard cutout in the shape of former L.A. Laker Earvin "Magic" Johnson, arguably the most famous living person infected with HIV, showing him holding a bottle of something called "My Defense," with his signature and the number of his jersey, 32. "This is My Defense," stated the advertisement for the "immune-enhancing" product sold by Mitchell Balbert's Natrol.

Beyond the specialty retailers, however, a key growth strategy of the industry has been to move out of the "ghetto" of health food and supplement stores to reach the average consumer at pharmacies and discount outlets, where whole aisles are now given over to echinacea, black cohosh, and the like. Candy and cough drops at checkout counters now compete for space with Cold-Eeze and Airborne, with no effort made to alert consumers to their unproved claims. At some CVS pharmacy counters, a thick guide to supplements, the *Natural Health Bible,* is available for shoppers to peruse, offering information that is often outdated, inaccurate, and unbalanced; and during the fall of 2005, CVS even had cardboard display cases at the end of aisles piled with "Dolivaxil Flu Season Defense," a French homeopathic remedy promoted in the store as helping to "stop the flu before it starts" and "formulated to resist the onset of flu symptoms," claims that could be considered dangerously misleading given the availability of proven flu vaccine and the potentially life-threatening risks of the illness among the frail and elderly.

Selling their products at pharmacies in this way accomplishes a key marketing goal for supplement manufacturers: overcoming customers' potential skepticism by placing them in the right context. "We are so much controlled by the context of our environment," says Donald A. Hantula, PhD, a professor of psychology at Temple University in Philadelphia who studies consumer behavior as director of the university's Decision Making Laboratory. "It's sort of like going to see a Disney movie and expecting to see good wholesome entertainment. When you walk into a pharmacy, aside from the Russell Stover candies, you expect to find stuff that's healthy. So when you see dietary supplements there, you expect them to be just more of the good stuff that will make you better."

For all their chic, modern packaging and "breakthrough" research, today's supplement salespeople owe much to the deft strategies first devised by the patent medicine manufacturers of more than a century ago—in fact, so do most companies today. According to the historian James Harvey Young, patent medicine manufacturers were among the first in the history of marketing to spend lavishly on advertising to build brand identity. They were among the first to use "before" and "after" photographs, offer money-back guarantees, and obtain the endorsements of celebrities (including the actors Edwin Booth and Sarah Bernhardt). They also pioneered a host of techniques that remain the special province of supplement manufacturers: they distributed books and pamphlets to explain and offer "proof" of their claims; they boasted of degrees from imaginary or unrecognized universities; and when any new scientific discovery engendered public interest, they jumped on the bandwagon with related products—for example, "radium impregnated" Radol, sold soon after the discovery of radiation by the Curies in 1898 and advertised as a "marvelous radiotized fluid" to cure cancer, or even plain old petroleum, which was marketed soon after its discovery in Pennsylvania as "THE MOST WONDERFUL REMEDY EVER DISCOVERED." In the same way, antioxidants and countless micronutrients are spun into products today and proffered to the public before studies can verify their true worth, or assess their danger.

Another classic strategy used to promote belief in alternative remedies is to sow disbelief and skepticism toward the medical establishment. In one example, described by Young in his book *The Toadstool Millionaires,* a "doctor" in an advertisement was quoted as saying: "BAD-EM SALZ? Yes, I used to prescribe it a great deal, but I stopped. Why? Simply because the patients didn't come back to me. If I had kept on they would all have been taking BAD-EM SALZ and getting well without my assistance!" The title of a recent bestselling book adopts the same conspiratorial strategy: *Natural Cures "They" Don't Want You to Know About.* But who are "they"? The author Kevin Trudeau, who never even attended college, has stated in interviews that "government agencies" and "entire industries" are devoted to keeping people sick. Thus, his lack of credentials as a health professional *are* his credentials, as he boasted to CBS *Early Show* co-host Harry Smith: "I'm not a medical doctor. I state that in the book. That's why I'm qualified to talk about health. Because I'm not a drug pusher. I'm not a pharmaceutical rep." Trudeau has even managed to turn his repeated prosecutions by the FTC, and the condemnation of his book as fraudulent by the New York State Consumer Protection Board, into a weird kind of triumph, evidence that he's the innocent victim of a witch hunt. Arthur Caplan, chair of the Department of Medical Ethics at the University of Pennsylvania, summed up Trudeau's marketing genius this way: "He's anticipated any backlash with his cuckoo conspiracy theory; he's built a firewall around himself."

Another marketing message—one of the industry's most powerful—
came into currency during the 1970s, when the FDA first started trying
to regulate vitamin potencies. The industry then began chanting a new
mantra: "freedom of choice." Let the consumer decide, they said. Big
Brother can't tell us how to live our lives. The message worked then, it
worked even better in the 1990s in support of DSHEA, and it continues
to work now, even among liberals who demand government oversight of
every other industry. But the supplement makers didn't invent the freedom of choice argument; they simply borrowed it from the sellers of automobiles and tires. As John Floberg, secretary and general counsel of the
Firestone Tire and Rubber Company, was quoted as saying back in 1965
in Ralph Nader's *Unsafe at Any Speed:* "I submit that the best standard, the
time-tested and proved standard and the appropriate free enterprise
standard of quality should be the one that has in the case of tires, as in
the case of other consumer products, worked most satisfactorily; namely,
the discriminating and sophisticated taste of the American consumer."
Remarkably, more than four decades after such rhetoric stopped working
for tire makers and car makers resistant to life-saving changes in their design and manufacture, the freedom of choice line remains a potent tool
for the very industry that claims as its raison d'être the health and well-
being of its customers.

◠ ◠ ◠

But why? One cannot really blame the supplement industry, after all, for
doing everything possible to persuade us to buy their products. That's
their job. The really interesting question is why their strategies have
worked on us—why, despite a century of unprecedented accomplish-
ments by science-based medicine, tens of millions of educated professionals who would be outraged if their children's schools stopped
teaching science are now seeking out dietary supplements that, science
tells them, are unproved, disproved, or dangerous. Why are we so eager
to believe?

That question has absorbed Wallace Sampson, MD, for more than
thirty-five years. Back in the early 1970s, Dr. Sampson had a thriving
practice as a cancer specialist in the Santa Clara valley area of California,
not far from San Francisco. One day, a middle-aged aerospace engineer—

a rocket scientist—whom Dr. Sampson was treating for stomach cancer failed to show up for an appointment, never to return. Soon after, a registered nurse and expert bridge player likewise being treated for stomach cancer also stopped showing up for her appointments, without explanation. Then an elderly woman who had breast cancer, and who had suffered a hip fracture that required her to use a walker, also stopped seeing him. Knowing that none of their cancers had been cured under his care, Dr. Sampson asked around to his fellow oncologists in the area, but learned that they weren't seeing any other specialist. It was a mystery—cancer patients don't normally stop showing up for treatment—until one day the nurse with stomach cancer dropped by unannounced to tell Dr. Sampson where she'd been: Tijuana, for treatment with laetrile, a chemical derived from apricot pits, which she insisted had cured her. Not long after, the elderly breast cancer patient came in, threw down her walker, and announced that she too had been cured in Tijuana with laetrile. The rocket scientist too revealed by telephone that he had gone to the same place. All three ended up dying of their cancers soon after, even while insisting that laetrile had extended their lives.

Curious yet cautious, open-minded yet unwilling to be converted without firm evidence, Dr. Sampson arranged to meet in San Francisco with Ernst T. Krebs, Jr., the son of the discoverer of laetrile and, by that time, its chief proponent. He went to lectures, met with patients, flew down to Tijuana, and boned up on his chemistry and statistics, all in an effort to figure out if indeed the stuff really worked. Finally he conducted a small study by interviewing thirty-three patients who had been diagnosed with terminal cancer but had forsaken standard treatments for laetrile. These he compared to twelve deceased patients selected from his files, who were matched for age, sex, and type of cancer. By the end of the study, all thirty-three of the laetrile patients were dead, yet all except one went to their graves convinced that laetrile had benefited them—despite the fact that, on average, they survived a shorter time than the patients who had received standard treatment. "Once I learned the biochemistry and realized it was impossible for laetrile to work," Dr. Sampson recalls, "I asked myself, how come all these people are believing this stuff?" The experience led him to later start, in 1997, the *Scientific Review of Alternative Medicine,* considered by many to be the most rigorous journal devoted to the subject. But the question he posed then continues to challenge academics, consumer advocates, and public health officials today.

There is not one answer to the question, but many—social, psychological, economic, and spiritual. Socially, for better or worse, herbs and vitamins have become part of today's health-conscious upper-class lifestyle that includes organic foods, yoga, red wine, and exercise. The largest organic grocery store chain in the country, Whole Foods, for instance, features a large selection of supplements, even advertising them in large posters on their windows, and nearly every issue of both *Yoga* magazine and *Vegetarian Times* features articles on herbs and other "natural" supplements. The fact that few supplements are actually healthful does not change the fact that they are part of the "healthy" lifestyle, a must-have dietary accessory.

Economically, supplements have come to be seen as a tonic to the influence of drug companies, in much the same way that Apple computers are seen by their ardent users as a shield against the evil empire of Microsoft. Supplements are the antidrug, representing everything that drugs are not. Where drugs are artificial, supplements are natural; where drugs are dangerous, supplements are safe; where drugs are developed by greedy, duplicitous pharmaceutical companies, supplements, at least the herbal ones, are hand-picked by family farmers. At least, that's the idea. And the news that drug companies are hiring former college cheerleaders to work as their sales reps has only further tarnished their bad reputation for unethically showering doctors with gifts, trips, and grants as inducements to prescribe their products. Marcia Angell, MD, the former editor in chief of the *New England Journal of Medicine,* published a withering critique of the $200 billion industry (ten times the size of the supplement business) in her 2004 book, *The Truth About the Drug Companies: How They Deceive Us and What to Do About It* (Random House). She points out that the drug industry has been the most profitable industry in the United States for decades, with prices growing 12 percent per year on average and with far more of its income spent on advertising and marketing than on new drug development. And news that pharmaceutical makers hid the risk of suicide in adolescents taking antidepressants, as well as the risk of heart attacks and strokes in patients taking Vioxx and other prescription painkillers, has only made their image worse. "There's a lot more public mistrust of drugs these days," says Eric Topol, MD, the former chairman of the department of cardiovascular medicine at the Cleveland Clinic, "and the Vioxx thing contributed to that greatly. It was on the market for four and a half years beyond when there was concern about its safety." A poll published in November of 2005 found that only 9 percent of consumers believe that drug makers are basically honest. And the distrust, some believe, is about much more than Vioxx. Much of it may be a backlash against direct-to-consumer commercials, first legalized in the early 1990s, that put prescription drugs on a level with dish detergent and diet sodas. By taking supplements, then, consumers are thumbing their noses at companies they don't believe have their best interests at heart. But the fact that some drugs have been unethically marketed does not change the fact that virtually all supplements are marketed with claims that are almost wholly without merit, and that they may be just as dangerous as prescription drugs.

Psychologically, supplements speak to us on many levels. For one, they give people a sense of control over one's body, far more than do prescription drugs. The very language we use regarding drugs is revealing: "patients" are "compliant" when they take the drugs that doctors have "prescribed." But it's a *person* who pops a supplement every morning, with no intervention from a doctor, pharmacist, or insurer. Doing so is a cheap and easy way to get a momentary burst of feeling in charge of one's life. Moreover, the simplicity and certainty of the assurances made by supplements salespeople feed into a foible of human psychology: a weakness for the sure thing.

"Do you want to hear a mechanic say he doesn't know how long it will take to fix your car, or even *whether* he can fix it?" asks Dr. Hantula of Temple University's Decision Making Laboratory. "Or do you want one who says, 'I'll have it done at five'?" In the same way, people faced with physicians explaining the uncertainties of a possible therapy, or hearing the long list of potential side effects in a drug advertisement, will tend to gravitate toward other products "guaranteed" to be safe and effective, even if that's not really the case. "I had two in-laws who both died of cancer," recalls Dr. Hantula. "At no time did any physician say, 'This is going to cure you.' They would say, 'We're going to try this and we hope it has the following outcomes, but we'll have to monitor and evaluate.' But for most people who are suffering, what do they want to hear? It takes a bit of sophistication to understand that there are no guarantees with any method." Mainstream medicine is also suffering, he says, because its days of grabbing headlines with sudden, clear-cut gains over ancient killers like polio, tuberculosis, diabetes, and whooping cough have given way to progress so slow it's often imperceptible. "A lot of things that were killing people two generations ago are not even an issue anymore," says Dr. Hantula. "The ones we have left are much harder, much trickier, and the solutions are not as grand. It's one thing to say, 'We're going to wipe out polio.' But now we have all of these other health things that plague us, and nobody's standing up to say, 'In two years we're going to wipe out cancer.' We can't. It's too hard. But people really like simple answers. People are impatient with 'We will continue to study the nature of cancer.' They feel like, 'Come on, you should have done that last week.' "

Another psychological factor behind people's faith in supplements—and one that has kept humans believing in all manner of ineffective cures for generations—is a logical fallacy called the illusory correlation. "The common cold, left untreated, gets better in five days to a week even if you do nothing," explains Dr. Hantula. "It's going to run its course. But if you take echinacea, you'll also get better. The problem is, your mind thinks that because you engaged in an action and you got the result, the echinacea *caused* you to get better from the cold. It's very self-reinforcing, but there are all kinds of things that seem to occur together yet have nothing to do with each other. It's almost like a magician's sleight of hand. It's how superstitions get built up."

Perhaps the most powerful psychological influence of all is the well known but still poorly understood placebo effect: the mind's remarkable ability to make one feel better, and even *get* better, after undergoing a treatment one believes in. A 1998 study of 303 men with enlarged prostates, for instance, found that *half* of those given placebos experienced symptom relief, including faster urine flow (and, ironically, 13.2 percent of those given a placebo discontinued the treatment and dropped out of the study because they were having significant adverse reactions—to a sugar pill). Another study, involving 340 severely depressed people given either St. John's wort, the antidepressant Zoloft, or a placebo, found that those given St. John's wort or Zoloft both gained significant relief—but that those who received the placebo improved even more. So pronounced is the placebo effect in complementary and alternative medicines, in fact, that in 2004, Stephen E. Straus, MD, the director of the National Center for Complementary and Alternative Medicine, coauthored a paper in the *Journal of the American Medical Association* arguing that it might be legitimate to give remedies that improve symptoms "solely or mainly by virtue of the placebo effect." But while it's comforting to know that virtually any pill given to people will make many of them feel better, permitting supplements to be sold based solely on the placebo effect would not only be dishonest: it would make a mockery of modern medicine. The very proposal suggests the desperation of those in the field to find a rational and ethical basis for continuing to promote remedies that simply have no other benefit.

Spiritual hunger also plays a role in many people's use of supplements, particularly for those who seek treatment from alternative care practitioners. When naturopaths burn incense and Chinese herbalists follow thousand-year-old traditions, they are invoking the age-old image of the "medicine man" that dates back not only to Native American healers and Egyptian high priests, but to Jesus. Indeed, the symbol of the American Medical Association and most medical associations around the world is the Asklepian, a serpent entwined around a staff, which is typically attributed to Asclepius, the ancient Greek demigod of medicine. The same symbol, however, was used in other ancient religions, and even the book of Numbers in the Bible describes a "serpent of brass" made by Moses and placed on a pole, which had healing powers. Human societies have always believed in a link between physical and spiritual well-being—indeed, it is a key tenet of Christian Scientists, who believe they must refuse medical care in favor of prayer to heal illnesses, and it even explains Tom Cruise's infamous harangue on the *Today Show* against Brooke Shields's use of antidepressants for postpartum depression, because his religion, Scientology, opposes the use of any psychiatric drugs. Many other people not affiliated with such religions are drawn to alternative medicine because it gives them a sense of connecting with the natural world as God created it. It is worth remembering, however, that the same Enlightenment tradition that led the Founding Fathers to insist on a strict separation between church and state also underlies the practice of science-based medicine practiced free from religious orthodoxy. And as much as people may find comfort in the spiritual trappings or message of alternative care practitioners—and surely many mainstream doctors could learn from their gentle, caring ways—the spiritual affiliation of a physician, company, product, or salesperson ultimately has no bearing on whether the ingredients inside a remedy, herbal or otherwise, are effective and safe.

○ ⊂⊃ ⊂

On September 17, 1997, the predictable outcome of the shark cartilage craze ignited by *60 Minutes* came to light when childhood cancer specialists at Alberta Children's Hospital in Calgary, Canada, reported in the *New England Journal of Medicine* on the case of a nine-year-old girl suffering from a brain tumor. After surgically removing the tumor, the doctors had recommended to the girl's parents that she receive both chemotherapy and radiation, which would give her better than a 50 percent chance of surviving the next three years. But in heartbreaking words, doctors led by Max J. Coppes, MD, PhD, director of the hospital's cancer center, described what happened. The parents, they wrote, "opted instead to treat their daughter with shark cartilage. Four months later, marked tumor progression was documented, and the patient subsequently died." While there was no reason to believe that shark cartilage caused the tumor's regrowth, the parents' decision to give the supplement to their daughter instead of letting her receive the chemotherapy and radiation certainly did. "We find it difficult to understand," the doctors wrote, "how conventional treatments for childhood cancer can be repudiated in favor of alternative approaches for which any evidence of efficacy is lacking."

All health decisions are profoundly personal and private matters. But for all the social, psychological, economic, and spiritual reasons that people believe in supplements—and they have every right to do so—none of those reasons justifies letting unscrupulous manufacturers exploit them. In a society where every mattress, tricycle, and nose-hair clipper undergoes rigorous government inspection, few consumers can comprehend that the herbs, vitamins, and memory boosters lining the shelves (not to mention wallets) of Wal-Mart, CVS, and GNC exist in a regulatory Wild West. Particularly when prestigious magazines, newspapers, and television shows tout their benefits; when deceptive advertisements are all over television, radio, and the Internet; and when marketers use every technique, new and old, to prey upon our weaknesses and desires, the real wonder is not that so many believe in and use supplements, but that *everybody* doesn't.

But there's one more reason we believe. It's not a *why,* but a *who:* the supersalesmen who have led us down the herb garden path by the force of their personality. It is time, then, to take a closer look: Who are these guys?

CHAPTER 10

LOOKING FOR MR. NATURAL

Nineteen days after Cooper Burkey's death from choking on a vitamin pill, the company that manufactured and marketed it, as well as the company's founder, settled unrelated charges by the Federal Trade Commission that they had made deceptive claims that their products could treat or cure asthma, allergies, arthritis, colds, cancer, high cholesterol, cardiovascular disease, Crohn's disease, diabetes, obesity, and more. Garden of Life, Inc., based in West Palm Beach, Florida, was founded in 2000 by Jordan S. Rubin. According to his books and Web sites, Rubin claims that he was near death at the age of nineteen due to a variety of ailments—"including intestinal parasites, abdominal pain, chronic diarrhea, liver problems, chronic fatigue, fibromyalgia, arthritis, prostate and bladder infections, irregular heartbeat, eye inflammation, and chronic depression"—when he met a nutritionist who told him that he needed to begin eating the "diet of the Bible." After following this diet and making a recovery worthy of Jack La Lanne, Rubin came to believe that his survival was "a true testament to the power of his faith in God and the revolutionary health program he calls The Maker's Diet." And what did this diet consist of? Milk and honey? Manna from heaven? No, it was something a little less predictable. "Dirt is so essential to health," he wrote in his book *Patient Heal Thyself,* that many illnesses "may be due to your lost connection to the soil." It's not the dirt itself that improves health, but the microorganisms he claims are found in dirt, and which, coincidentally, he sells in a variety of supplements. After a stipulated final order was filed in the U.S. District Court for the Southern District of Florida on March 8, 2006, Garden of Life and Jordan Rubin agreed to pay $225,000 in consumer redress as part of the settlement, and to make no more unsubstantiated claims that their products treated or cured any ailment.

Rubin is hardly the only supplement salesman to wear his religion on his sleeve. Consider Valerie Saxion, vice president of Silver Creek Laboratories of Fort Worth, Texas, and author of *Every Body Has Parasites* (Bronze Bow Publishing). "God gave us herbs, He gave us the good things," she told the audience at the Las Vegas meeting of the National Nutritional Food Association in July of 2004. "The way I feel, I am a Christian. I do believe there's one God—people call Him different names—but I do believe Jesus is the son of God, and I do believe He created us, that He gave us the things on this Earth that we need to survive. The body is made to heal itself, I truly believe."

A frequent guest on Christian-oriented television shows, Saxion claims that 85 percent of Americans have intestinal parasites that can be cleansed with herbal enemas. Her company sells such a product, ParaCease, containing seventeen herbal ingredients, including the dangerous stimulant laxative cascara sagrada, determined by the FDA in 2002 to be unsafe and ordered by the agency to be removed from all over-the-counter drugs. However, since dietary supplements are not drugs by virtue of DSHEA, the ruling left companies like Saxion's free to continue selling it. Exactly what God has to do with enemas (or what she calls "the cleanse") is a mystery, but Saxion's belief in their power to improve health is total. She told the story of a friend who suffered from acid reflux for years. After three weeks of "doing the cleanse," as she put it, "he vomited up a whole handful of parasites." Saxion hurried to explain that the man didn't literally vomit into his hand, but into the toilet. "It was a bright orange," she said. "Once it hit the water, it burst, and what looked like a hundred little parasite eggs came out. He never had acid reflux ever again."

Undoubtedly the most famous figure to mix religion and supplements is the televangelist Pat Robertson, founder of the Christian Broadcasting Network. In the early 1990s he founded a multilevel marketing company selling vitamins and herbs, Kalo-Vita, which went out of business in 1995. Then, in August of 2001 he began promoting a free recipe on his show, *The 700 Club*, for what he called "Pat's Age-Defying Shake," which includes protein powder, safflower oil, and vinegar. Soon after, he started promoting "Pat's Age-Defying Antioxidants," a do-it-yourself recipe of high-dose vitamins, minerals, and other supplements. He wrote in an accompanying booklet that CBN receives "over 2 million calls per year, many of which involve some type of sickness or disease. I repeat what the Bible states, 'My people perish for lack of knowledge.' God wants us to be healthy, and so many of the illnesses that plague us today can be avoided or dramatically alleviated. There are benefits to be derived from taking my Age-Defying Shake and these Anti-Oxidant Vitamins—you will feel more energy and be much healthier." In the summer of 2005, he began selling the shake at GNC stores at a price of $21.99 for nine servings. Almost immediately, the Trinity Foundation, an evangelical media watchdog group, criticized Robertson for misusing his ministry's tax-exempt, nonprofit status to sell the shake. In May of 2006, ESPN commentator Clay Travis pointed out that the CBN Web site was claiming that because of his shake, Robertson could leg press 2,000 pounds—more, Travis pointed out, than the all-time Florida State University record of 1,335 pounds.

There is certainly nothing wrong with believing that one's work is heavenly inspired. Generally speaking, however, such beliefs in a company's founder are rightly seen as irrelevant to the value of that company's products and services. Who cares, after all, about the religious beliefs of Bill Gates? Yet dietary supplement salespeople routinely make much of their beliefs and personal biographies. And in an industry where neither scientists nor the government can vouch for the safety or efficacy of their products, the character and integrity of the salespeople who say "trust me" merits our consideration. Indeed, their shenanigans demand it.

⌁ ⌁ ⌁

One of the more remarkable things about the supplement industry is just how many of its leading figures are convicted felons. Maybe it shouldn't be surprising—after all, what's a Wild West without outlaws? But in modern American industry, the criminal backgrounds of supplement manufacturers is without parallel. As noted earlier, Gregory Caton, founder of the company that sold one of the products that burned off Sue Gilliatt's nose, had been previously convicted of felony counterfeiting. Michael Ellis and Michael Blevins, founders of Metabolife, were busted together for making methamphetamine, a crime for which Blevins served five years in prison. Robert Occhifinto, founder of the company that manufactured the Stackers taken by Todd Lee before his death, was previously convicted of importing hashish and served eighteen months in federal prison after supplying ephedra to a methamphetamine dealer.

And then there is Kevin Trudeau, who for years now has been a frequent presence on cable television infomercials. In 2005, Trudeau self-published a book that became a number one best seller, *Natural Cures "They" Don't Want You to Know About*. Before getting into the supplement business, Trudeau was indicted in 1988 on seven counts of larceny for depositing $80,000 in worthless checks; he pleaded guilty and served fewer than thirty days. In 1990 he was indicted again, this time for charging $122,000 on credit cards that weren't his own; he again pleaded guilty and served nearly two years in prison. Accused in 1996 by Illinois of operating a pyramid scheme at a company called Nutrition for Life, he settled the case by paying a fine of $10,000. Charged soon after by the Federal Trade Commission of running false and misleading infomercials for "Doctor Callahan's Addiction Breaking System," "Eden's Secret Nature's Purifying Product," a "mega memory system," and a "hair farming system" that was supposed to "finally end baldness in the human race," he settled in 1998 by paying $500,000. In 2003 the FTC charged him again for making false and misleading infomercials for coral calcium, which he claimed could cure cancer. The next year he agreed—in the harshest penalty ever extracted by the FTC against any advertiser—to pay $2 million and to never again sell any health product in any setting, or to make or appear in any infomercial to sell *anything,* with one exception: he could exercise his First Amendment right to write a book, and he could promote it. That's what he did, and by early 2006 the book had sold 5 million copies. To the news media's credit, Trudeau came in for serious criticism in print and on television, yet the drubbing had as little effect on sales of his book as bad reviews have on many other blockbusters. In fact, in mid-2006 he came out with a sequel, *More Natural "Cures" Revealed,* which in May entered the *New York Times* list of best-selling hardcover advice books at number eight.

Compared to Trudeau, A. Glenn Braswell is far less well known, but he has undoubtedly sold far more supplements through the *Journal of Longevity,* which at its peak was mailed to 20 million people each month, almost as many as the widest-circulation magazine in the world, AARP's *Modern Maturity.* Beginning in the 1970s, Braswell sold dozens of products through direct-mail flyers that promised to promote men's hair growth and enlarge women's breasts. The failure of any of them to actually work incurred the wrath of the U.S. Postal Service, which lodged 138 complaints of false representation against him—a record. His use of phony before-and-after photographs in his mailers eventually resulted in a guilty plea of mail fraud. Along with a conviction on tax evasion and perjury, Braswell was sentenced in 1983 to three years in prison and five years' probation, but ended up receiving parole after just seven months. He also pleaded no contest to charges that he had burglarized the home of a former employee and was sentenced to two years' probation, running concurrently with his other sentences. To settle charges brought by the Federal Trade Commission, his companies paid $610,000 and were barred from making any future claims without adequate scientific evidence.

But Braswell soon bounced back, founding a company with the innocuous name of GB Data Systems, which sold supplements through ten or so corporate subsidiaries and published the *Journal of Longevity.* Although it contained articles that looked as though they were authored by independent experts, they were actually written by company executives, simply to tout the company's products. One of its biggest sellers was Gero H3 Anti-Aging Pill, which supposedly "Stops Aches, Pains, Fatigue, Depression," "Improves Memory, Skin Tone and Sex Drive!" and "Reduces Chance of Heart Attack by 83%!" The company also claimed, "People Taking Gero H3 Lived 29% Longer!" But successful as such claims might have been in getting people to buy his products, they were also plainly illegal under DSHEA, because they asserted the power to heal or treat a disease, when the company had no evidence that Gero H3 could do anything whatsoever.

Perhaps fearing the reaction of the FDA or FTC, Braswell began to show signs of wanting to turn over a new leaf. He hired a respected financial turnaround wizard, Ted Ponich, as his chief operating officer and number two man in 1996 with the express purpose of toning down the over-the-top claims and bringing the company into the mainstream of supplement marketers. To lure him in, Braswell offered Ponich an interest-free $750,000 loan on a home on Los Angeles's Mulholland Drive, and paid for a lease on a new Corvette. Then, in a further move toward respectability, in 1998 Braswell donated $25,000 to George W. Bush's campaign for reelection as governor of Texas, and went on to donate nearly $200,000 more to Republican campaigns in the next two years, including $125,000 to the Republican Party of Florida. He could afford it, as GB Data Systems had grossed some $250 million in 1998.

But by year's end, Ponich and the company's number three executive, the chief financial officer Mike O'Neil, realized that Braswell was not serious about ending the company's illegal practices, with regard not only to the unsubstantiated claims being made for its products but also to Braswell's Enron-like accounting tricks to avoid paying taxes. Shortly after Thanksgiving, Ponich met with Braswell for a showdown over the company's direction. "Either this company gets cleaned up," he told his boss, "or I will personally turn you in to the government authorities."

Just over a month later, in January of 1999, Braswell fired Ponich, O'Neil, and four other department heads. Ponich, with O'Neil's backing, went to the IRS, the FDA, the FTC, the Postal Service, and other agencies to tell them of Braswell's illegal activities. Braswell responded by suing them both. Then, shortly after five p.m. on Monday, October 23, 2000— a month before a trial against Braswell was set to begin with Ponich as a witness—Ponich and a friend died in a mysterious single-car crash on Mulholland Drive. O'Neil decided to stop cooperating with authorities in pending cases against Braswell, and Braswell then dropped his libel suit against O'Neil.

A few months later, on January 12, 2001, Braswell's high-powered attorney, the former U.S. attorney Kendall Coffey, sent a letter to Hugh Rodham, President Clinton's brother-in-law, asking for his help in seeking a pardon for Braswell's previous convictions. Rodham negotiated a fee of $230,000 and forwarded to Clinton advisors a letter from Coffey calling Braswell a "visionary" with an "exemplary record of business accomplishments." A week later, on January 19, the pardon was granted. Clinton later denied knowing that Rodham had been paid, saying he was "deeply disturbed" to learn of it, and Rodham eventually returned the $230,000 after facing much criticism. The pardon, however, stood.

But that didn't stop the investigations that Ponich had set in motion before his untimely death. In January of 2003, Braswell was arrested in Miami on charges of tax evasion and was jailed without bail. On September 13, 2004, Braswell was sentenced to eighteen months in prison for tax evasion, with credit for time served, and ordered to pay $10 million in fines, back taxes, and interest. In 2006, he also agreed to pay $1 million, turn over $3.5 million in assets, and stop nearly all direct-mail marketing and all unsubstantiated health claims to settle FTC charges that he had been "peddling empty promises to consumers battling serious illnesses," according to Lydia Parnes, director of the FTC's Bureau of Consumer Protection. But the payments were peanuts for a man whose companies had grossed an estimated $1 billion.

◯ ▭ ◯

Colorful as rascals like Braswell and Trudeau may be, there is no question that as the industry has grown into its present mammoth size, it has come to be dominated by buttoned-down corporate executives—the suits, if you will—with close ties to the chemical, pharmaceutical, and agribusiness conglomerates their customers are often trying to avoid. But even these corporate chieftains have had serious run-ins with the law.

A window onto their world opened during the last week of October of 2004 at the luxurious Lansdowne Resort outside Washington, D.C., when the Council for Responsible Nutrition (CRN), the supplement industry's most influential and exclusive trade group, convened its annual meeting. The attendees included three senior managers from Wyeth, the pharmaceutical giant that bought Solgar Vitamin and Herb Company in 1998, now the third-largest supplement company in the United States, with 2003 sales of $480 million. Steve Furcich, president of the Natural Health Nutrition division of Archer Daniels Midland Co. (ADM), was there; so was David Christensen, senior counsel of Bayer HealthCare, maker of One-A-Day multivitamins. BASF Corp., better known for its chemicals and plastics divisions, sent Mike Coyle, business director of human nutrition, and Greg Thies, director of government relations. Cadbury Adams, maker of Certs, Dentyne, and Bubblicious, sent Norma Skolnik, senior director of regulatory affairs (Americas), presumably because of its new product, a line of cough drops called Halls Defense, which includes vitamin C, zinc, and echinacea. A representative was there from Cargill—another agribusiness giant, and the world's largest privately held company. And so was Carolyn E. Moore, PhD, director of nutrition and health at the Beverage Institute for Health & Wellness, an arm of the Coca-Cola Company that supports, according to its Web site, "research to help better understand the role that beverages can play in diets and health."

"Minute Maid Heartwise was one of my projects," Dr. Moore said. "That's the kind of thing Coca-Cola is interested in doing more of in the area of health and wellness. Heartwise has free sterols, vitamin E and B vitamins. It's evolving, new science." One of the reasons that Coca-Cola formed the institute, she said, was to "dispel myths" and "communicate science-based reports to the public." Such as, for instance, "How does hydration improve health?"

Of course, companies devoted primarily to supplements attended as well, including Herbalife, Shaklee, Nutrition 21, Weider Nutrition, General Nutrition Centers, Pharmavite (owner of Nature's Resource and Nature Made) and Leiner Health Products. The country's largest supplement manufacturer, NBTY, had four of its top executives on hand, including its president, Harvey Kamil. With $1.65 billion in sales in 2004 from brands including Nature's Bounty, Vitamin World, Puritan's Pride, Rexall Sundown, and MET-Rx, NBTY is among the 1,000 largest companies in the United States.

Together, the 125 attendees heard Mike Green, CRN's director of government relations, boast of how their group had killed a California bill that would have required the reporting of all serious adverse events to the state. "The legislation would have been burdensome for the California Department of Health, resulting in a flood of insignificant and meaningless results," Green said. "CRN recognized the potential fallout for the industry if this bill had passed. We hired a California lobbyist, Randy Pollack. We put a plan in place. We built a strong coalition of CRN member companies and California groups. We held a California lobbying day. We had a presence at hearings. We mounted a letter-writing campaign. By presenting a strong, unified front, we defeated this onerous legislation."

Of course, they did not present quite as strong and unified a front in that instance as did BASF, ADM, Hoffman-LaRoche, and the nineteen other companies in seven countries that controlled more than 90 percent of the bulk vitamin and mineral market in the 1990s. Known as Vitamins Inc., the companies were found to have formed a global price-fixing cartel that jacked up the prices of almost every vitamin and mineral sold in the United States and around the world. When the assistant attorney general Joel Klein announced a settlement of the case on May 20, 1999, he stated, "The vitamin cartel is the most pervasive and harmful criminal antitrust conspiracy ever uncovered. It lasted almost a decade and involved a highly sophisticated and elaborate conspiracy to control everything about the sale of these products. These companies fixed the price; they allocated sales volumes; they allocated customers; and in the United States they even rigged bids to make absolutely sure that their cartel would work. These companies have agreed to pay the largest criminal fines in antitrust history—nearly three quarters of a billion dollars in all. The enormous effort that went into maintaining this conspiracy reflects the magnitude of the illegal revenues it generated as well as the harm it inflicted on the American economy."

⊂⊃ ⊂⊃ ⊂⊃

Some in the supplement industry, it must be admitted, are doing their best to raise their standards. Such a one is Mitchell Balbert, president of Natrol Inc. With revenues of about $80 million a year, his company was listed as the country's thirty-fifth-largest supplement manufacturer in 2003 by *Nutrition Business Journal*. Bald, middle-aged, affable, and with enough of a sense of humor to have a photo in his office of the episode from *I Love Lucy* in which Lucy did a commercial for a product called Vitameatavegamin, Balbert's practices are as good as or better than anyone's in the industry, and his perspective is refreshingly, well, bland.

"I'm not a nutritionist," he said one morning in August of 2004 at his company's headquarters on the outskirts of Los Angeles. "I'm not a chemist. By trade I'm a salesman, okay? I'd like to say I'm a reasonable businessman. Which is one of the reasons why I personally champion the implementation of an industry-wide adverse event reporting system. I think that's a very meaningful step in helping to reestablish credibility." That summer, the ephedra scare that had lost the industry so much credibility had been all over the news, and one of the very first products his company had marketed was Natrol High, which contained ephedra (although, Balbert said, they never received a single report of an adverse event from one of their customers).

After founding the company in 1980, Balbert rode the post-DSHEA boom in supplements with sober enthusiasm. "In the second half of the nineties, the industry showed dramatic growth—what could be characterized as the golden age of dietary supplements," he said. "The industry blossomed in ways that it couldn't have without DSHEA. Clearly our company grew as well."

Balbert was eager to show off the state-of-the-art testing laboratories his company has invested heavily in. Genia Khudagulyan, director of quality assurance and quality control, wore a white jacket as she pointed out the two new high-performance liquid chromatography machines for analyzing ingredients and a $120,000 device that can detect heavy-metal contaminants down to ten parts per million.

Khudagulyan, who previously worked for a large pharmaceutical company, admitted she had been initially reluctant to join a supplement company. But, she said, "I figured I was willing to bring this company up close to the standards of a pharmaceutical. This is the way it should be. Whether it's required or not, our kids are taking these products. I'm happy now, because I got all the support from Mitchell. We're bringing this up close to pharmaceutical level—very close. I don't think the majority of supplement companies are doing this testing. I don't think ninety percent are. I feel better that we are doing it. At least we can sleep at night."

Although quality control is a big step, the lack of contaminants doesn't mean the herbal ingredients on the label have been proven safe or effective. In 1998, the firm purchased the Laci LeBeau line of teas, including the Super Slimming Tea that contains the herbal stimulant laxative senna and came with a number of severe adverse incidents in its brief history. In 1991, thirty-seven-year-old June Grell of California died unexpectedly in her sleep after drinking the tea for a few months; doctors involved in the case had concluded that the senna had caused severe cardiac arrhythmia. Soon after, twenty-two-year-old Debbie Helphrey of Fort Lauderdale also died after the tea caused an electrolyte imbalance that led to fatal arrhythmia, according to her death certificate. In 1993, a report in the *American Journal of Gastroenterology* had coined the term "Laci LeBeau Syndrome." In 1995, a special working group of the FDA had heard reports of up to sixty adverse events, including five deaths, that had been associated with stimulant laxative teas. The group recommended that warning labels be placed on all such products, and the current label used by Natrol does warn of the potential risks and recommends against taking it for more than ten days straight unless advised by a doctor.

When his company was considering whether to buy the product line, Balbert said, "We had both a comprehensive legal review and a comprehensive science review of the product, the ingredients, and the formula. At that time we were a public company, and I wasn't going to buy a product line that would cause ill will or ill health. We had to make sure we were making intelligent business decisions. The answer we got from lawyers and scientists was that the product was safe to use as directed." Referring to the six years since Natrol bought the Laci LeBeau line, he said, in language that seemed carefully worded, "To the best of my knowledge, we have had no adverse reporting that ultimately ended up in any form of litigation. And we sell a ton of it."

Christopher Grell, an attorney who has specialized in litigation involving dietary supplements since the death of his wife, June, conceded that senna is used as an ingredient in many laxatives, including the over-the-counter drug Senokot. "The difference," he said, "is that Senokot is sold as a *drug,* with drug warnings and FDA approval." A tea containing senna, he said, is particularly dangerous because if brewed too long the natural laxatives can reach higher levels than are safe. And, he pointed out, "The FDA has a proposed rule that would ban senna because of its potential carcinogenic effect. It's already banned several other herbs that were used in the same kind of dieters' tea. Unfortunately, because the drug laws do not apply, there are still dietary supplements that contain ingredients banned for use in drugs but can still be used in dietary supplements."

The marketing strategies for certain Natrol products have also raised concerns. In September of 2004, Balbert agreed to pay $250,000 to settle charges made by a California district attorney that Natrol had made false and misleading advertising claims for a chitosan-based weight-loss product. The DA's investigation found no scientific evidence that chitosan causes fat to be "bound" or "trapped" in the digestive tract, or that it results in appreciable weight loss. The investigation also found levels of lead in the chitosan supplements that exceeded state limits.

Yet Balbert and his company do struggle mightily to maintain standards that exceed those currently required by the FDA, or are exercised by many other supplement companies. "I hate being painted with the same brush that the black knights are being painted with," he said. "I'm scared to death that reporters will paint the whole industry based upon the wackos that are truly out there. They should be regulated out of business. But you want to be careful you don't regulate the white knights out of existence too."

○ ▭ ⊂⊃

Of all the "white knights" on the supplement scene today, only one has inherited the mantle of prestige and cultural influence once worn by Adelle Davis, enjoying her reputation for expertise and healthful common sense, taking on her media role as the voice of a movement—not to mention selling books by the millions. Described by *Publishers Weekly* as "America's best-known complementary care physician," hailed by the *San Francisco Chronicle* as "the guru of alternative medicine," and nicknamed in a *Time* magazine cover story "Mr. Natural," Dr. Andrew Weil is as famous for his views as for his appearance: bald, white-bearded, and slightly overweight, the very picture of a guru.

But for all his best sellers, sold-out lectures, and appearances on *Oprah* and *Larry King Live,* Dr. Weil's background, unknown to most of his millions of readers and Web site visitors, is not quite what one might expect from someone modestly self-described in the subtitle of his own book as "America's most trusted medical expert." His very first media appearance—on December 14, 1968, in no less a spot than the front page of the *New York Times*—was on a subject that defined the first fifteen years of his career and has, by his own admission, influenced everything he has since done: marijuana. In a tiny study carried out in a Harvard laboratory, where he was attending medical school, Dr. Weil gave marijuana (obtained from the Federal Bureau of Narcotics and rated for potency by a U.S. Customs laboratory) to nine young men who had never before taken it but agreed to smoke it for the study, as well as to nine who had been regular users. The new users were first given a training session in which they were taught to smoke the marijuana "properly," and were then put through three sessions of three hours each: one with a gram of marijuana rolled into a cigarette, another with a half-gram, and a third with just tobacco. The regular users were given the full gram all three times. He found that although all the regular users said they felt "high" after smoking the full gram of marijuana, only one of the nine new users did. And while all nine of the first-timers showed a small but significant drop in their performance on some mental and physical tests after the full gram (even though they didn't feel high), the regular users did not show a performance decline (even though, paradoxically, they did feel high). On the basis of that, Dr. Weil concluded in his study that marijuana is "a relatively mild intoxicant with minor, real, short-lived effects." Although the subjects' hearts did beat faster after smoking, he told the *Times,* "Medically, it's quite harmless."

Upon graduating from Harvard Medical School and interning at Mt. Zion Hospital in San Francisco's Haight Ashbury neighborhood, Dr. Weil began what was supposed to be a two-year stint with the National Institute of Health. He quit after a year, however, because of objections to his work with marijuana. He then set to expanding on the topic that had garnered him such early media renown, and the result was his first book, *The Natural Mind,* published in 1972. An exploration of how hallucinogenic drugs can "unlock" the mind, the book proposed that humans have an innate need to alter their consciousness. The seventh chapter, "A Trip to Stonesville," asserted that "stoned thinking" allows people to have more profound, intuitive insights than can be achieved by traditional rational thinking. "To the straight mind," he wrote, "faith healing is held in contempt ... despite the abundant evidence of cures." He even went so far as to celebrate psychosis. "Psychotics are persons whose nonordinary experience is exceptionally strong," he wrote. "Every psychotic is a potential sage or healer.... I am almost tempted to call psychotics the evolutionary vanguard of our species."

While such romantic notions of mental illness enjoyed a fad in the early 1970s, they have long since been relegated to the history of psychology as naive, even harmful myths that stand in the way of getting desperate patients and their families the help they need to regain functional lives. Yet Dr. Weil insisted in an interview in 1998 that he still holds fast to such views: *The Natural Mind,* he said, "came from my own experience, which I've always drawn on. I feel very confident about that book. It's just been reissued in a new edition, twenty-six years after it was first published. I didn't find the need to make changes. I wrote a little bit of a new preface to it. I talked about the fact that these ideas have really held up over time and I still consider them very useful."

He followed up *The Natural Mind* with two more books exploring similar themes, including the 1983 *From Chocolate to Morphine: Everything You Need to Know About Mind-Altering Drugs,* coauthored with Winifred Rosen. Their intent, he said in an interview, "was to write a book that presented factual, unbiased information about all categories of drugs, both legal and illegal—medical, recreational, over-the-counter—that might affect the mind, so that young people could make up their own minds as to what they wanted to do about them." He went on, "A prominent senator from Florida stood up on the floor of the Senate and waved the book around and said that this was a very dangerous book, because it was neutral, that it didn't tell people to not use substances. And that's exactly what I aimed for; I wanted to put out neutral information."

Even as he metamorphosed into an all-purpose alternative medicine guru, beginning with *Health and Healing* in 1983, he maintained his stance as a conveyor of "neutral information," with one foot in the mainstream medical world and the other in the alternative universe. As he told one interviewer in 1997, "I really think I'm in the middle. Sometimes I'm attacking traditional medicine, sometimes I'm defending it; sometimes I'm defending alternative medicine and sometimes attacking it, so I think I'm pretty even-handed in my criticism." In 1998, he told another interviewer, "I think that my voice is very much listened to as a source of information, and seen as being trustworthy, neutral. I'm not selling people things. I'm only selling information to the public. And I try to make that the best-quality information that I can find."

But both claims—that his attitude toward alternative medicine is middle-of-the-road, and that he was selling only information—turn out, upon inspection, to be untrue. Here, after all, is a man whose 1996 best seller, *Spontaneous Healing,* was filled with stories of people who survived despite dire medical prognoses, and sometimes after ignoring standard medical care—people like Eva Forrester, who, he wrote, refused radiation and chemotherapy after undergoing surgery for breast cancer: "Eva embarked on a course of natural healing under the guidance of a chiropractor/naturopath." While we all have the right to choose our own medical care, Eva's likelihood of surviving after her decision was greatly reduced, as chemotherapy has been shown to "substantially improve" survival for most types of breast cancer, according to NIH, and studies of postoperative radiation has shown it can cut the long-term risk of relapse from about one third without it to as low as 10 percent with it. Yet in his book, Dr. Weil celebrated the fact that Eva, who worked at a health food store, was encouraging other women to follow her example. "It is a fact of life in America of the nineties," he wrote, "that health food store clerks have replaced pharmacists as dispensers of practical advice to many people, especially those with difficult problems.... I have often watched Eva Forrester play this role from behind the counter of the New Life Health Center. She stands in front of shelves of vitamins and supplements and engages clients with an open, nonjudgmental, comforting manner. She explains patiently the basics of natural healing, of helping the body rely on its own resources."

But encouraging women to avoid life-saving medical care after breast cancer, or supporting the practice of having untrained clerks dispense medical advice at health food stores, certainly isn't middle-of-the-road. Nor is there anything moderate about the view that miracles and magic are fundamental aspects of medicine. Health and illness, he has written, are "manifestations of good and evil, requiring all the help of religion and philosophy to understand and all the techniques of magic to manipulate." Such views may explain why his books and Web site recommend remedies for which scientific evidence is weak, including high-dose vitamin E to prevent heart disease, self-hypnosis to remove warts, and evening primrose oil for psoriasis and eczema. (As the Center for Science in the Public Interest has noted, "Virtually all of the well-designed scientific studies show that evening primrose oil is ineffective for dermatitis, psoriasis, eczema, brittle nails, and PMS.") Thus, the recommendation that remained on his Web site until 2004 to use bloodroot for skin cancer, the very recommendation that put Sue Gilliatt on the path that ended in the loss of her nose, is not surprising. And when one reads the title of an adoring 1996 profile of him in the *New York Times*—"A Shaman's Tools: Ma Huang and Bloodroot Paste"—it is high time to ask: What really is the difference between Dr. Andrew Weil, Harvard graduate, and Clark Stanley, Snake Oil King?

Certainly, the good doctor is now in the business of moving product. Behind his carefully cultivated appearance of impartiality, and despite his 1998 profession that he is not in the business of "selling things," Dr. Weil has made a major business of offering his own brand of premium-priced supplements to consumers, which he only hinted at in a 2005 *Time* magazine cover story when he stated, "I take a good daily multivitamin-multimineral supplement, one that I formulated myself." In fact, he sells an entire line of supplements under the brand name "Dr. Weil Select." Shoppers can buy a sixty-day supply of his "Daily Antioxidant for Optimum Health," containing the high doses of beta carotene and vitamin C shown in studies to increase the risk of premature death, for $43.99. Or one can buy thirty days' worth of his "Memory Support," including the gingko biloba that has been shown not to improve memory, for $56.10. In fact, none of the dozens of products he sells has been conclusively proven to do anything more than to enrich Dr. Weil, or at least his Weil Foundation, to which he has pledged to donate the after-tax profits from the sale of his products. But despite signing a deal with Drugstore.com that paid his company $3.9 million in royalties between September 2003 and August 2004, as well as $465,000 to Dr. Weil personally as an "honoraria" for him to promote the businesses, his foundation paid out only a single $5,000 grant between 2002 and 2004, according to a review of its tax returns by the Center for Science in the Public Interest. In 2005 it picked up the pace, awarding $60,000 to "integrative medicine" organizations in Arizona, Maine, Oregon, and Texas, and in early 2006 gave another $30,000 to the Consortium of Academic Centers for Integrative Medicine. But CSPI's senior nutritionist, David Schardt, remains critical: "Consumers should know that when they buy any supplements recommended by Andrew Weil on his and Drugstore.com's Web sites, Weil's company is collecting a sales commission of up to twenty-five percent on every bottle. Even if some of this money eventually trickles down to his foundation, that's still a pretty big incentive to push lots of vitamins and herbs, even where the evidence is dubious."

For better or worse, though, Dr. Weil is as good as it gets in the wild and wooly world of supplements. "Mr. Natural" is today's "Mother Nature." After all, when it comes to credibility that stands up to scrutiny, one must remember that not even Adelle Davis lived up to Adelle Davis's reputation.

CHAPTER 11
PROOF

Growing up poor in rural Iowa during the 1940s, Tom Harkin, a coal miner's son, found little reason to put much faith in mainstream medicine. His mother, a Slovenian immigrant, died when Harkin was ten. His brother Frank became deaf at the age of nine. During the 1970s, while Harkin was serving as a proudly liberal Democrat in the U.S. House of Representatives, two of his sisters died from breast cancer. So in 1991, during his second term in the Senate, it shouldn't have surprised anyone that when he was offered an unconventional treatment for his hay fever allergies, Harkin was willing to give it a try.

"I went on this very tough regimen of taking a lot of bee pollen, sometimes as much as sixty pills a day," Harkin later recalled. Although bee pollen had by then been linked to many cases of severe allergic reactions—including anaphylactic shock and memory loss—Harkin reported no problems. Instead, he said, "Literally on about the tenth day, all of a sudden my allergies just left. Well, that's when I began to think, 'We've got to have somebody looking at these different approaches.' "

As it happened, Harkin at that moment had more power to get somebody to look at those different approaches than just about anyone in the United States. As chairman of the Senate subcommittee in charge of health-care appropriations, Harkin held the purse strings for the National Institutes of Health. And he wasn't much bothered that Royden Brown, the man who provided him with the bee pollen, had just paid a $200,000 fine to the Federal Trade Commission for making unproved claims that the supplement could do everything from curing heart disease to improving one's sex drive.

In October of 1991—just as the FDA commissioner David Kessler was beginning the crackdown on supplement claims that would lead Gerry Kessler to begin the great struggle for DSHEA—Harkin opened a bold new front in the war for government support of the industry's interests. He pushed through Public Law 102–170, providing $2 million to NIH to establish an office to "investigate and validate . . . unconventional medical practices." As small as the $2 million was in comparison to NIH's overall budget of $10 billion, its significance could hardly be overstated: after more than a hundred years of battling the purveyors of herbal and other alternative remedies, the U.S. government was bringing them into the fold. It was only the first crack in the dam, but for NIH, with all its scientific authority, to give alternative medicine even a weak embrace rather than its usual slap in the face was revolutionary. What DSHEA would do for public acceptance, Harkin's little gambit would soon begin doing for scientific respectability.

Known for a short while as the Office of Unconventional Medicine, it quickly settled on a less easily lampooned name, the Office of Alternative Medicine (OAM). A full year passed before its first full-time director was appointed in October of 1992, Joseph J. Jacobs, MD. Having studied medicine at Yale and Dartmouth and obtained an MBA from the Wharton School of Business, Dr. Jacobs brought the added perspective of being a Native American, part Mohawk and part Cherokee, who had grown up seeing herbal remedies used in healing ceremonies, and had studied the work of medicine men while serving as a pediatrician on a Navajo reservation in New Mexico. He wore a blue blazer and black loafers, kept a bundle of dried herbs attached to an eagle feather on his desk, and exuded an easygoing charm.

"I describe my role as the captain of the starship *Enterprise*," he told the *New York Times* soon after his appointment. "We're going where no one has gone before," he told *Time*.

As his budget quickly grew, doubling to $4 million by 1994, Dr. Jacobs tried to maintain a sense of humor about the skepticism that his office drew from more staid researchers, at one point even suggesting that the office's phone number be changed to 1–800–PEYOTE. But he soon discovered that Harkin was not laughing, particularly not about Jacobs's insistence on bringing the same rigorous, scientific methods to studying alternative remedies that the rest of NIH brought to studying drugs. In an article he wrote at the time, Harkin criticized what he called "the unbendable rules of randomized clinical trials," and went on, "In my much-publicized victory over allergies through the use of bee pollen, did I need someone to show me exactly how that was accomplished in order to experience the results I did? Of course not! And it is not necessary for the scientific community to understand the process before the American public can benefit from these therapies."

Over Dr. Jacobs's objections, Harkin succeeded in convincing Donna Shalala, then secretary of Health and Human Services, to appoint four of his hand-picked candidates to the eighteen-member board overseeing OAM. One was Frank Wiewel, leader of a group called People Against Cancer, which arranged trips outside the United States for people seeking remedies, such as laetrile, that were illegal in this country due to being dangerous, disproved, or both. Another was Ralph W. Moss, who published People Against Cancer's newsletter. Third was Gar Hildenbrand, executive director of the Gerson Institute, which recommended, among other things, coffee enemas as a way to prevent and treat cancer. And fourth was the friend of Harkin's who had first told him about bee pollen: Berkley Bedell, the former six-term congressman from Iowa who believed he had been cured of prostate cancer by a man who had twice been convicted of practicing medicine without a license in Europe.

As pressure in the office mounted between those who wanted to put alternative therapies to the test and those who wanted them simply accepted without testing, at least one member of the advisory board who had not been appointed by Harkin began complaining publicly. Dr. Barrie Cassileth, then an adjunct professor of medicine at the University of North Carolina, said at the time, "The degree to which nonsense has trickled down to every aspect of this office is astonishing. It's the only NIH activity where people can come along and say with a straight face,

'It's not DNA that is at the heart of cellular functioning but ABC,' and people will say, 'He's right!' It's the only place where opinions are counted as equal to data."

Harkin's aides frequently called Dr. Jacobs to demand that he fund a study of one or another of the senators' pet theories—including in one instance when an aide told him to issue a $200,000 grant for the study of bee pollen to Royden Brown, the man who had provided Harkin with the bee pollen that had supposedly cured his hay fever, and who had previously been fined by the FTC for making bogus claims. At a hearing, Harkin asked why Brown's bee pollen study was not getting funded. Dr. Jacobs testified that he had actually gone to Brown's manufacturing facility in Arizona. "When I was there, I was suffering really bad from allergies. . . . I took his therapy and became nauseous and almost vomited. . . . I tried the bee pollen. It did not work for me."

Harkin then demanded to know at the hearing why a study for which he had set aside $750,000 to test antineoplastons—substances isolated from human urine that were supposedly capable of curing cancer—had not yet begun. Before an overflow crowd in Room 192 of the Senate's Dirksen Office Building, Dr. Jacobs tried to explain that OAM was legally required to get the collaboration of at least one of NIH's large institutes to conduct any study, but that the National Cancer Institute had so far refused to do so with antineoplastons, believing them to be without merit.

Plainly dissatisfied with the response, Harkin pulled out the brass knuckles. "I'm faced with a problem here," he told Dr. Jacobs. "I intend to see this office move forward, and I will do whatever it takes. To the extent that I have any information and believe that there is foot-dragging going on in this office, that you are not being aggressive enough in pursuing the mandate we've given that office, then you will hear from me. We've had enough time and now we have to start going ahead aggressively."

The breaking point came in July of 1994, when Harkin appeared on national television with the father of a girl suffering from leukemia who accused Dr. Jacobs of blocking her access to antineoplastons. It wasn't true—New York State was taking away the medical license of a doctor who wanted to treat the girl with the substance, and Dr. Jacobs had no power over a state licensing board—but for Dr. Jacobs the accusation was the last straw. The next day, when a Harkin aide called to discuss the matter, the usually lighthearted administrator blew up on him.

"Quite frankly, fuck you all," Dr. Jacobs told him. "I don't give a shit what happens. I'm leaving this job. If I don't get out of here, I'm going to have a heart attack."

Harkin's appointees on the advisory board were overjoyed. The party pooper was gone. (He went on to a well-regarded career running state medical agencies in Vermont and New Jersey.) Wiewel, the board member who led People Against Cancer, expressed the hope that OAM would now be freed to study unconventional remedies by the unconventional methods they had been calling for, without the scientific rigmarole. "The office is not only supposed to look at alternative ideas, but to look at them in innovative, alternative ways, and this is where we hit a snag with Dr. Jacobs," he said at the time.

◯ ◯ ◯

But the office itself was hitting a snag as power brokers at multiple levels of the federal bureaucracy grew increasingly uneasy about its ever-worsening reputation for being a haven for witch doctors doing voodoo science. With the Republicans' takeover of the Senate in the 1992 elections, Bill Frist of Tennessee, on his way to becoming majority leader, had taken over Harkin's chairmanship of the Senate subcommittee in charge of health-care appropriations. "There's a fear that the peer review there [at OAM] won't be as rigorous as at other institutes," Frist said at a hearing. Dr. Harold Varmus, the Nobel Prize–winning researcher who took over the helm of NIH in November of 1993, proposed spending cuts two years in a row and stricter oversight for the office. And at a time of belt-tightening imposed by the Republicans, some in the House of Representatives even wanted to see OAM gone for good.

Harkin rolled over the objections with help from many of the same lawmakers who were proving pivotal in the fight, then under way, for DSHEA, including Representative James Moran, Democrat of Virginia. When Moran's daughter, Dorothy, developed brain cancer, he and his wife developed a "vitamin and nutritional supplement program" for her. "[It] not only helped her withstand chemotherapy," Moran testified at a

House hearing, "but also bought us some time to strengthen Dorothy and wait until she was a little older before undergoing radiation treatments." One of the supplements they gave her, in fact, was shark cartilage. "Every parent of a child facing a serious illness should be able to make the kinds of choices we made about pursuing alternative and complementary therapies," he said.

As a result, far from withering, OAM's budget nearly doubled again between 1994 and 1996, when it reached $7.8 million, and more than doubled once more by 1998, when it hit $19.5 million. As if that wasn't enough, Harkin then managed a coup that would have been unthinkable seven years earlier when the office first crept into existence. In October of 1998 he succeeded in elevating the office into a full-fledged center, not as big as one of the institutes (such as the National Cancer Institute or National Institute on Aging), but on a par with the Center for Information Technology, established in 1964, and the Center for Scientific Review, formed all the way back in 1946 to oversee the review of grant proposals. In 1999, the budget for the new National Center for Complementary and Alternative Medicine (NCCAM) was a staggering $49.9 million—almost twenty-five times the amount that Harkin had secured for the office in 1991.

With greater size came greater expectations and demands for credible proof that something—anything—actually worked. Politicians overseeing NIH's appropriations—including Frist; Senator Arlen Specter, Republican of Pennsylvania; and Representative John Porter, Republican of Illinois—were under increasing pressure from prominent scientists to force the *enfant terrible* of NIH to grow up. Paul Berg, PhD, a Nobel laureate in chemistry and professor of biochemistry at Stanford University Medical Center, wrote to Frist to say that "quackery will always prey on the gullible and uninformed, but we should not provide it with cover from the NIH." D. Allan Bromley, PhD, a Yale professor, president of the American Physical Society, and former science advisor to the first President George Bush, also wrote to Frist, saying, "When the Office of Alternative Medicine was created in 1992, I think most of us assumed that its mandate would be to critically evaluate practices that lie outside mainstream medicine. Unfortunately the OAM has emerged as an undiscriminating advocate of unconventional medicine. It has bestowed the considerable prestige of the NIH on a variety of highly dubious practices, some of which clearly violate basic laws of physics and more clearly resemble witchcraft than medicine." Leon Jaroff, founder and first managing editor of *Discover* magazine, wrote an op-ed in the *New York Times* calling the office a "bee pollen bureaucracy" and "Tom Harkin's folly."

In response to such pressures, Stephen E. Straus, MD, formerly chief of the Laboratory of Clinical Investigation at the National Institute of Allergy and Infectious Diseases, was brought in as the new director, and he immediately set to cleaning house. Out went the "alternative" ways for assessing alternative therapies. In came the rigorous scientific methods that Harkin's cronies had once resisted. The only thing that didn't change was the budget's rapid rise. In the first four years under Dr. Straus's management, it again more than doubled, reaching $104.6 million in 2002.

"I think there's very little skepticism left," Dr. Straus said in an interview published in the *Scientist* in December of that year. "Over the past few years, the debate went from 'Why would anyone want to study these things?' to 'How can you study these things?' to 'What are the studies showing?' "

But the studies—more than 700 of them published in the first four years after Dr. Straus's arrival—were generally small and hampered by the same variability and contamination of herbal products plaguing consumers. One of them was the notorious study of BeneFin shark cartilage in terminal cancer patients, described earlier, that had to be stopped early when only 83 of the expected 600 patients enrolled and no benefit was found in those who did. Meanwhile, money was being poured into getting larger studies off the ground, training researchers, creating a huge Web site, publishing review articles, collaborating with other institutes at NIH, and starting up academic centers at universities across the country devoted to the study of what was now being called complementary and alternative medicine (CAM). A national infrastructure, in other words, was rising up around the study and use of dietary supplements.

The outpouring of work kept the critics at bay until late in 2001, when Saul Green, PhD, the former chairman of the Mammalian Antitumor Factors Research Labs at Memorial Sloan-Kettering Cancer Center in New York, published the results of an exhaustive review he'd undertaken of NCCAM's studies. "To my knowledge," he wrote in the *Scientific Review of Alternative Medicine*, "and based on a review of abstracts published by the OAM/NCCAM, no report stated that a treatment did not work. In the past nine years, no negative result has been published, nor have any of the methods studied been shown to work to the satisfaction of the medical science community." In other words, none of the positive studies were big enough or well designed enough to prove that the supplements being studied truly worked. And on the flip side, when the studies failed to find the hoped-for results, the NCCAM reports always stopped short of declaring the treatment to be of no value. If 10 milligrams of an herbal extract didn't work, perhaps 20 milligrams would—or perhaps a different method of extracting the herb was necessary. When California regulators tested the vaunted supplement PC-SPES and found that its apparent effects on prostate cancer were due to prescription drugs that had been illegally added, NCCAM announced that it would permit three out of its four ongoing studies of the supplement to continue—including, incredibly, one being conducted by Sophie Chen, the owner of the company that manufactured (and doctored) the PC-SPES. "The laboratory studies will seek to learn the cellular and molecular mechanisms of action of the herbs as opposed to the drug ingredients that contaminated the product," announced NCCAM, apparently unable (or unwilling) to give up the belief that PC-SPES had any effects other than those from the added drugs.

Later in 2002, Wallace I. Sampson, MD, editor of the *Scientific Review,* called for Congress to shut down NCCAM based on its failure to produce results and the many conflicts of interest that existed. "Ten individuals account for 20% of NCCAM awards," he wrote. "Two individuals originally on the Advisory Council that approves NCCAM policy were awarded over $4 million and $5 million in repeated awards." Even the chairman of the panel formed by NCCAM in 2002 to assess the academic research centers receiving NCCAM funds came from one of the very centers the panel was supposed to review. Such incestuous relationships, Dr. Sampson argued, cast a shadow of ethical and scientific doubt over the entire enterprise.

But just as the chorus of criticism was growing to a howl, Dr. Straus finally began to deliver on his promise to bring scientific objectivity to NCCAM's efforts. On April 10, 2002, the *Journal of the American Medical Association* published a study, funded in part by NCCAM, showing that an extract of St. John's wort was no better than a placebo at relieving major depression. And as displeasing as the results were to the supplement industry and its supporters, in fact they gave Dr. Straus the credibility in the eyes of scientists that he had been desperate for. "Our commitment is to apply exacting scientific methods to studying popular complementary and alternative medicine practices and to publish the results of such studies in critical peer-reviewed journals, so that the public and practitioners can make the most informed decisions about them," Dr. Straus said in a printed statement. "This study represents one of our first 'down payments' on this commitment." Later that year, when researchers from the Netherlands published the first report that St. John's wort interfered with the chemotherapy drug irinotecan, Dr. Straus took the step of coauthoring an editorial stating that although many cancer patients were trying herbal remedies, "it would be prudent for patients and their oncologists to appreciate that, no matter how beneficial some approaches may appear to be, they are not all safe."

The first and, still to this day, only major NCCAM-funded study to show benefit of any alternative remedy in a large, randomized study was published on December 21, 2004, in the *Annals of Internal Medicine*—but it was about acupuncture rather than a supplement. In the study, 570 people with arthritic knees were given either acupuncture or a sham procedure that felt like acupuncture but wasn't. After twenty-six weeks, those who received the real acupuncture felt and moved slightly better than those who received the sham procedure. But speaking on behalf of the Arthritis Foundation, David Felson, MD, a rheumatologist at Boston University, said that while the study was well designed, "the effect is almost so small as to be ... undetectable. Individual patients are going to have a hard time getting noticeable benefit from this treatment."

In search of benefits even that slight for supplements, Dr. Straus redoubled the center's efforts. "Because NCCAM's early research demonstrated some inconsistency and contamination of commercial products used in research," he wrote in a budget document, the center had now "established new policies and procedures to guide further research on botanicals. In April 2005 ... NCCAM issued a policy requiring newly funded researchers to provide evidence of the quality of their study materials, submit selected samples for independent testing, and justify proposed dosing."

Yet hundreds of small studies of remedies already proven not to work, or of peculiar treatments with no rational hope of benefit, continued to receive funding. One such study—still under way—involves a remedy for pancreatic cancer called the Gonzalez Protocol, in which patients are given "up to 150 pills daily in the form of dietary supplements such as magnesium citrate, papaya . . . vitamins, minerals, trace elements, and animal glandular products. Coffee enemas [are] also administered daily." (The Johns Hopkins Web site includes the Gonzalez Protocol on a list of unproven and potentially dangerous cancer treatments, and NIH's Office for Human Research Protection concluded in 2002 that the informed consent forms for the study "did not list the risk of death from coffee enemas.") Another ongoing study is examining the effect of mistletoe—not the decorative American kind, but a supposedly medicinal European type—injected into solid tumors, based on some European studies that even NCCAM concedes were poorly designed. Still another recent study funded by the center examined whether people's level of the stress hormone cortisol changed in response to harp music.

With its budget for fiscal year 2007 pegged at $120,554,000, the cumulative tab for the center since Harkin established its predecessor OAM back in 1991 is now $853.6 million and counting. Having finally stopped growing—its 2007 budget was actually a few million less than its 2005 budget—the center has basically leveled off at a flat $120 million per annum for the past few years. That means that by 2008, the citizens of the United States will have spent just shy of a billion dollars on the little program that Senator Harkin brought into existence.

And what have we gotten in return? Just lately, as it happens, we have finally gotten quite a bit, although none of it turned out to be what Harkin and his supporters had been hoping for. In the seven months stretching from July of 2005 to February of 2006, three major NCCAM-funded studies provided proof that some of the most revered and widely used dietary supplements—echinacea, saw palmetto, and the combination of chondroitin and glucosamine—were all, ultimately, ineffective.

⊂⊃ ⊂⊃ ⊂⊃

Back during the patent-medicine era, Meyer's Blood Purifier claimed that its echinacea could treat rheumatism, headaches, stomachaches, sores, bites, wounds, dizziness—just about everything, it seemed, but the one ailment for which echinacea is now used: the common cold. The *Journal of the American Medical Association* tried to debunk those claims in an editorial published on February 27, 1908, followed by an article in November 1909 titled "Echinacea Considered Valueless." But by 2002, echinacea was by far the most popular herbal remedy sold in the United States, used by 7.6 percent of adults. Then, on December 3, 2003, *JAMA* published a study of 407 children between the ages of two and eleven—the largest study that had yet been done on echinacea—and concluded that it was ineffective in relieving symptoms and in fact increased the risk of rash. "Despite multiple subanalyses," the authors noted, "we did not find any group of children in whom echinacea appeared to have a positive effect." Another major study, in March of 2005 in the journal *Clinical Infectious Diseases,* likewise found no benefit, with an accompanying editorial calling the $300 million spent each year on echinacea a "major unjustifiable cost of health care at a time when legitimate health care costs are escalating."

Four months later, NCCAM weighed in on July 28, 2005, with a major study published in the *New England Journal of Medicine.* Even bigger and better designed than the one in *JAMA,* the NCCAM-funded monster involved 437 adults in the most exasperatingly careful, thorough study ever performed on any herbal remedy. The researchers prepared their own echinacea extract, and then gave either a 60 percent pure extract, a 20 percent pure extract, or a placebo to see if they could detect a dose response, with fewer colds in those given the stronger doses. They then gave some of the volunteers the treatments before spraying a cold virus into their noses, and others for a few days after the virus had been sprayed, to see whether it worked better at preventing colds or suppressing the symptoms once they began. Then they kept each of the 437 volunteers alone in individual hotel rooms for a full week to see what happened.

They found nothing: no statistical difference between those who received a placebo or echinacea on their rates of developing a cold, their severity of subjective cold symptoms, their volume of nasal excretions (yes, they can measure such a thing), the number of cold viruses found in a sample of their blood, the concentration of immune system leukocytes (a type of white blood cell) found in swabs of their nose, or the concentration of another immune system cell, interleukin-8. Even Dr. Straus agreed that it was time to give up the ghost. "We've got to stop attributing any efficacy to echinacea," he told the *New York Times.* Predictably, the American Herbal Products Association formally complained about what it called Dr. Straus's "gratuitous" commentary, stating: "It is essential that all such communications are factual and do not mislead the public." In response to the criticism, NCCAM changed its Web site to "correct" the "erroneous" statements Dr. Straus had made.

Nearly seven months passed before the results of the next major study funded by the center were published on February 9, 2006, again in the *New England Journal of Medicine*. Saw palmetto sales by then were estimated to be about $134 million, according to *Nutrition Business Journal*, making it the third most popular herbal supplement in the United States. With one of the supplement industry's best reputations, even among some doctors, for being safe and effective, it was then taken by about 2.5 million U.S. men, including Senator Orrin Hatch, to relieve the symptoms of benign prostate hyperplasia (BPH), in which the prostate's size increases, putting pressure on both the bladder and the urethra, increasing the urge to urinate while making it more difficult to do so. The study of 225 men, however, found it to be no better than placebo.

"If you look at the change in symptoms over time between the two groups, it was almost identical," said the leader of the study, Peter Bent, MD, assistant professor of medicine at the University of California, San Francisco. "There was no statistically significant difference at any time point during the study." He did find, however, a clue as to why some previous smaller, less well designed studies had found signs of benefit from saw palmetto. "This is a very pungent herb," he said, "and it took our research team a long time to create a placebo that convincingly duplicates its strong smell and taste. We suspect that prior trials didn't adequately address that problem." In other words, men in previous studies might have been able to accurately guess which they were getting: the smelly saw palmetto or the tasteless placebo.

Unsurprisingly, a spokesman for the Council for Responsible Nutrition called the findings "puzzling." Dr. Andrew Shao, the trade group's vice president, hypothesized that perhaps "exclusion of those patients with mild symptoms from the study may have reduced the ability to detect the benefits . . . seen in other trials. Future trials need to explore in more detail the response of those with both mild and moderate symptoms." Yet two other recent, well-designed trials—one by researchers at Columbia University, another by an Australian group—have likewise found no benefit. Of even greater concern is that prostates can become enlarged not only because of BPH, but also (less frequently, but far more danger-ously) because of an infection or prostate cancer. Self-medicating with saw palmetto can therefore delay diagnosis and treatment of prostate cancer, the most common cancer, other than skin cancer, in American men, seriously increasing their risk of death.

But Dr. Straus was not willing to concede that his center's study had proven anything about saw palmetto one way or another. Rather, he told the *Wall Street Journal*, NCCAM was funding yet another study to see if a higher dose of saw palmetto worked. In an unusually revealing quote, he said, "Our goal is not to debunk things."

Two weeks later, he would have more explaining to do when the third major NCCAM-funded study in a row came out finding little benefit for a popular supplement. Glucosamine and chondroitin, sold separately or together as a combination product, are the most widely used "specialty supplements" (meaning they are neither herbs, vitamins, nor minerals) in the United States. Derived from the cartilage of cows and other ani-mals (although not from sharks), they are taken by at least 5 million Americans over the age of fifty to relieve arthritis pain, generating sales totaling about $1 billion, according to *Nutrition Business Journal*. Even President Bush was using it in the summer of 2005 for knee pain, but by the time of the new study's publication on February 23—yet again in the *New England Journal of Medicine*—a spokesperson said the president had switched from jogging to mountain biking and no longer needed it.

The new study was by far the biggest and best ever conducted on the substances. It involved 1,538 people with arthritic knees randomly as-signed to take either glucosamine alone, chondroitin alone, both to-gether, the painkiller Celebrex, or a placebo for six months. No statistically significant difference was seen between those taking any of the supplements and those taking placebo, but the study indicated why so many people think they benefit from it: a whopping 60 percent of those taking just a placebo said they felt better. The only sign of real ben-efit from the supplements came from an analysis of just the patients with moderate to severe pain, for whom those taking the glucosamine-chondroitin combination reported slightly less pain compared to those taking placebo. However, the number of patients in that category was rel-atively small, and experts have generally put little credence in such "sub-group analysis," because one or another subgroups of patients in any study, if sifted through carefully enough, will turn out—simply by chance—to have fared better following a treatment.

Accordingly, the press was almost unanimous in characterizing the study as showing that the treatments failed. *USA Today,* the *Dallas Morning News,* the *Seattle Post-Intelligencer,* Reuters, and *Forbes* all came out with headlines that were variations on the one offered by the Associated Press: "Supplements Fail to Ease Arthritis." The editorial accompanying the study in the *New England Journal of Medicine* came to a similar conclusion, stating that on the basis of the new results, "it seems prudent to tell our patients with symptomatic osteoarthritis of the knee that neither glucosamine hydrochloride nor chondroitin sulfate alone has been shown to be more efficacious than placebo for the treatment of knee pain."

But NCCAM's press release tried to put a positive spin on the study in its headline: "Efficacy of Glucosamine and Chondroitin Sulfate May Depend on Level of Osteoarthritis Pain." And the audacious Council for Responsible Nutrition turned the study's main finding on its head. "Study Shows Supplements Relieve Osteoarthritis Pain," stated the main headline of the trade group's press release, with the subhead adding, "Combination of Glucosamine and Chondroitin Helps Patients Suffering the Most."

Clearly, this last of the three major NCCAM studies has left open some room for debate. And who knows: maybe one day a large, well-designed NCCAM study of a supplement will actually find clear evidence that one works. But after fifteen years and nearly a billion dollars of disappointment, the question is, why should the American taxpayer keep feeding this beast, when other arms of NIH are desperate for funds to study truly promising treatments for heart disease, stroke, diabetes, Alzheimer's disease, and more?

As with nearly every other question that people might ask about supplements, the answer comes down to money and politics. According to a search of the database maintained by the Center for Responsive Politics (CRP), Senators Harkin and Hatch have received far more in political donations from employees, family, and political action committees of companies in the supplement industry than have any other politicians in the United States. Between 1992 and 2006, Senator Hatch received $208,650 in such donations and Senator Harkin took in $150,880. In fact, either Hatch or Harkin has been the number one recipient of supplement-industry funds during every two-year cycle tracked by CRP since 1992 except two: in 1998, when Representative Brian P. Bilbray, Republican of California, received $31,750 (much of it from Metabolife after he wrote letters to federal administrators defending the company), and in 2002, when Representative Ernest J. Istook, Republican of Oklahoma, received $42,000 (after he co-sponsored a bill that would have made purchases of dietary supplements tax deductible). But even those figures may underestimate the amounts given, as a separate search on CRP's database shows that individuals and PACs associated with just two supplement companies, Starlight International and Herbalife, have given Harkin at least $141,310 since 1993—all but $9,570 of the money he's supposedly received from the entire industry. (CRP explains such apparent inconsistencies on its Web site by noting, "Sometimes it's hard to make apple-to-apple comparisons across some of the pages in a candidate's profile.") What's more, a close reading of Harkin's list of individual donors between 2000 and 2004 reveals that he received at least an additional $28,625 from individuals associated with Herbalife—spouses, children, and such—who did not disclose that association.

But it hasn't been all about money for Harkin. In the view of Dr. Jacobs, the first director of OAM, "He's a politician who panders. I think Harkin jumped on the bandwagon. He was a political opportunist."

⊂⊃ ⊂⊃ ⊂⊃

Luckily, the search for proof of safety and efficacy of dietary supplements has not been limited to work funded by NCCAM. Even as Harkin's folly has burned through close to a billion dollars to reach conclusive (if negative) evidence on just three supplements, scientists, consumer-protection groups, and other government agencies independent of NCCAM's sphere of influence have reached consensus on the risks and benefits of dozens of the most popular supplements on the market today. Their conclusions are based not only on hundreds of well-designed, difficult-to-dispute studies, but on thousands of real-world reports from patients, physicians, and poison centers in the United States and abroad.

In May of 2004, just weeks after the FDA's much-publicized ban on ephedra went into effect on April 14, the highly respected monthly magazine *Consumer Reports* published a cover story warning: "The supplement marketplace still holds hidden hazards for consumers, especially among products that aren't in the headlines." After consulting with experts nationwide, the group published what it called the "Dirty Dozen," a list of the twelve most dangerous supplements on the market. At the top of the list was the only product categorized as "definitely hazardous": aristolochia, the herb that caused Beverly Hames's kidney failure.

Next were five supplements under the category of "very likely hazardous," due to FDA warnings, reports of serious adverse effects in studies, or bans in other countries. Only one of the supplements in this category, androstenedione, or "andro," has been banned in the United States (by Congress in 2004). Three of the others—comfrey, chaparral, and germander—are herbs linked to liver damage, cancer, or death, yet they remain widely available in health food stores. The fifth is kava, which, as noted in chapter 8, has been seeing reports of severe adverse reactions grow as its use spreads.

The remaining "Dirty Dozen" all fell into the category of "likely hazardous," because of adverse-event reports or risks that were then considered only theoretical. Since that time, however, one of them—bitter orange, which has come into wide use as a stimulant to replace ephedra in weight-loss products—has been linked by the FDA to seven deaths and eighty-five adverse reactions. Another, organ and glandular extracts, still poses a theoretical risk of mad cow disease, particularly from brain extracts, yet remains on the market. And the herb lobelia, already banned in Italy and Bangladesh due to reports of breathing difficulty, rapid heartbeat, low blood pressure, diarrhea, dizziness, and possible deaths, likewise remains legal in the United States.

Pennyroyal oil, another on the list, was reported in a 1996 study in the *Annals of Internal Medicine* as the cause of four poisonings, including one death, at a single hospital. As a group, essential oils of all kinds have been linked to 78,750 adverse events reported to the American Association of Poison Control Centers between 1983 and 2004, including 10,135 that required treatment in a hospital (among them was the Long Island eighteen-month-old whose mother gave him eucalyptus oil for a fever) and six deaths. A 2001 report in the *Journal of Paediatrics and Child Health* concluded: "Although essential oils have been used to treat coughs due to colds, reports in the literature document that they can be harmful when ingested. Parents and caregivers should be aware of the life-threatening risks of ingestion."

The last two supplements on the *Consumer Reports* list were yohimbe and scullcap. The former, a powder made from the bark of a West African tree, has long been used as an aphrodisiac. In fact, the active alkaloid, yohimbine, has been a prescription drug in the United States for decades—the only medication doctors had for treating impotence prior to the approval of Viagra in 1998. Proven to relax blood vessels and to stimulate the central nervous system, yohimbine has been shown in some small studies to improve sexual performance. But the handful of randomized, controlled trials published in the past decade have reached conflicting conclusions, and in 1993, doctors from Wayne State University reported the case of a forty-two-year-old African-American man who, after taking yohimbine, developed a severe allergic skin rash, kidney failure, and lupus. Seizures, heart attacks, and death have also been reported. It's also been shown to increase anxiety in people prone to panic disorder. Even more worrisome, however, is that the amount of active yohimbine in supplements can vary from as little as one tenth of a part per million to as much as 489 parts per million, according to an FDA study. For those determined to try one of those little packets sold at convenience stores, the FDA offers this warning: "Yohimbe should also be avoided by individuals with hypotension (low blood pressure), diabetes, and heart, liver or kidney disease. Symptoms of overdosage include weakness and nervous stimulation followed by paralysis, fatigue, stomach disorders, and ultimately death."

Scullcap, the last of the "Dirty Dozen," is derived from the root of a plant long used both in traditional Chinese medicine to treat everything from epilepsy to cancer, and in North America as a relaxant. But it has been linked to liver damage in two reports from Norway, and to pneumonia in a report from Japan. The Web site of Memorial Sloan-Kettering Cancer Center cautions, "Signs of scullcap toxicity include stupor, confusion, and seizures." And it was one of the eight herbal ingredients in the now-banned PC-SPES. But for NCCAM, it seems, the fat lady never sings: it has funded at least four studies of scullcap in the past few years to look for its effects on skin cancer, colon cancer, and cardiovascular disease.

Scullcap is hardly the only dangerous or disproved supplement that NCCAM continues to study. Ginkgo biloba, despite the side effects and lack of proven benefits cited in chapter 8, was the subject of three studies funded by the center in 2005. Garlic was the subject of two NCCAM-funded studies that year, despite the negligible benefits and considerable dangers found in a recent review by the Agency for Healthcare Research and Quality (AHRQ). The center also funded three studies in 2005 on ginseng, despite a 2002 review in the *Annals of Internal Medicine* that concluded, "Well-conducted trials do not support the efficacy of ginseng to treat any condition." As the country's second most popular herb, taken by 4.5 percent of U.S. adults, ginseng enjoys a venerable history but suffers from a stunning lack of supporting scientific evidence. Sometimes sold as an aphrodisiac, other times to improve stamina, energy, concentration, or mood, ginseng has shown none of these effects when put to the test in well-designed studies. But it has been linked to vaginal bleeding, severe headaches, and insomnia, and has been found to interfere with blood-thinning medications. To make matters worse, ConsumerLab.com reported in 2003, after testing a number of commercial products, that "a high amount of the pesticide hexachlorobenzene—a potential human carcinogen—was found in one of five products labeled as containing 'Korean Ginseng.' Levels of two other pesticides, quintozene and lindane, were also above acceptable levels. Another product that failed the new testing was a liquid 'Chinese Ginseng' sold in single-dose bottles. Despite being labeled 'EXTRA STRENGTH' this product contained less than 10% of the expected ginsenosides."

At least it could be said that the evidence for SAM-e, marketed for the relief of depression and arthritis, is not uniformly bad. In 2002, AHRQ published a review of 102 studies—most of which turned out to be small and of widely varying quality. Even so, the agency tentatively concluded that evidence for SAM-e's ability to relieve depression was "statistically as well as clinically significant and is equivalent to a partial response to treatment." It also found evidence of a modest benefit on the pain of osteoarthritis. But in 2001 the FDA sent letters to two manufacturers of SAM-e, advising them that the agency had "significant concerns about the potential for consumers who have certain diseases or conditions to experience serious adverse effects with the use of SAM-e. For example, the scientific literature . . . suggests that persons who have a bipolar major affective disorder (manic-depressive disease) may experience mood switching from depression to hypomania when supplemented with SAM-e." Studies have also found that SAM-e has neuropsychiatric effects that could pose "potential serious risks" for people taking other drugs with similar properties. In addition, as little as 400 milligrams of SAM-e daily has been shown to cause heartburn, nausea, and other gastrointestinal complaints. But given AHRQ's findings of potential benefit, perhaps it makes sense that in 2005 NCCAM funded five studies on it.

Not even NCCAM, however, could conduct studies on all the 29,000 dietary supplements recently estimated by the FDA to be on the market today. Just for preventing heart disease, for instance, there's coenzyme Q10, a naturally occurring antioxidant promoted by countless Web sites, despite an April 2000 study in the *Annals of Internal Medicine* finding no benefit for heart patients (not to mention that the only randomized trial in cancer patients showed that it actually decreased the effectiveness of doxorubicin, a drug used to treat cancer). There is conjugated linoleic acid, an unsaturated fatty acid pitched as an antioxidant that just might be the next miracle supplement—despite the spate of recent studies in prominent journals showing that it actually promotes oxidation. There's flaxseed oil, found in the refrigerated sections of nearly all health food stores and promoted for containing ALA, a type of omega-3 fatty acid, even though the best thing that AHRQ could say after reviewing the evidence for ALA is that it *may* help reduce deaths from heart disease, "but to a much lesser extent than fish oil." There's guggul, the resin of the mukul plant, grown in northern India and promoted as an effective cholesterol-lowering supplement despite an August 2003 study in the *Journal of the American Medical Association* finding no benefit on the patients' cholesterol, triglyceride, or HDL (the so-called good cholesterol) and a 5 percent rise in LDL, the bad cholesterol, compared to a 5 percent *drop* in LDL on the patients who took a placebo. What's more, six of the patients taking guggul developed a hypersensitivity skin rash, compared to none in the placebo group. Then there is red yeast rice, which contains a compound identical to lovastatin, the active ingredient in the statin drug Mevacor—which is why the FDA considers it a drug, not a supplement, and has warned against the rare but life-threatening reactions it can cause in muscles and kidneys. And finally, the latest supplement shown to have no benefit for preventing heart disease is policosanol, a natural substance produced by the waxy coating of sugar cane and promoted for years as a cholesterol-lowering agent by a single research group in Cuba (where sugar cane is, coincidentally, a leading export crop), but shown in a study published on May 16, 2006, in the *Journal of the American Medical Association* to have no effect on cholesterol whatsoever.

But perhaps scientific proof is beside the point to the supplement industry, which has even gone so far as to market a supposedly safe alternative to L-tryptophan (which itself can still be bought online in violation of federal law). The product 5HTP is claimed to have the same effects that L-tryptophan supposedly had on insomnia, depression, obesity—even on attention deficit disorder. But a 1998 study in the journal *Nature Medicine* found that samples from six manufacturers had some of the same chemical impurities as those in L-tryptophan that caused so many deaths and injuries. In April of 1999, Renee Kleemeier of suburban Colerain Township, Ohio, bought a bottle of 5HTP at a local GNC. She took it at bedtime for ten days just to help her get a good night's sleep. Within days, she began experiencing severe shortness of breath, coughing, and wheezing. Over the summer the symptoms worsened and landed her in the emergency room several times. On November 8, 1999, she was admitted to Mercy Franciscan Hospital for heart failure. She remains critically ill.

⬭ ⬭ ⬭

At the end of the day, then, has no supplement been found to be both safe and effective for its intended use? Can the news really be all that grim for a $21 billion industry?

In fairness, two supplements do look promising for the average person, although both of them actually appear normally in the diet, unlike most of the products that fall under the heading of "dietary supplements." First, as noted in chapter 7, vitamin D does seem beneficial for the average person, especially African-Americans, people of all races living in the North during the winter months, and anyone who rarely goes outside. Second are the omega-3 fatty acids derived from fish oil, another combination product that President George W. Bush takes. In October of 2000, in response to a lawsuit filed by a manufacturer that wanted permission to make health claims for omega-3 fatty acids, the FDA decided, for the first time, to permit what it called a "qualified" health claim, something it had never permitted for any supplement. Until then, the FDA permitted a claim only when it concluded that there was "significant scientific agreement" behind it—something no supplement had ever managed to achieve. But finally the agency decided that it would allow a "qualified" claim if the evidence was "suggestive but not conclusive." Such was the state of knowledge, the FDA concluded, for the ability of omega-3 fatty acids (typically obtained from fish oil but also found in flaxseed and canola oils) to prevent heart disease. Two of the components of omega-3 fatty acids—EPA and DHA—appear to be responsible for most of the benefits, the agency noted. Even so, it stated: "FDA recommends that consumers not exceed more than a total of 3 grams per day of EPA and DHA omega-3 fatty acids, with no more than 2 grams per day from a dietary supplement." But in April of 2004, AHRQ got into the act, concluding after an exhaustive review of the evidence that "fish oil can help reduce deaths from heart disease." Although omega-3 fatty acids "do not alter total cholesterol, HDL cholesterol, or LDL cholesterol, evidence suggests that they can reduce levels of triglycerides," the agency stated. Even here, though, the jury is still very much out. On June 14, 2006, the *Journal of the American Medical Association* published the largest double-blind study of fish oil yet conducted, but found no benefit.

Still, for now anyway, fish oil and vitamin D appear to be a decent bet for the average adult. Let it be recorded, then, lest anyone suggest that not a single dietary supplement has been found to be both safe and effective for the masses despite Mr. Harkin's billion-dollar search for proof: of the 29,000 products now on the market, two look pretty darn good.

CONCLUSION
WHAT WE CAN DO

Perhaps it is only predictable, cynics might say, that an editorial in the *New England Journal of Medicine* called DSHEA "misguided"; that the *Washington Post* called it a "truly terrible federal law"; that the *San Jose Mercury News* called it "one of the worst pieces of legislation passed during the Clinton administration"; or that the *New York Times* nicknamed it the "Snake Oil Protection Act." It is perhaps more surprising and credible that two independent federal bodies have similarly criticized it, although in more measured language. The Institute of Medicine, created and funded by Congress to be an independent expert advisor on medical matters, concluded in 2004 that because of DSHEA, "The constraints imposed on the FDA with regard to ensuring the absence of unreasonable risk associated with the use of dietary supplements make it difficult for the health of the American public to be adequately protected." Likewise, the Office of the Inspector General of the U.S. Department of Health and Human Services titled its April 2001 report about the adverse-event reporting system created by DSHEA "An Inadequate Safety Valve." Even *Consumer Reports,* which normally confines itself to rating tangible items like washing machines and automobiles, was moved to state that DSHEA "opened up a loophole big enough to be exploited by anyone." When Charles Bell, program director of Consumers Union, which publishes *Consumer Reports,* testified before John McCain's Senate Commerce Committee, he said that DSHEA "opened the floodgates to thousands of untested herbal products and handcuffed the Food and Drug Administration from performing any meaningful oversight over what has since developed into a multibillion-dollar industry." Things have even reached the point where New York State has been urged to take matters into its own hands. In October of 2005, the New York State Task Force on Life and Law urged the state to move into the breach created by DSHEA by empowering the state health department to ban unsafe supplements and require manufacturers to report serious adverse events. But passage of such a plan looks unlikely, and in any case, the crisis in regulating supplements is a national matter, not a local one.

What, then, should be done? Most of the steps outlined below are recommended by Consumers Union, leading newspaper editorial boards and the Institute of Medicine, to name a few, and many are already being undertaken by Europe, Canada, and other countries. The Codex Alimentarius Commission, created in 1963 by the United Nations and World Health Organization to create food standards to protect consumer health, has been working for more than a decade to set safe upper limits for vitamins and minerals, and to define permissible health claims. The European Union Directive on Food Supplements, a set of regulations which went into effect on August 1, 2005, requires all adverse events to be reported to the government, permits sales of only those supplements for which at least some safety data is available, mandates extensive warnings on labels, and generally allows only one active ingredient in any product. Canada's Natural Health Products Directorate is likewise phasing in premarket approval for all supplements, registration of all manufacturers, and good manufacturing standards. According to Phil Waddington, who is running Canada's program, "The United States does stand out in the global marketplace in how it regulates its products."

Here, then, are thirteen steps the United States can take to bring its supplement marketplace in line with the rest of the world, and propel it into the twenty-first century.

1. Establish seed-to-shelf quality controls.

Nearly a hundred years after Congress passed the Pure Food and Drug Act of 1906, it is simply inexcusable that supplement manufacturers have been given a free pass to operate outside the fundamental principle that all drugs should be, at the very least, pure and of reliable potency. Although authorized by DSHEA to establish good manufacturing practices (GMPs), the FDA has waited more than ten years to do so. In October of 2004, Commissioner Crawford promised to issue the long-awaited regulations by year's end, but as of May 2005, his promise remained unfulfilled. With no manufacturing standards in place, manufacturers have proven themselves woefully unable to produce reliable products, with countless studies showing potencies ranging from 0 to 500 percent of the labeled amount, as well as containing many unlabeled contaminants. Even when the FDA eventually implements standards (as they surely will do sooner or later), Dr. Tod Cooperman of ConsumerLab.com emphasizes that they will be modeled on the relatively lax standards governing foods, not the far tighter standards for manufacturing drugs, because DSHEA deemed supplements to be foods.

In its 2005 report on complementary and alternative medicine, the Institute of Medicine said it was concerned about the quality of supplements in the United States. "There is little product reliability," the report concluded. "In addition to the confusion that this introduces to the consumer, the lack of reliable and consistent products is a challenge to the research and clinical practice communities. Without consistent products, research is extremely difficult to conduct or generalize. Furthermore, without high-quality research, evidence-based clinical recommendations cannot be made to guide patients." The academy recommended that Congress establish "seed-to-shelf quality control."

2. Require that supplements be registered with the FDA.

When the Office of Inspector General reviewed all the complaints the FDA had received about supplements from 1994 to 1999, what it found verged on the bizarre: "FDA could not determine the identity of the manufacturer for 32 percent (1,153 of 3,574) of the products involved in the reports. FDA does not know the city and states where the manufacturer is located for 71 percent (644 of 904) of the manufacturers in its database. FDA does not routinely contact the supplement manufacturer when it receives an adverse event on its product. One of the reasons FDA gives for not contacting the manufacturer is that it cannot locate many of them.... In one instance, FDA received two reports of comas associated with a product, but when field inspectors tried to track down the manufacturer, they found a post office box belonging to an owner who had since moved and closed the account." It took the Bioterrorism Act of 2002 to finally require supplement manufacturers to register with the FDA, but how many have actually done so is unknown. And still to this day, no law requires them to tell the FDA which products they make, or even what the ingredients are. The Dietary Supplement and Awareness Act, introduced in 2005 by Representatives Waxman, Davis and Dingell, would close this loophole, while making it slightly less impossible for the FDA to ban dangerous supplements. But without greater public support, its chances for passage look dim.

3. Require clearer, more complete labels.

Presently, many supplement labels omit ingredients that are in a "proprietary blend," or use obscure botanical names to lend their product an exotic appeal. Few include the kind of safety warnings found on all drug labels. It would seem the soul of sense to follow the recommendations made in a *New England Journal of Medicine* editorial in December of 2002: "The labels of dietary supplements should contain a list of constituents that unambiguously identifies herbs by their botanical and common names. Information about possible adverse effects, including the potential for herb-drug interactions, should be included."

4. Require manufacturers to report serious adverse events to the FDA.

In March of 2000, Alexander M. Walker, MD, former chairman of epidemiology at the Harvard School of Public Health, delivered to the FDA a study it had commissioned him to conduct. He calculated that the agency was receiving reports on less than 1 percent of all the adverse events caused by supplements. In 1999, for instance, the FDA received just 460 reports of adverse events caused by dietary supplements. That same year, U.S. Poison Control Centers received approximately 13,000 such reports.

How many reports of adverse events did the FDA receive from manufacturers in the years between 1993 and 2000? *Fewer than ten,* according to the Inspector General report. In contrast, 90 percent of the adverse events reported to the FDA on drugs come directly from manufacturers, who are legally required to report all reactions to prescription drugs.

Both the Inspector General and the Institute of Medicine recommended that manufacturers be required to report all "serious" adverse events to the FDA. Senator Dick Durbin introduced a bill in 2004 to require just that, and the *Star-Ledger* of New Jersey reported in August of 2006 that a deal for passage of the bill was near. In the meanwhile, the Inspector General report also urged the FDA to better inform health professionals and consumers about its adverse-event reporting system for dietary supplements. (To report an adverse event, consumers can call the FDA, toll free at any time, at 1–800–FDA–1088, or go online at www.fda.gov/medwatch.)

5. Require pre-market proof of safety.

The supplement industry has done a superb job of convincing consumers that it would be somehow un-American to require them to prove that their products are safe before putting them on sale. Instead, as the case of ephedra has demonstrated, the industry—and current federal law under DSHEA—demands that the government spend millions of taxpayer dollars on testing to prove that a supplement is dangerous, despite the fact that doing so, in many cases, would amount to unethical human testing. Europe and Canada both now require at least some proof of safety before allowing supplements to be sold. No one is calling for a Spanish Inquisition or the kinds of multimillion-dollar studies required for new drugs. But some minimal standard—even if it amounts to a simple review of the medical literature and traditional usage—must be established for U.S. companies to make their case to the FDA that their product is safe before it goes on sale. Those products already on the market could be given a grace period, as Canada has granted.

6. Replace NCCAM with an expert panel to review safety and efficacy.

The National Center for Complementary and Alternative Medicine was a boondoggle when Senator Harkin created its forerunner, the Office of Alternative Medicine, with passage of a $2 million bill in 1991. Nearly a billion dollars later, it has turned into a kind of perpetual motion machine, endlessly going in circles to study the same supplements over and over again in ever greater detail, rarely seeing the forest through the ginkgo trees. Besides proving a few supplements to be of no value, its main achievement to date has been to create a national network of academics whose entire careers are now devoted to the study of supplements—and dependent on its handouts. It is time to shut the thing down. Let NIH spend the $120 million per year it's been pouring into NCCAM to fund studies whose goals are to investigate remedies not because they're considered alternative or complementary but simply because they're promising.

And what of those supplements with truly uncertain value? A model for deciding their worth was established back in 1962, when Congress decided that it was no longer enough for drugs to be proven merely safe; henceforth, they also had to be proven effective for the claims made. In just three years, between 1966 and 1969, the National Academy of Sciences completed the awesome task of reviewing the evidence for the 3,000 to 4,000 drugs that had been on the market prior to 1962, tossing out those for which the evidence was lacking.

The FDA has already contracted with the National Academy of Sciences to describe a process for developing research summaries, or monographs, that would review the safety and efficacy of supplements—a process that is already under way in Europe and Canada. The Office of the Inspector General has noted that "FDA could require manufacturers to adhere to the monographs in the future," presumably selling only those supplements, and making only those claims, endorsed by the monographs.

Such a process would certainly take years of careful work. As Phil Waddington describes the situation now facing Canada's Natural Health Products Directorate: "We've got thousands of applications. We've told people it's going to take years. It's not like we're pretending it will be done Thursday." Contentious as such a process would surely be in the United States, it must begin. Those supplements found effective for treating or preventing any disease should be put on an equal footing with drugs and reimbursed by insurance companies, Medicare, and Medicaid.

7. Empower the FDA to set maximum safe doses.

There is no rational reason for vitamins and minerals to be sold at doses proven to be dangerous. They pose a public health threat, particularly to innocent children. Anyone determined to take dangerously high doses can endure the inconvenience of having to take multiple pills. Senator Proxmire's 1976 bill to prohibit the FDA from setting maximum safe doses of vitamins and minerals was wrong then, and it is wrong now.

8. Increase funding of the FDA.

The FDA's funding for all of its activities related to dietary supplements in fiscal year 2001 was $6 million. That year, it had the equivalent of forty-six full-time employees devoted to dietary supplements. In 2002, in a report to Congress, it estimated that 158 million consumers were using supplements and stated that "the dietary supplement industry is one of the fastest growing industries in the world." The agency estimated that it would need up to $65 million per year—about ten times as much as it was getting—to implement a strategic plan it had developed for fulfilling the requirements of DSHEA. That plan, it should be noted, presumed no changes in DSHEA, and no increased regulatory authority. When Cynthia T. Culmo of the Association of Food and Drug Officials testified before the Senate in 2002, she repeated one of her suggestions for improved regulation of supplements three times: "Fund FDA! Fund FDA! Fund FDA!"

But by 2004, the agency's supplement division remained, as *Consumer Reports* put it, "understaffed and underfunded, with about 60 people and a budget of only $10 million to police a $19.4 billion-a-year industry. To regulate drugs, annual sales of which are 12 times the amount of supplement sales, the FDA has almost 43 times as much money and almost 48 times as many people."

If Congress takes no other action on supplements, it should immediately give FDA the money it needs to carry out the pathetically minimal mandates of DSHEA.

9. Require child-resistant packaging.

Under DSHEA, the FDA has no authority to require child-resistant packaging of supplements that can and do kill young children every year.

While not all supplements pose a danger when ingested by children in large amounts, some, including iron, clearly do. In January of 2003, the medical journal *Lancet* published an analysis of 489 reports of adverse reactions to supplements as reported to eleven U.S. poison control centers in 1998. After finding that 70 percent of the events involving preadolescents were "unintentional," the researchers concluded: "These data warrant concern about the absence of child-resistant packaging for dietary supplements." If even one of the four or five deaths of toddlers that still occur each year due to iron supplements could be prevented, it would be well worth the inconvenience of requiring the same child-resistant packaging on potentially dangerous supplements that have long been required for drugs.

10. Limit multiple ingredients.

The *Lancet* study described above also found that 51 percent of the cases reported to poison control centers involved substances that had more than one ingredient. "Use of multiple ingredients seemed to be associated with a larger number of symptoms, as well as with more severe outcomes," the researchers found. The dozens of ingredients crammed into some supplements make a mockery of the entire industry, while also making it impossible for anyone to figure out which might be helping or hurting consumers. The European Union generally permits only single-ingredient products, and the United States should do likewise.

11. Ban high school coaches from promoting sports supplements.

A 2001 survey by the Blue Cross and Blue Shield Association concluded that more than 1 million U.S. students in high school and junior high had taken performance-enhancing sports supplements. That same year, Texas became the first state in the country to pass a law making it illegal for public school employees to distribute, sell, or market supplements for student athletes. In 2002, a survey of high school and college coaches conducted for GNC, the supplement retailer, found that 43 percent recommend such products to their athletes. That November, the National Federation of State High School Associations issued the following statement: "All student-athletes and their parents/guardians should consult with their physicians before taking any supplement product. In addition, coaches and school staff should not recommend or supply any supplement product to student-athletes." Illinois, Michigan, and California have now passed bills similar to Texas's. A law banning coaches and teachers from hawking supplements should be national.

12. Limit where supplements can be sold.

A hundred years ago, America's pharmacists had mixed feelings about patent medicines: they knew that most of them were ineffective or dangerous, yet the products were also among their best sellers. Eventually, though, drugstore proprietors came to realize that the patent medicines were undermining their credibility and destroying their customers' faith in everything they sold. Pharmacies today should reach the same conclusion and stop selling all supplements that are unproved and dangerous— and that's nearly all supplements. Their trade associations, at the very least, should take a stand against the sale of these products. And the very idea that delis, grocery stores, and gas stations are in the business of selling dietary supplements is a violation of common sense, unless one considers it a good idea that the same retailers sell cigarettes.

13. Hold media accountable.

While awaiting the aforementioned legislative fixes, the nation's news media can take action of its own. To repeat the statement made by Pamela Jones Harbour, commissioner of the Federal Trade Commission: "Media outlets should be responsible for not running false advertising. They should demand substantiation for the claims they allow to run on their air, and if they don't, the media should be called to account by consumers." The FTC has noted that advertisements for diet supplements making obviously false claims still appear regularly in mainstream newspapers, magazines, and television commercials.

But advertisers aren't the media's worst problem; reporters and editors also need to do a better job of fully informing consumers about supplements. For one, they should stop routinely quoting the Council for Responsible Nutrition, which is merely a trade group promoting their members' products, despite its attempts to position itself as a purveyor of the "science behind the supplements." In fact, its own Web site describes its mission as "enhancing confidence among media, healthcare professionals, decision makers and consumers." The group likes to boast about how often it's quoted in the major news media whenever a scientific study dares to cast doubt on the benefits of a supplement. While it's perfectly legitimate to seek comment from CRN on policy issues, it's inexcusable to give them a voice on matters of science. Reporters in search of balance in their health articles should seek comment from independent research scientists, not from paid spokespeople.

But a deeper problem afflicts the media's coverage of dietary supplements. From L-tryptophan to echinacea, from Airborne to shark cartilage, virtually every supplement has ridden a wave of popularity generated by press coverage as favorable as it was fatuous. Journalists must recognize the danger their seemingly benign stories pose to consumers who rely on them, no matter how "objective" or "accurate" they may try to be, because products that have undergone no serious scientific or regulatory scrutiny exist only in the realm of opinion, not fact. They must strive to seek independent sources and be wary of manufacturers bearing "research" that is often bought and paid for to promote their products. So long as our government refuses to fulfill its fundamental duty to provide for the welfare of citizens, the media must exercise its role as watchdog.

⬭ ⬭ ⬭

In the final analysis, however, it is not the fault of manufacturers, or Congress, or coaches, or the media that America has become a Supplement Nation. The fault lies with us. It is we, the people, who have allowed ourselves to be bamboozled. In an age of postmodern cynicism toward experts, doctors, politicians, and reporters of every stripe, we have made a special exception for the claims of supplement manufacturers—precisely because they prey upon our skepticism toward all other sources. "The doctors and the drug companies are just trying to keep you from getting the inexpensive, life-saving, natural remedies that really work," they proclaim. That was their ingenious argument of a hundred years ago, when they were selling snake oil and Peruna and Dr. Williams' Pink Pills for Pale People, and it's their same argument today. They have hijacked our skepticism and convinced us that health can be found in a pill, so long as the label tells us that the pill is "natural." Is it a coincidence that our obsession with "natural" supplements has come precisely at a time when Americans are more removed from nature than ever before, eating more fast food, watching more television, parked in front of computer screens and growing more obese?

Michael R. Harris, the historian of pharmacy, puts it this way: "Most of these supposedly life-extending supplements, people take them because they promise health without having to do the work. They keep forgetting the basics: don't smoke, eat properly, and exercise. My whole career has been trying to educate people to swallow less, think more. Every time you swallow something you take a chance of a side effect. The thing is, you have to pay your dues. You don't get stimulated endlessly without the body reacting against it. Any time you swallow something short of water—and if you drink too much water, you can have a problem—someone is going to react negatively to it, I don't care what the substance is or where it comes from. But we're in a cycle now where we believe that Mother Nature won't harm you—that if it's natural, it's safe."

Despite the tragedies of L-tryptophan and ephedra, despite the tainting of Olympic careers and the death of a professional baseball player and thousands of other Americans, the pendulum of history has yet to swing back against so-called natural dietary supplements. Without a significant course correction, it is difficult to imagine that another major tragedy will not strike again. But as with the years of unheeded warning for the devastation that a category 5 hurricane could inflict on New Orleans, it just may take a Katrina-size event to awaken the public to the dangers that supplements pose. One can only wonder how many deaths will be chalked up to natural causes before the pendulum at last swings back.

ACKNOWLEDGMENTS

Before thanking those who have helped me with this book, I wish first to acknowledge the millions of Americans whose deep faith in dietary supplements may be offended by it. I respect their right to care for their health, and the health of their children, as they think best. My only concern has been with the right of manufacturers to lie and mislead them.

I first came to learn about the curious and colorful world of supplements in the course of writing articles for *Pharmacy Practice News* and the *New York Times*. It has always been an honor and pleasure to work with my editors at those newspapers, David Bronstein and Erica Goode, respectively.

I would not have undertaken *Natural Causes*, nor would I have been able to complete it, without the wise counsel and support of Jane Dystel and Miriam Goderich, literary agents extraordinaire. They have stood by me and guided me for years, through thin and thinner.

When I was initially hesitant to take on such a controversial subject, one of my brothers, Michael, gave me a much-needed push by telling me to stop worrying and start writing.

This book simply would not have been possible without the decades of investigative work by Stephen Barrett, MD, as described in the source notes. I—along with millions of other Americans whose well-being he has worked tirelessly to protect—owe him an enormous debt of thanks.

I was incredibly lucky to have had Ann Campbell as my editor. Her countless requests for more information, a tighter structure, or just a better word, always made the book better. Thank heaven she didn't accept the first draft, or the second, or the third. Thanks, too, to her former and current assistants, Ursula Cary and Laura Lee Mattingly, and to everyone else at Broadway.

Sarah Despres and Anna Laitin, aides to Representative Henry Waxman, were uniquely helpful in pointing me to knowledgeable individuals within and outside the government.

My wife, Alice, and my daughter, Annie, endured nearly two years of my working nights, weekends, vacations, and holidays as bills piled up and the lawn went unmowed. Alice stayed up until 2 a.m. one night proofreading the final manuscript. I can't thank them enough, or love them more.

Our dear friends Michael and Anne Mernin listened to me yammer ad nauseam about the book as it progressed, always managing to look interested.

The gifted photographer Rob Fraser kindly agreed to shoot me for the book jacket in exchange for a 60-Second Novel, and even Photoshopped my nose hairs.

Many supplement manufacturers and their advocates showed great kindness and class in speaking with me, chief among them Gerry Kessler and Mitchell Balbert. I do not like what they sell, but I found much to like and admire about them personally.

I am indebted to the hundreds of physicians, toxicologists, nutritionists, pharmacists, journalists, historians, advocates, legislators, government employees, attorneys, and others who spoke with me about their experiences and their research.

Most of all, I thank the victims and their families—including Sue Gilliatt, Ruth Alterman, Phil Howry, Camille Lee, and Beverly Hames—who shared their unhappy stories with me in the hope that others might avoid such tragedies.

NOTES

Though he is never mentioned in the preceding pages of this book, Stephen Barrett, MD, was in fact an indispensable source of information in my research and writing, as indeed he has been the entire country's leading source about the supplement industry for more than three decades. Many of the books, experts and Congressional testimonies to which I have referred were lent or suggested to me by Dr. Barrett. He allowed me to photocopy documents from his files, and reviewed the final manuscript for errors. (All errors remaining are mine alone.) Dr. Barrett is perhaps best known to the public as the founder of www.quackwatch.org, which offers thousands of carefully researched and footnoted articles, many of them containing documents unavailable anywhere else, on supplements and other unproved remedies, as well as on the unsavory individuals and business practices behind them. He is also a founder, vice president, and a board member of the National Council Against Health Fraud, and has written and edited dozens of books. Among his many honors and awards is the 1984 FDA Commissioner's Special Citation Award for Public Service. For anyone interested in keeping up on the supplement industry, the weekly e-mailed newsletter he edits, Consumer Health Digest, is must reading; a free subscription can be had by sending a blank e-mail to chdigestsubscribe@ssr.com.

PROLOGUE: SUE GILLIATT'S NOSE

Sue Gilliatt's story first came to my attention from the Web site of WISH television, the Indianapolis affiliate of CBS, in content based on the station's two-part news broadcast on November 25 and 26, 2003. Sue spent hours talking with me by telephone. She gave me permission to speak with the attorney John Muller, and authorized him to send me the extensive legal file on her case. Sue then spent much of an afternoon meeting with me at her home in Indianapolis. By telephone I interviewed the assistant United States attorney Larry J. Regan, who prosecuted the case against Gregory Caton. Mr. Caton was unavailable for interview, due to being jailed, but I was able to speak by telephone with his wife, Cathryn. I also spoke by telephone with Rev. Dan Raber; the police chief Corey

Parker of Abbeville, Georgia, as well as the clerk who answered his telephone; and with a spokesperson for Georgia's Composite State Board of Medical Examiners. I made many requests, both by telephone and e-mail, to interview Andrew Weil, MD, but he declined through his administrative assistant. A wealth of news reports, Web site postings, and legal filings further contributed to my account of Sue's story.

3   *A 1998 survey*   Cited in David M. Steinberg, Roger B. Davis, Susan L. Ettner, et al, "Trends in Alternative Medicine Use in the United States, 1990–1997," *JAMA* 280 (November 11, 1998): 1569–75.

Another survey published that same year   See Vicky A. Newman, Cheryl L. Rock, Susan Faerber, et al, "Dietary Supplement Use by Women at Risk for Breast Cancer Recurrence," *Journal of the American Dietetic Association* 98 (2003): 285–92.

she got a hit from the Web site   The brief article on bloodroot was posted on Dr. Weil's site at www.drweil.com/app/cda/drw_cda.html-command=TodayQA-questionId=4038-pt= Question, where I accessed it on January 13, 2004, copied it onto my computer, and printed it out. The article has since been removed from the site.

7   *On September 15*   Dates of all of Sue's outgoing long-distance telephone calls were confirmed by her telephone billing records.

8   *A study presented in October 2005*   The study, "Initiation of Complementary and Alternative Medical Therapies by Cancer Patients During Radiation Therapy," led by Neha Vapiwala, MD, a radiation oncologist at the University of Pennsylvania in Philadelphia, was presented on October 16, 2005.

9   *On her medical record*   From a computer printout of Dr. Rehme's treatment notes, dated October 1, 2001.

According to Alpha Omega's brochure   Mail-order catalog dated Summer/Fall 2001, "Alpha Omega Laboratories' Amazing Herbal Discoveries."

11   *Caton pled guilty*   This information was provided by the assistant United States attorney Larry J. Regan, who handled the case, and was also described by Tabetha LeDoux, a manager at Alpha Omega, in a letter posted online at www.newmediaexplorer.org/chris/2003/ 09/25/the_alpha_omega_story_ another_fda_scam.htm.

But the résumé on his Web site   See www.gregcaton.com.

in February of 1997   See news report on the Web site of the Reporters Committee for Freedom of the Press, "Judge Awards $133 Million, Permanent Gag Order Against Author," at www.rcfp.org/news/1997/0324f.html.

12   *"50 Reasons Why I Am a Vegetarian"*   See www.soybean.com/50rea.htm.

But by September of 2003   I surmised this by the fact that agents of the FDA and FTC raided Caton's offices to investigate on September 17, 2003.

Sharon Lee of Mexia, Texas   The attorney Peter Malouf in Dallas, who represented Sharon, spoke with me by telephone. A report about her case, by reporter Ginger Allen, also appeared on the CBS TV affiliate in Dallas on December 11, 2003.

On Wednesday, September 17, 2003   The date was noted in a posting on Caton's Web site, www.altcancer.com.

13   *ten guns, ten thousand rounds of ammunition*   From my interview with the attorney Peter Malouf.

In May of 2004   This information was first relayed to me by Sue Gilliatt, from a letter she received from the victim witness coordinator of the U.S. Attorney's Office. The information is now posted online at www.cancertreatmentwatch.org/reg/caton.shtml.

The summer of 2005   See Associated Press: "Doctor Accused of Aiding Man Who Disfigured Cancer Patients," August 14, 2005, and "Georgia Healer Targeted over Cancer Treatment,"

August 29, 2005. Details of the medical board's charges are posted at www.casewatch.org/board/med/march/march.shtml.

He settled a lawsuit   In a statement on his Web site, www.cancerx.org, Raber asserts that he has "refused to settle the case," accuses Sue and her attorney of using "dirty tactics," and states that "his product did not and could not harm Gilliatt or any one else."

16   *a staggering 62 percent of Americans*   This figure comes from an Ipsos-Public Affairs telephone survey of 1,000 U.S. adults, with the results weighted to represent the U.S. population. The survey was commissioned by the Council for Responsible Nutrition and released on October 25, 2004, during the trade group's annual conference.

One fourth of U.S. adults   Cited by the National Center for Health Statistics, "Complementary and Alternative Medicine Use Among Adults: United States, 2002," May 27, 2004.

According to Grant Ferrier   The figures and quotes come from an e-mail Mr. Ferrier sent me on May 18, 2006.

Herbs are now added to a beer   The company unveiled its new beer B^E, containing caffeine, guarana, and ginseng, on October 4, 2004.

vitamins and other "heart healthy nutrients"   Mars, Inc., announced the release of CocoaVia on September 14, 2005. The product contains "a patented blend of heart-healthy cocoa flavanols and cholesterol-lowering plant sterols from soy," as well as "calcium and a mix of heart-healthy nutrients including folic acid, vitamins B-6, B-12, C, and E," the company announced.

herbs and vitamins are loaded into   The syrups, called Rhino Blasts, are available in a limited number of Carvel shops and at many other retail outlets, according to the supplement manufacturer Rhino Naturals, Inc., of Rancho Santa Margarita, California.

the National Center for Complementary and Alternative Medicine (NCCAM) . . . has already expended nearly a billion dollars   This figure comes from my tabulation from a variety of official government reports over the years. For a full explanation of how I reached this figure, please see the notes for chapter 11, which examine the history of NCCAM in detail.

17   *President George W. Bush's 2005 budget request*   The request was made in a statement to the Senate Subcommittee on Labor-HHS-Education Appropriations on April 1, 2004, by Stephen E. Straus, MD, director of NCCAM.

As of 2005   I performed this search myself in January of 2005.

with the possible exception of fish oil and vitamin D   This broad conclusion, shared by many scientists and critics of the supplement industry but hotly disputed by its supporters, is really what this whole book is about. It is ultimately my own conclusion, based not on any single document or interview but on two years of interviews with hundreds of people and my review of thousands of studies and reports of government agencies, medical societies, and consumer organizations, many of which are listed in these notes.

Vitamin E . . . progesterone . . . multivitamins . . . iron   The evidence regarding these supplements is considered in detail in chapters 7 and 8.

18   *the American Association of Poison Control Centers*   I tabulated the data from twenty-two yearly reports of the AAPCC, which have appeared each September in the *American Journal of Emergency Medicine* since 1984, and are available online at www.aapcc.org/poison1.htm.

Metabolife . . . had received   See U.S. General Accounting Office, "Report to the Chairman, Subcommittee on Wellness and Human Rights, Committee on Government Reform, House of Representatives: Dietary Supplements, Review of Health-Related Call Records for Users of Metabolife 356," submitted in March of 2003, and available online at www.fda.gov/ohrms/dockets/dailys/03/May03/050803/95n-0304-rpt0008-GAO%20report.pdf.

In April of 2004   This information was provided to me "on background only" by a public information officer at the FDA in an e-mail dated April 8, 2004, while I was working on an article for the *New York Times* about the agency's ban on ephedra.

But a March 2000 study   The chilling, carefully documented report has never been published, but an electronic copy of it was provided by Dr. Walker's office. "The Relation Between Voluntary Notification and Material Risk in Dietary Supplement Safety," dated March 9, 2000, further states that its "pessimistic evaluation of reporting efficacy is supported by direct experience . . . Our present methods of detecting adverse effects through voluntary reporting depend on coincidence, luck, and sometimes tragedy."

19   *a survey of U.S. adults*   Cited in the 2004 survey, described above, commissioned by the Council for Responsible Nutrition.

    68 percent of Americans believe   The survey, "Anti-Aging Medicine, Vitamins, Minerals and Food Supplements," conducted for the International Longevity Center, was based on 1,010 telephone interviews with a nationwide cross section of adults surveyed in October of 2002.

CHAPTER 1: THE RATTLESNAKE KING

23   *American consumers could buy*   Containers of this and other snake oil remedies have been offered for sale on eBay in recent years. Copies of the eBay offers, including photographs and descriptions of the containers, were provided to me by Bill Riggle, a collector and amateur historian of patent medicines who lives in Jeffersonville, Indiana. Mr. Riggle also provided me with a complete copy of the FDA's file on Clark Stanley, which he obtained from the agency before it sent its collection to the Library of Congress.

    In a fifty-page booklet he published in 1897   A facsimile reproduction of the booklet "The Life and Adventures of the American Cowboy, by Clark Stanley, Better Known as the Rattle Snake King," was published in England by Pryor Publications in 2003. This and other colorful historic works can be ordered online at www.pryor-publications.co.uk.

24   *President Teddy Roosevelt would attend one*   Roosevelt described the experience himself in his 1916 book, *A Book-Lover's Holidays in the Open* (Charles Scribner's Sons, New York), devoting an entire chapter to his account. The book is reprinted in full, free for the reading, at www.bartleby.com/57/.

25   *the only surviving interview of Stanley*   This account was given by Stanley during a hearing on August 23, 1916, held by the USDA in Boston. A transcript of the hearing was kept in the Stanley file held by the FDA until it was transferred to the Library of Congress.

26   *On the day Columbus first set foot*   I came upon the quote from Columbus's journal at www.tobacco.org/History/Tobacco_History.html.

    The historian Michael R. Harris spoke to me by telephone on many occasions, offering many helpful insights and suggestions for further research.

27   *In 1632, Catholic Jesuits who had gone to Peru*   The well-known history of quinine, also called Jesuit's bark, is widely described in encyclopedias, including the Catholic Encyclopedia, online at www.newadvent.org/cathen/08372b.htm.

    more than one fourth of modern medicines   American Cancer Society Web site at www. cancer.org/docroot/MBC/content/MBC_6_2X_Understanding_Dietary_Supplements.asp? sitearea=MBC.

    My account of William Withering's discovery of the use of foxglove is drawn primarily from an excellent article by Jeremy M. Norman, "William Withering and the Purple Foxglove: A Bicentennial Tribute," *Journal of Clinical Pharmacology* 25 (October 1985): 479–483.

28   *In 1630, Nicholas Knapp of Massachusetts Bay*   This and many other facts and quotations in this chapter are drawn from James Harvey Young's invaluable and encyclopedic masterpiece, *The Toadstool Millionaires: A Social History of Patent Medicines in America Before Federal Regula-*

tion, originally published in 1961 by Princeton University Press, Princeton, New Jersey, and now available in its entirety online at www.quackwatch.org/13Hx/TM/00.html.

30   *The claims of the patent medicines*   In addition to *The Toadstool Millionaires,* these examples are also drawn from a beautifully illustrated book by Adelaide Hechtlinger, *The Great Patent Medicine Era; Or, Without Benefit of Doctor,* 1970, Grosset & Dunlap, New York.

31   "The Great American Fraud," originally published as a series of articles in *Collier's Weekly* by the reporter Samuel Hopkins Adams, was published as a book in 1905 by the American Medical Association. A facsimile reproduction of the book was published in April of 1997 by Rosemary Jacobs, who made me a gift of one.

33   *On January 9, 1915*   From the FDA's Clark Stanley file, now held by the Library of Congress.

35   *The swing of the pendulum*   Much of this history of the FDA comes from the agency's Web site, at www.fda.gov/oc/history/.

CHAPTER 2: MOTHER NATURE

I was surprised to find that no biography of Adelle Davis has been published; her fascinating life and immense importance in the history of nutrition cry out for one. The only biographical information I could find came from news reports in magazines and newspapers of the day, the most extensive of which was "Supernutritionist," by Daniel Yergin, the *New York Times Magazine,* May 20, 1973.

37   *"You could say my interest in nutrition began"*   Quoted in Yergin, "Supernutritionist."

   born in an Indiana farmhouse at three in the morning   See Jane Howard, "Earth Mother to the Foodists," *Life* October 22, 1971.

   "for the simple reason that there was a blizzard"   Quoted in Yergin, "Supernutritionist."

   "My interest in nutrition was neurotic"   Ibid.

   Even before she could read   All the information in this sentence is from Howard, "Earth Mother."

   "for baking bread and canning things"   See Jacqueline King, "Adelle Davis, 68, Carries on Nutrition War," *Allentown (Pa.) Call-Chronicle,* November 19, 1972.

   she had stopped going by Daisie   See Ronald M. Deutsch, *The New Nuts Among the Berries: How Nutrition Nonsense Captured America,* Bull Publishing (Palo Alto), 1977.

38   *"Vitamin Davis," they called her*   Yergin, "Supernutritionist."

   The very notion of vitamins   The information in this paragraph on the history of vitamins can be found in many encyclopedias, including at www.wikipedia.org/wiki/Vitamin.

   After two years at Purdue   Yergin, "Supernutritionist," and King, "Adelle Davis."

   Davis moved to New York   Yergin, "Supernutritionist."

39   *Walter Campbell, commissioner of the nascent FDA*   Quoted by James Harvey Young, *The Medical Messiahs: A Social History of Health Quackery in Twentieth-Century America,* Princeton University Press, Princeton, New Jersey, 1967, and available in its entirety at www.quackwatch.org/13Hx/MM/00.html.

   In those days, as she recalled years later   Quoted in Howard, "Earth Mother."

   Davis soon returned to California   See Yergin, "Supernutritionist."

   "not intended to be merely a cookbook"   See Adelle Davis, *Let's Cook It Right,* Harcourt Brace Jovanovich, New York 1947.

40   *"It's impossible to get a high cholesterol level"*   Quoted in Howard, "Earth Mother."

"a single adult to develop cancer"   See Adelle Davis, *Let's Get Well*, Harcourt, New York, 1965.

One day, young George came home   See Enid Nemy, "Adelle Davis: 67 and Going Strong," *New York Times*, June 14, 1971.

References to Adelle Davis, *Let's Have Healthy Children*, first published in 1951 by Harcourt Brace Jovanovich, New York, are from the paperback edition published by Signet, New York, 1972.

All references to *Let's Eat Right to Keep Fit*, first published in 1954 by Harcourt Brace Jovanovich, New York, are from the paperback edition published by Signet, New York, 1970.

42   *"Alcoholism, crime, insanity, suicide"*   Quoted in Jean Wixen, "Adelle Davis: 'Let the Doctors Harp...'" *San Francisco Chronicle*, December 6, 1973.

"The whole food industry is a cruel thing"   Quoted in King, "Adelle Davis."

"You have to remember that I'm bucking"   Quoted in Yergin, "Supernutritionist."

"guru"   See King, "Adelle Davis."

"prophet"   See Martin Weil, "Adelle Davis, Diet Advocate, Dies," *Washington Post*, June 2, 1974.

43   *Gordon Schectman, a researcher*   Schectman wrote an exhaustive review of Davis's writings in an unpublished paper, "Adelle Davis and Atherosclerosis: An In-Depth Critique," prepared for the Institute of Human Nutrition at Columbia University, August 1974. A copy of the paper was provided to me by Stephen Barrett, MD.

Russell Randall, MD   Quoted in Yergin, "Supernutritionist."

44   *"She's making people aware"*   Quoted by James Trager, "What Adelle Davis and Others Say About Eating Right," *Family Circle*, February 1972.

Gladys Emerson ... signed a letter of protest   See "U.C.—Adelle Davis Flap Flutters," *Oakland Tribune*, March 22, 1973.

Edward Rynearson, MD, professor emeritus of medicine   Dr. Rynerason's statements, and Davis's reply, were quoted in Wixen, "Adelle Davis."

The first was Eliza Young   Although the case was widely reported in the media at the time, my account is based on the original lawsuit filed by Eliza's mother in the Supreme Court of the State of New York on September 8, 1971, and on the order approving compromise of the claim filed in the Superior Court of the State of California on September 27, 1976. Copies of these documents were provided to me by Stephen Barrett, MD.

45   *The second child injured by Davis's advice*   See Stephen Barrett, "The Legacy of Adelle Davis," posted on his Web site at www.quackwatch.org/04ConsumerEducation/davis.html.

J. I. Rodale was scheduled to appear   The death of Rodale during a taping of *The Dick Cavett Show* has been widely recounted, with many conflicting accounts. I reviewed many news accounts of the circumstances to form my account here.

46   *"I had the craziest letter"*   Quoted in Yergin, "Supernutritionist."

"I was shocked"   See Adelle Davis, "How I Discovered I Have Cancer—And What Caused It," *National Enquirer*, February 20, 1974.

47   *sales of vitamins, minerals, and other supplements rose 40 percent*   Cited by Jane Brody, "For Good Nutrition: Balanced Diet vs. Vitamin Pills," *New York Times*, July 7, 1982.

Ernest T. Krebs, Jr.   Wallace Sampson, MD, editor of the *Scientific Review of Alternative Medicine*, spent a couple hours on the telephone with me describing his meetings with, and knowledge of, Krebs, whose promotion of laetrile prompted Dr. Sampson's initial interest in alternative remedies in the 1970s.

The FDA had fired the first shot   An invaluable resource on the history of events leading to passage of the Proxmire bill can be found in *Food Supplement Legislation, 1974: Hearings Before the Subcommittee on Health of the Committee on Labor and Public Welfare, United States Senate,* U.S. Government Printing Office, Washington, DC, 1974. The book provides a transcript of the hearings regarding Senate bills 2801 and 3867, held on August 14 and 22, as well as copies of newspaper articles and historic records provided by witnesses and senators.

Of this group's past and present officers   Richard D. Lyons, in "Disputed Health Lobby Is Pressing for a Bill to Overturn Any Limits on Sales of Vitamins," *New York Times,* May 14, 1973.

A House staffer knowledgeable in health legislation   Ibid.

48   *Whereas three quarters of the public had said in polls*   Cited by Bill Schneider, "Cynicism Didn't Start with Watergate, but the Scandal Has Had a Long-Lasting Impact on Public Confidence in Government," CNN, June 17, 1997, published online at www.cnn.com/ALL POLITICS/1997/gen/resources/watergate/trust. schneider/.

"The Food and Drug Administration"   Quoted on page 2 of the Proxmire bill hearings book.

49   *First up to defend his bill, was Proxmire*   See page 10 of the hearings book.

50   *Alexander M. Schmidt . . . began by entering into the record*   See page 36 of the hearings book.

the second speaker was Senator Bob Dole   See page 828 of the hearings book.

51   *Following Dole to the witness table*   See page 830 of the hearings book.

To answer that question came Sidney Wolfe   See page 893 of the hearings book.

Wolfe then introduced Anita Johnson   See page 897 of the hearings book.

52   *none brought more independent . . . credentials than Marsha N. Cohen*   See page 920 of the hearings book.

CHAPTER 3: WHOLESOME AS A GLASS OF MILK

54   The information on Paul L. Houts and many other victims of L-tryptophan is derived from their testimony at a hearing, *FDA's Regulation of the Dietary Supplement L-Tryptophan,* held before the Human Resources and Intergovernmental Relations Subcommittee of the Committee on Government Operations of the House of Representatives on July 18, 1991, and published by the U.S. Government Printing Office, ISBN 0–16–038309–9.

Paul L. Houts couldn't have been healthier   See page 30 of the L-tryptophan hearings book.

56   *another of the hundreds of thousands . . . Frances L. Thompson*   See page 24 of the hearings book.

Dorothy C. Wilson's doctor prescribed her L-tryptophan   See page 12 of the hearings book.

Ruth Alterman was enjoying the prime of her life   I interviewed Dr. Alterman and her husband, Carl, at their home in the autumn of 2004. Their son, the political journalist Eric Alterman, alerted me to her experience via e-mail.

58   *Tamar Stieber . . . was bit by the journalism bug*   Ms. Stieber spent hours on the telephone explaining how she broke the L-tryptophan story, and she sent me a collection of her Pulitzer Prize–winning articles for the *Albuquerque Journal,* published between November 7, 1989, and February 13, 1990.

60   *Dr. Ron Voorhees . . . told Stieber*   See Tamar Stieber, "Three N.M. Women Contract Unusual Medical Syndrome," *Albuquerque Journal,* November 7, 1989.

61   *Ron Voorhees, the health official who had warned Stieber*   See Lawrence K. Altman, MD, "How

Medical Detectives Identified the Culprit Behind a Rare Disorder," *New York Times,* November 28, 1989.

It was Esther M. Sternberg's morning to drive   I interviewed Dr. Sternberg by telephone on a number of occasions.

65   *a supplement to the Journal of Rheumatology*   See Esther M. Sternberg, "Correspondence," *NEJM* 337 (October 30, 1997), 1314–19. In the same "Correspondence" section in the October 30 *NEJM,* the editor of the *Journal of Rheumatology,* Duncan A. Gordon, responded to Dr. Sternberg's charges, defending both the researchers who wrote the L-tryptophan studies he published and his journal's editorial process. "In my opinion," he wrote, "their reports and our editorial process qualify as unbiased peer review."

67   *Mitch Zeller, counsel to the subcommittee*   Mr. Zeller spent a couple of hours speaking by telephone with me about his experiences.

Next to speak was Dr. Richard J. Wurtman   See page 74 of the L-trytophan hearings book.

69   *Douglas L. Archer, PhD, the agency's deputy director*   See page 95 of the hearings book.

The problem, he explained, could be tracked back to 1972   In addition to Dr. Archer's comments in the hearings book about the consequences of the FDA's error on the GRAS listing, Mitch Zeller also did his best to help me understand the byzantine background of the regulatory history.

which is exactly what a company called Schiff Vitamins did   The history of this case was described in testimony by Douglas L. Archer, PhD, then the deputy director of the FDA's Center for Food Safety and Applied Nutrition, at the House hearing, "FDA's Regulation of the Dietary Supplement L-Tryptophan," on July 18, 1991.

Schiff insisted it had merely relied on   See *United States v. An Article of food . . . Schiff Natural L-Tryptophane,* No. 77–768 (D.N.J. Nov. 30, 1977).

CHAPTER 4: KESSLER VS. KESSLER

72   *David A. Kessler pursued an education and career*   Although I was able to interview two senior FDA officials who served under him, Dr. Kessler himself turned down my many requests for an interview. Biographical information about him is widely available on the Web sites of the FDA and the University of California, San Francisco, School of Medicine, where he now serves as dean.

on Thursday, October 11, 1990   See Susan Heller Anderson, "New Yorker Nominated to F.D.A," *New York Times,* October 13, 1990.

the agency he was being handed   For this characterization, including the quotes from Ted Kennedy and Sidney Wolfe, see Philip J. Hilts, "New Chief Vows New Vitality at F.D.A," the *New York Times* article of February 27, 1991.

73   *"I do not think we ought to wait the regular time"*   See *Legislative Issues Related to the Regulation of Dietary Supplements:* (ISBN 0–16–043659–1) Hearing of the Committee on Labor and Human Resources, United States Senate . . . October 21, 1993," U.S. Government Printing Office, Washington, DC, 1994, Testimony of Senator Metzenbaum begins on page 10 of the book.

Metzenbaum and his colleagues   See "Kessler Confirmed as Head of FDA," *Washington Post,* October 31, 1990.

74   *"The magnitude of the death and permanent injury"*   The quotes from Mitchell Zeller are based on my telephone interviews with him.

In the view of Representative Henry Waxman   My quotes from Rep. Waxman are from an interview he gave me at his Washington, DC, office.

76 *the one senator they believed to be their most reliable advocate*   Despite many phone calls and e-mails to his press officers in Washington and Utah over a one-year period, as well as an unscheduled visit to his Senate office in Washington, Orrin Hatch never spoke with me. Nor did Loren Israelson, a former aide who is now executive director of the Utah National Products Alliance.

70 percent of its population is Mormon   Cited in an excellent article by Stephanie Mencimer, "Scorin' with Orrin," *Washington Monthly,* September, 2001.

"Active Mormons abstain from alcohol, coffee, tea, and tobacco"   Quoted by Guy Gugliotta, "Unlikely Allies, Harkin and Hatch Aid Industry," *Washington Post,* December 25, 2000.

"I really believe in them"   Statement of Sen. Hatch introducing the Dietary Supplement Regulation Moratorium Act of 1993, per Congressional Record of November 20, 1993.

The supplement industry has also given   The figures on Senator Hatch's contributions from supplement companies, as well as from the senator's financial disclosure for 2003, are based on my own analysis of figures from the database maintained by the Center for Responsive Politics on its Web site, www.opensecrets.org.

he wrote a huffy letter to the editor   *Los Angeles Times,* February 27, 1993, page 7.

77 *Hatch's son Scott began working*   See Chuck Neubauer, Judy Pasternak and Richard T. Cooper, "A Washington Bouquet: Hire a Lawmaker's Kid," *Los Angeles Times,* June 22, 2003.

"Elliot Knessler"   FDA Web site, www.fda.gov/oc/commissioners/kessler.html.

he drew page one headlines by sending federal marshals   See Warren E. Leary, "How Fresh Is Fresh? Citing Labels, U.S. Seizes Orange Juice," *New York Times,* April 25, 1991.

78 *"In the district offices and in the consumer affairs office"*   Quoted in Marian Burros, "Dietary Supplements: Let the Buyer Beware," *New York Times,* October 16, 1991.

79 *Soon Dykstra was receiving death threats*   *National Journal,* July 24, 2003.

Kessler's doppelganger lived much of the year   Gerald A. Kessler showed me great hospitality by spending the better part of a day with me in October of 2004 at his Circle K Ranch, showing me around the place, answering every question I asked, and then taking me out for a late lunch with his lovely companion, the actress Meadow Williams, and refusing my offers to pay my share. Details of his biography and much about the campaign he led to win passage of DSHEA are based on what he told me that day.

81 *On the morning of February 22*   My account of the big meeting at Gerry Kessler's ranch is based on the interviews I conducted with those who attended it, including Gerry; Allen Skolnick, then president of Solgar Vitamins and Herbs; Doug Greene, founder of New Hope Communications (which publishes industry newspapers and runs its biggest trade show); and Jack Martin, then an aide to Senator Orrin Hatch.

83 *The April–May 1992 issue of* Health Store News   A copy of the issue was provided to me by Stephen Barrett, MD.

84 *Kessler had taken a keen interest*   See Lena Williams, "F.D.A. Steps Up Effort to Control Vitamin Claims," the *New York Times* on August 9, 1992. Additional information on the incident can be found on the Quackwatch Web site at www.quackwatch.org/04Consumer Education/Nonrecorg/aqa.html.

85 *Wright soon began selling videos*   But just four months after the raid, Wright signed a legal document consenting to the destruction of the L-tryptophan bottles seized by FDA agents, and even agreed to pay related court costs and fees. See United States of America, plaintiff, v. 103/100 capsule bottles containing L-tryptophan, defendant. No C91–1445. U.S. District Court for the Western District of Washington at Seattle. Consent decree, August 20, 1992.

"If there is any plausible excuse"   The May 11, 1992 editorial in the *Seattle Post-Intelligencer* is quoted in Lena Williams, "F.D.A. Steps Up Effort to Control Vitamin Claims."

A week later, the Times *ran a correction*   See "Correction: F.D.A. On Vitamin Policy," *New York Times,* August 16, 1992.

86   *Hatch told the* Washington Post   See Carole Sugarman, "House Gives Vitamin Makers a Break," *Washington Post,* October 7, 1992.

"Write to Congress today or kiss your supplements goodbye!"   A copy of the undated brochure produced by the group formed by Gerry Kessler, the Nutritional Health Alliance, was provided to me by Stephen Barrett, MD, whose room full of files on alternative medicine offers a treasure trove of material to future historians. Gerry Kessler told me during my interview with him, "That's my line; I wrote it."

On August 15, 1992, his words were echoed   See Lena Williams, "F.D.A. Steps Up Efforts to Control Vitamin Claims." I could find no other press account of the event, and all of the celebrities who appeared at it declined my requests for interviews.

87   *"Health Freedom Kit"*   A copy of one of the kits was provided to me by Stephen Barrett, MD.

"No other law has ever received as much"   See R. William Soller, PhD, "Regulation in the Herb Market: The Myth of the 'Unregulated Industry,' " *HerbalGram* 49 (2000): 64–67. A number of sources I interviewed said they had heard that more letters had been sent to Congress regarding this legislation than over any other matter, including the Vietnam War, but this article is the only published piece I could find that contained an actual figure. In truth, both assertions—that 2 million letters were sent and that they amounted to more than had been sent regarding the Vietnam War—are guesses, as no figures are kept by Congress. Still, the view that the public outcry on the legislation was unlike anything seen before or since was shared by everyone I spoke to, including Rep. Henry Waxman.

88   *On a Tuesday evening late in October of 1992*   See Jeff Kramer, "Waxman Takes Flak on FDA Bill, Economy," *Los Angeles Times,* October 22, 1992.

89   *At the first encounter of the two Kesslers*   My account of the meeting is based on what Gerry Kessler told me, as David Kessler would not comment.

90   *At times, Gerry and the young attorney he'd retained*   Mr. Martinez spoke with me by telephone about his recollection of those days, including the confrontation with Rep. Synar.

Gerry followed Hatch and Richardson's advice   I interviewed Tony Podesta by telephone, and he confirmed details of meetings in which he participated.

91   *Later honored along with Kessler by* Natural Foods Merchandiser   See Mitchell Clute, Vicky Uhland, Bryce Edmonds, et al, "25 Who Fortified Supplements," April 1, 2004.

a heated debate at Waxman's hearing   See *Regulation of Dietary Supplements: Hearing Before the Subcommittee on Health and the Environment . . . House of Representatives . . . July 29, 1993, Serial No. 103–57,* U.S. Government Printing Office: Washington, DC, 1994, ISBN 0–16–043518–8.

93   *He pointed to the label of Ultra Male*   A copy of Ultra Male's label listing all the noted ingredients is reproduced on page 300 of the hearings book, and a current listing of the ingredients was accessed online on May 20, 2006, at www.vitaminshoppe.com/store/en/browse/sku_detail.jsp?id=NT-1447.

94   *a one-minute commercial began airing*   A copy of the Mel Gibson commercial, as well as the lengthier videotaped interviews with other celebrities, is held in the James H. Quillen Papers of the Archives of Appalachia, East Tennessee University, listed as tape 375 under the title "Health Free Task Force 'Message to Congress'; October 1993."

95   *The commercial had actually been made*   Mr. Mooney spoke with me by telephone about his experience doing so.

96   *Speaking early in Kennedy's Senate hearing*   See *Legislative Issues Related to the Regulation of Dietary,* ibid.

98   *But Waxman managed to block the renewal*   See Alan C. Miller, "Waxman's Dose of Regulation Angers Makers of Supplements," *Los Angeles Times,* December 6, 1993.

    on December 29, the FDA   See Irvin Molotsky, "U.S. Issues Rules on Diet Supplement Labels," *New York Times,* December 30, 1993.

    With both Kennedy and Waxman holding up the bills   See Alan C. Miller, "The Potent Politics of Vitamins: The Industry has launched a controversial campaign against FDA regulations. It's had surprising impact," *Los Angeles Times,* July 2, 1994.

99   *By early October, the full Senate had passed the bill*   See Philip J. Hilts, "Bill Allowing Vitamin Claims Wins Approval," *New York Times,* October 8, 1994.

    Richardson, Harkin, and Hatch called a meeting   My account of these final maneuvers is based on the interviews I conducted with Doug Greene, Gerry Kessler, Jack Martin, Tony Martinez, Tony Podesta, Bill Schultz, Allen Skolnick, and Rep. Henry Waxman.

101   *President Clinton read from a statement*   Both Gerry Kessler and Tony Podesta confirmed Mr. Podesta's role in writing the first draft of the statement. The president's signing statement is collected in *Public Papers of the Presidents, William J. Clinton, 1994,* volume 2, pages 1872–73, U.S. Government Printing Office, Washington, DC. It can be accessed online at www.gpoaccess.gov/pubpapers/search.html.

CHAPTER 5: ANCIENT CHINESE REMEDY

104   *Julie Puett Howry*   My account of Julie Puett Howry's death is based on lengthy telephone interviews with her husband, Phil Howry, and with Cynthia T. Culmo, the pharmacist who served as director of the state health department's Drugs and Medical Devices division.

105   *"Out of a table of six at lunch the other day"*   This quote, like many other details of Texas's attempts to deal with the outbreak of deaths and injuries due to ephedra, comes from a series of well-researched articles written by Dick Stanley of the *Austin American-Statesmen.* This quote in particular appeared in his article of May 1, 1994, "Stimulant Suspected in Austin Death."

106   *On May 12, just over two weeks after Howry's death*   See Dick Stanley, "Popular Pep Pill Banned by State," *Austin American-Statesman,* May 13, 1994.

    a Travis County district judge issued a temporary injunction   These facts, and the quote from distributor Barbara Whisenant, are from another article by Dick Stanley, "Consumers, State Divided over Herb," *Austin American-Statesman,* May 23, 1994.

    Then, on May 30 . . . fifty-four-year-old Judith Whisenhunt   See Dick Stanley, "Six Wrongful-Death Suits Challenge Pep/Diet Pill," *Austin American-Statesman,* April 20, 1996.

107   *The Chinese, he said, had used it*   Quoted by Dick Stanley in "Consumers, State."

    "most of these have been on the market for four thousand years"   Hatch's statement was made during the Senate hearing on October 21, 1993, and appears on page 60 of the book of transcripts of that hearing published by the government, *Legislative Issues Related to the Regulation of Dietary Supplements* (ISBN 0–16–043659–1).

    The discovery of ma huang   Background information on the mythical Shen Nong can be found online at Encyclopaedia Britannica, www.britannica.com; as well as in an article on People's Daily Online, "Herbal Leaves Stand for Harmony Between Man and Nature," at english.people.com.cn/200601/19/eng20060119_236670.html.

    According to a memoir written years later   See George B. Koelle, "Carl Frederic Schmidt, July 29, 1893–April 4, 1988," at newton.nap.edu/readingroom/books/biomems/cschmidt.pdf. The first scientific report on ephedrine by Drs. Schmidt and Chen, "The Action of Ephedrine, the Active Principle of the Chinese Drug Ma Huang," was published in 1922 in the *Journal of Pharmacology and Experimental Therapeutics* 24: 339–57.

109 *"Elsinore pill"*   See Axel Malchow-Moller, "Ephedrine as an Anorectic: The Story of the 'Elsinore Pill,' " *International Journal of Obesity and Related Metabolic Disorders* 5 (1981): 183–87.

In 1983, however, the FDA played party pooper   See Sidney M. White, "Ephedra—Scientific Evidence Versus Money/Politics," *Science* (April 18, 2003): 437.

the state health commissioner David Smith decided   See "Age Restriction for Stimulant Withdrawn," *Austin American-Statesman*, June 2, 1994.

110 *It finally reached a settlement with the maker of Formula One*   See Stanley, "Six Wrongful-Death Suits."

on March 31, 1995, the department proposed rules   This and other facts in this paragraph come from my interview with Cynthia Culmo.

But by October of 1995, the agency had grown sufficiently alarmed   See "Minutes of the Special Working Group on Food Products Containing Ephedrine Alkaloids of the FDA Food Advisory Committee," at www.cfsan.fda.gov/~dms/ds-ephel.html.

111 *Robert Occhifinto, for instance*   See congressional hearings held on July 23 and 24, 2003, the full text of which can be found online at energycommerce.house.gov/108/Hearings/07242003hearing1036/print.htm.

Michael Ellis and Michael Blevins   Many of the details on the founding of the company come from Seth Hettena's riveting feature for the Associated Press, dated October 16, 2004. A copy of it, under the headline "Metabolife: Its Rise and Fall," was accessed on the Web site of the *Seattle Times* on May 27, 2006, at seattletimes.nwsource.com/html/business technology/2002065218_ drugdiet17.html.

112 *In August of 1996, the FDA convened*   A transcript of the FDA's Food Advisory Committee hearings on August 27 and 28, 1996, is online at www.fda.gov/ohrms/dockets/ac/96/transcpt/3210t2.pdf.

in September of 1997, Governor Bush appointed   See Michael Weisskopf, "Bush's Diet-Drug Problem," *Time*, May 22, 2000.

It was then that the death threats   Cynthia Culmo described these threats to me during our interview.

113 *In the hallway outside*   Phil Howry gave me this account of his conversation with Reyn Archer.

As its first key lobbyist, Metabolife   See Weisskopf, "Bush's Diet-Drug Problem."

114 *On June 4, 1997, the FDA announced*   See the Federal Register for that date, a copy of which is kept on the FDA Web site at www.cfsan.fda.gov/~lrd/fr97064a.html.

The GAO concluded that the reports of injury and death   See the GAO report of July 1999, "Dietary Supplements: Uncertainties in Analyses Underlying FDA's Proposed Rule on Ephedrine Alkaloids," available online at www.gao.gov/cgi-bin/getrpt?GAO/HEHS/GGD-99-90.

115 *Back in Texas, the department of health*   See Texas Department of Health news release dated January 12, 1999, "Board of Health Approves Proposed New Rules for Ephedrine Products," online at www.tdh.state.tx.us/news/b_new259.htm.

this too appeared to pass muster   See Texas Register, volume 25, number 27, at www.texinfo.library.unt.edu/Texasregister/pdf/2000/0707is.pdf.

Bush's secretary of Health and Human Services, Tommy G. Thompson, was approached   See Weisskopf, "Bush's Diet-Drug Problem." Cynthia Culmo also confirmed these facts.

Sales of Metabolife 365 had by then   See Guy Gugliotta, "Dietary Supplement Makers Flex

Muscle; $15 Billion Industry Fends Off Attempts to Regulate Ephedra over Health Risks," *Washington Post,* December 25, 2000.

The same could be said in California   Ibid.

116   *during a deposition for a court case*   The deposition of Dr. Winters was taken on July 19, 2004, for a civil lawsuit in California lodged by Mark Hagen and Gina Hagen against AST Sports Science and other firms.

     But upon retiring, he did become an expert witness   See disposition of Dr. Winters taken on July 19, 2004.

     President Bush's appointment of Dan Troy   See Michael Kranish, "FDA Counsel's Rise Embodies US Shift," *Boston Globe,* December 22, 2002.

117   *Troy refused a request by one of the agency's top officials*   This information was provided to me by the official on the condition that I not disclose his identity.

118   *By then, between 12 and 17 million people*   Stated by Rep. James C. Greenwood of Pennsylvania in his opening remarks for the hearings he chaired on July 23 and 24, 2003, in *Legislative Issues.*

     On May 26, Illinois became the first state   See Associated Press, "Ephedra Bill Signed In Illinois," May 26, 2003.

     Born on March 4, 1981, Todd James Lee   My account of the death of Todd Lee is based on interviews I conducted in Oklahoma and by telephone with his mother, Camille; his sister, Shayna; his girlfriend, Kristie Runion; his stepfather, Karl Power III; his onetime supervisor at Williams-Sonoma, Wendy Musgrove; and with documents provided to me by Camille.

122   *the House Subcommittee on Oversight and Investigations held a hearing*   See House hearings on July 23 and 24, 2003, in *Legislative Issues.*

125   *By the end of 2003, according to sources*   Again, these sources spoke on the condition that their identity not be revealed.

     On December 30, McClellan announced   See FDA press release "FDA Announces Plans to Prohibit Sales of Dietary Supplements Containing Ephedra," December 30, 2003.

     stores and Web sites rushed to move as much product as they could   I reported these incidents for the *New York Times* in an article published on April 11, 2004, "As Ephedra Ban Nears, a Race to Sell the Last Supplies."

126   *by March of 2005 the company faced three class-action lawsuits*   See Janet St. James, "Ingredients in TrimSpa Remain Unclear," WFAA-TV, Dallas, March 2, 2005.

     the new Xenadrine contained bitter orange peel   Reported on its own Web site and labels at the time, Xenadrine's new ingredient also drew the attention of news reports and studies, including one that found that a single dose of Xenadrine EFX, containing bitter orange and caffeine, raised patients' blood pressure and heart rate as much as ephedra did. See Christine Haller, Neal L. Benowitz, P. Jacob III, "Hemodynamic effects of ephedra-free weight-loss supplements in humans," *American Journal of Medicine,* 118 (September 2005): 998–1003.

     the FDA revealed that it had received reports   The FDA gave me this information in response to questions I posed for my *New York Times* article "As Ephedra Ban Nears."

     By then, the Annals of Pharmacotherapy *had reported*   See Aleda M. Hess and Donald L. Sullivan, "Potential for Toxicity with use of Bitter Orange Extract and Guarana for Weight Loss," (May 2004) 38: 812–16.

127   *an additional four ephedra-related deaths*   I reported this in "As Ephedra Ban Nears."

     At ten-thirty in the morning on Monday, April 12   I covered this hearing for the *New York Times* for an article published on April 13, 2004, "Judge Clears the Way for US Ban on Ephedra."

128   *The FDA filed an appeal on June 13*   See *Nutraceutical Corp. and Solaray, Inc. v. Lester Crawford,*

D.V.M., Acting Commissioner, U.S. Food and Drug Administration, et al., No. 2:04CV409TC (C.D. UT).

the loser would likely want to appeal   Mr. Emord spoke with me by telephone.

129   *a company selling something called Eca Fuel*   My wife, Alice, forwarded a copy of the Eca Fuel e-mail she had received. I then accessed the company's Web site at www.ecafuel.com on October 28, 2005. The site now promotes another ephedra product, Tabolizer.

In February, he was indicted on charges   See Seth Hettena, "Metabolife Founder Ellis Indicted on Charges of Illegally Having Guns, Ammunition," Associated Press, February 9, 2005.

The company filed for Chapter 11   See Terri Somers, "Future of Operations in San Diego in doubt," *San Diego Union-Tribune,* November 8, 2005.

In October, the company pleaded guilty   See Seth Hettena, "Metabolife Pleads Guilty in San Diego to Filing False Tax Returns," Associated Press, October 5, 2005.

"It just boils down to greed"   Quoted in ibid.

Occifinto's company, NVE, also filed for bankruptcy protection   See Greg Saitz, "Stacker 2 Maker Files for Chapter 11," *Star-Ledger* (N.J.), August 11, 2005.

131   *"If FDA can't take a supplement"*   Kennedy's statement was widely quoted in the media, including at www.citizens.org/ephedra-ban-overturned.

"This decision leaves no doubt"   Bruce Silverglade's quote is from a press release of the Center for Science in the Public Interest, found at www.cspinet.org/new/200504152.html.

"Nobody has shown me the need"   Quoted in Glen Warchol and Robert Gehrke, "Ephedra Ban Lifted by Judge in Utah," *Salt Lake City Tribune,* April 15, 2005.

On December 14, 2004, the U.S. secretary of labor   See U.S. Department of Labor press release for that date: "U.S. Secretary of Labor Elaine L. Chao Announces New Appointments at OSHA."

132   *he had also lobbied Texas officials*   Molly Ivins, "Henhouses Overstaffed with Foxes," column on AlterNet.org posted on January 20, 2005, at www.alternet.org/columnists/story/21041/.

CHAPTER 6: WHAT'S REALLY IN THAT BOTTLE?

135   *The largest herbal extraction facility*   I visited the facilities of Pure World in October of 2004.

137   *Beverly Hames's unwanted education*   I met with Beverly at her home in Portland, spoke with her many times by telephone, and reviewed records of her case. I also met with and interviewed the naturopath Mitchell Stargrove and with Beverly's doctor, William M. Bennett; and I spoke by telephone with Subhuti Dharmananda.

139   *"Homeopathic remedies do not have any toxicity"*   Mitchell Stargrove told me this during an interview I conducted in his office. Such views may explain why homeopathic remedies have been used by 7.3 million people in the United States, accounting for $453 million in sales in 2003, up 13 percent over the year before. But toxic reactions reported to the American Association of Poison Control Centers have grown fivefold in the past fifteen years, jumping from 1,052 in 1989 to 5,359 in 2003, including 508 that required hospitalization that year and 4 considered life-threatening. All told, six people have died over those fifteen years as a result of homeopathic treatments. In February of 2006, the maker of Zicam Cold Remedy, labeled a homeopathic product, agreed to pay $12 million to settle 340 lawsuits brought by users who claimed their sense of smell and taste had been reduced or destroyed after taking the zinc-containing spray. But the company admitted no responsibility, and continued its radio advertisements featuring endorsements by Rush Limbaugh. As for the efficacy of home-

opathic remedies, the National Center for Complementary and Alternative Medicine states: "Systematic reviews have not found homeopathy to be a definitively proven treatment for any medical condition. A number of its key concepts do not follow the laws of science (particularly chemistry and physics)."

142 *other cases of kidney diseases*   See Jean-Louis Vanherweghem, M. Depierreaux, C. Tielemans, et al, "Rapidly Progressive Interstitial Renal Fibrosis in Young Women: Association with Slimming Regimen Including Chinese Herbs," *Lancet* 341 (February 13, 1993): 387–91.

"Stephania and Magnolia Bark: Targets of a Misdirected Investigation"   A printed copy of this manuscript by Subhuti Dharmananda, stating that it was "prepared for the American Botanical Council," was provided to me by Beverly Hames.

143 *In January of 1994, Dr. Vanherweghem published an addendum*   See M. Vanhaelen, R. Vanhaelen-Fastre, P. But, et al, "Identification of Aristolochic Acid in Chinese Herbs," *Lancet* 343 (January 15, 1994): 174.

Dharmananda wrote an addendum   Dharmananda, "Stephania and Magnolia Bark."

Dharmananda felt concerned enough   This paragraph describing Dharmananda's actions and knowledge is based on the deposition he gave on February 23, 1998, in the civil suit brought by Beverly Hames.

144 *He wrote hundreds of articles*   Many of these articles can be found online at the Web site of the Institute for Traditional Medicine, at www.itmonline.org.

147 *Catherine Ulbricht . . . says that it's difficult*   I interviewed Dr. Ulbricht by telephone.

A survey published in the British Journal of Cancer   See Ursula Werneke, J. Earl, C. Seydel, et al, "Potential Health Risks of Complementary Alternative Medicines in Cancer Patients," 90 (2004): 408–13.

148 *Karen A. Wolnik, director of the Inorganic Laboratory Branch*   Dr. Wolnik sent a memorandum on FDA letterhead reporting her results, titled "Summary of Results: Samples of 127744/45 and 128397 through 128406," on June 27, 2001, to her colleague Constance Hardy. A copy of the memo was provided to me by Beverly Hames.

according to a report by the Belgian doctors   See Joëlle L. Nortier, Marie–Carmen Muniz Martinez, Heinz H. Schmeiser, et al, "Urothelial Carcinoma Associated with the Use of a Chinese Herb (Aristolochia fangchi)" *NEJM* 342 (June 8, 2000): 1686–92.

In an editorial accompanying the NEJM *report*   Dr. Kessler's accompanying editorial, "Cancer and Herbs," appeared on pages 1742–43 of ibid.

149 *The herb was quickly banned*   See *Consumer Reports*, "12 Supplements You Should Avoid," May 2004.

Even Dharmananda was finally convinced   See his article at www.itmonline.org/arts/aristolochia.htm.

On May 16, 2000, the agency wrote a letter   See "Letter to Industry—FDA Concerned About Botanical Products, Including Dietary Supplements, Containing Aristolochic Acid," online at www.cfsan.fda.gov/~dms/ds-botl1.html.

On April 9, 2001, the once-proud agency   See "Letter to Industry Associations Regarding Safety Concerns Related to the Use of Botanical Products Containing Aristolochic Acid," online at www.cfsan.fda.gov/~dms/ds-botl4.html.

According to Richard Ko   I interviewed Dr. Ko by telephone.

According to Arthur P. Grollman, MD   I interviewed Dr. Grollman by telephone on three occasions.

150 *William Martens Lee . . . estimates that about forty*   Dr. Lee gave me his estimate of the number of herb-linked cases of liver failure during a telephone conversation.

The herb, after all, is one of the oldest known   I found information on the history of aristolochia from a variety of online encyclopedias and historical texts.

151   *Xiaomei Li . . . published an editorial*   See "Aristolochic Acid Nephropathy: What we know and what we have to do," *Nephrology* 9 (July 2004): 109.

On July 20, 1999, Jerry Oliveras   A full transcript of the FDA's hearing on dietary supplements is online at www.fda.gov/ohrms/dockets/dockets/99n1174/tr00002.rtf.

152   *In September of 2000, doctors writing in the journal* Pediatrics   See Cynthia Moore, MD, and Robert Adler, MD, "Herbal Vitamins: Lead Toxicity and Developmental Delay," *Pediatrics* (September 2000): 600–602.

New York City health commissioner Thomas R. Frieden warned   See Richard Pérez-Pena, "Dominican-Made Powder Remedy Is Poisonous, Health Officials Say," *New York Times*, November 6, 2003.

153   *The FDA investigated the product*   See press release "FDA Warns Consumers About Use of Litargirio," at www.fda.gov/bbs/topics/ANSWERS/2003/ANS01253.html.

a survey they had made of products   See Robert B. Saper, Stefanos N. Kales, Janet Paquin, et al, "Heavy Metal Content of Ayurvedic Herbal Medicine Products," *JAMA* 292 (December 15, 2004): 2868–73.

154   *The FDA issued a nationwide alert*   See FDA Talk Paper, "FDA Initiates Seizure of Ginseng Because of Potentially Risky Pesticide Residues," December 16, 2004.

Lois Swirsky Gold . . . reported on her online check   See Gold, "Aristolochic Acid, an Herbal Carcinogen, Sold on the Web After FDA Alert," *NEJM* 349 (October 16, 2003): 1576–77.

ConsumerLab.com analyzed dozens of children's multivitamins   See www.consumerlab.com/results/multivit.asp.

155   *Lawrence R. Schiller . . . recently told the Drug Enforcement Administration*   I interviewed Dr. Schiller by telephone.

a supplement called Sleeping Buddha   See "FDA Warns Consumers Against Taking Dietary Supplement 'Sleeping Buddha,'" FDA press release, March 10, 1998. For this and other press releases regarding products listed in this paragraph, see www.fda.gov.

156   *PC-SPES, marketed to promote 'prostate health.'*   The best article I know of describing the PC-SPES debacle was written by Justin Gillis in the *Washington Post* on September 5, 2004, "Herbal Remedies Turn Deadly for Patients."

publication of a study . . . in the New England Journal of Medicine   See Robert S. DiPaola, Huayan Zhang, George H. Lambert, et al, "Clinical and Biologic Activity of an Estrogenic Herbal Combination (PC-SPES) in Prostate Cancer," *NEJM* 339 (September 17, 1998): 785–91.

On September 23, 1999, his Committee on Government Reform   A transcript of the hearing, titled "Fighting Prostate Cancer: Are We Doing Enough?" can be found at www.access.gpo.gov/congress/house/house07ch106.html.

157   *John Meyer of Sonoita, Arizona*   See Gillis, "Herbal Remedies."

158   *In a study published in October of 2001*   See Mark C. Weinrobe and Bruce Montgomery, "Acquired Bleeding Diathesis in a Patient Taking PC-SPES," *NEJM* 16 (October 18, 2001): 1213–14.

"you have a three out of four chance"   I interviewed Tod Cooperman, MD, president of ConsumerLab.com, by telephone.

159   *In October of 2004, Commissioner Crawford promised*   He made this promise before the Council for Responsible Nutrition's annual meeting, which I attended.

160   *In January of 2003, the U.S. swimmer Kicker Vencill*   The Associated Press reported on Vencill's successful lawsuit against the supplement maker on May 13, 2005.

Similar cases occurred during and preceding the 2000 Olympics   An excellent account of the supplement industry's effects on Olympic athletes can be found in Stephanie Mencimer's "Scorin' with Orrin," in the September 2001 *Washington Monthly.*

161   *"Jovanovic told the* New York Times   See Lynn Zinser "Just Say Yes: U.S.O.C. Hires a Maker of Nutritional Supplements and Requires Testing," November 16, 2005.

it decided . . . to create an education campaign . . . said Gary I. Wadler, MD   I interviewed Dr. Wadler by telephone.

the USOC announced   See Zinser, "Just Say Yes."

CHAPTER 7: ONE A DAY

163   *Cooper Burkey had stopped*   Cooper's parents declined to be interviewed for this book. I relied on reports of Cooper's death from New York–area newspapers. See Albert Amateau, "Boy Chokes on Pill," *The Villager,* February 22–28, 2006; Alex Schmidt, "Tribeca Boy Dies Choking on Pill," *Downtown Express,* February 24–March 2, 2006; Mark Bulliet and Joe McGurk, "Four-Year-Old Tribeca Boy Chokes to Death on Pill," *New York Post,* February 17, 2006; Kerry Burke and Carrie Melago, "Two Young Kids Die in Separate Incidents," *New York Daily News,* February 17, 2006; Murray Weiss, "Pill Was a Monster," *New York Post,* February 18, 2006; "Paid Notice, Deaths: Burkey, Cooper Chandler," the *New York Times,* February 22, 2006.

big believers in the benefits of whole foods   See Frederick Kaufman, "Psst! Got Milk?" *The New Yorker,* November 29, 2004.

164   *According to the National Maternal-Infant Health Survey*   See Stella M. Yu, Michael D. Kogan and Peter Gergen, "Vitamin-Mineral Supplement Use Among Preschool Children in the United States," *Pediatrics* 100 (November 1997): e4, at www.pediatrics.aappublications.org/cgi/content/full/100/5/e4.

165   *The most recent and thorough survey*   See Kathy Radimer, Bernadette Bindewalde, Jeffrey Hughes, et al, "Dietary Supplement Use by US Adults: Data from the National Health and Nutrition Examination Survey, 1999–2000," *American Journal of Epidemiology* 160 (2004): 339–349.

"Most people need a multivitamin"   Jeffrey Blumberg's quote can be found at www.on health.webmd.com/script/main/art.asp?articlekey=56712.

"A well-formulated vitamin"   Chris Rosenbloom's quote can be found at www.site65 .com/health65/library/medicineandyou/vitamins/dvit001. html.

A 2004 article   Found online at www.hsph.harvard.edu/nutritionsource/vitamins.html.

according to the American Academy of Pediatrics   See *Caring for Your School-Age Child: Ages 5–12,* from the American Academy of Pediatrics (Bantam, New York, 1999).

166   *Even the American Dietetic Association*   This position was adopted by the ADA's House of Delegates on October 29, 1995, reaffirmed on September 28, 1998, and remained in effect until December 31, 2004.

a panel of thirteen experts   See the draft statement of the panel at www.consensus.nih.gov/2006/MVMDRAFT051706.pdf.

"Most of the vitamin supplements consumed"   Dr. Benjamin Caballero spoke with me by telephone.

Look at the 2005 Dietary Guidelines for Americans   A copy can be found at www.health. gov/DietaryGuidelines/.

167   *Another nationally prominent nutritionist*   Dr. Robert M. Russell spoke with me by telephone.

The first time the words vitamin *and* antioxidant *appeared together*   I searched the *Times'* historical database, available online at www.nytimes.com.

only then were the results published in the New England Journal of Medicine   See the Alpha-Tocopherol, Beta-Carotene Cancer Prevention Study Group, "The Effect of Vitamin E and Beta Carotene on the Incidence of Lung Cancer and Other Cancers in Male Smokers," *NEJM* 330 (April 14, 1994): 1029–35.

168   *academic researchers in California and Texas*   See Jane E. Brody, "Making a Case for Antioxidants," *New York Times*, April 20, 1994; D. L. Tribble, J. J. M. V. D. Berg, P. A. Motchnik, et al, "Oxidative Susceptibility of Low Density Lipoprotein Subfractions Is Related to Their Ubiquinol-10 and Alpha-Tocopherol Content," *Proceedings of the National Academy of Sciences* 91 (February 1, 1994): 1183–87; I. Jialal, C. J. Fuller, B. A. Huett, "The Effect of Alpha–Tocopherol Supplementation on LDL Oxidation," *Arteriosclerosis, Thrombosis, and Vascular Biology* 15 (1995): 190–98.

169   *the first randomized, placebo-controlled study*   See the Alpha-Tocopherol, Beta-Carotene Cancer Prevention Study Group, "The Effect of Vitamin E."

170   *The Physicians' Health Study*   See Charles H. Hennekens, Julie E. Buring, JoAnn E. Manson, et al., "Lack of Effect of Long-Term Supplementation with Beta Carotene on the Incidence of Malignant Neoplasms and Cardiovascular Disease," *NEJM* 334 (May 2, 1996): 1145–49.

The Carotene and Retinol Efficacy Trial   See Gina Kolata "Studies Find Beta Carotene, Used by Millions, Doesn't Forestall Cancer or Heart Disease," *New York Times*, January 19, 1996. For a follow-up study, see Gary E. Goodman, Mark D. Thornquist, John Balmes, et al, "The Beta-Carotene and Retinol Efficacy Trial, *Journal of the National Cancer Institute* 96 (December 1, 2004): 1743–50, which found that the harmful effect of beta carotene persisted, but to a lesser degree, for at least five years after people in the study had stopped taking it.

Similarly disappointing results   A press release from the Institute of Medicine describing the findings of its report on antioxidants can be found online at www4.national academies.org/news.nsf/isbn/0309069351?OpenDocument.

In October of 2004 the British medical journal Lancet   See G. Bjelakovic, D. Nikolova, R. G. Simonetti, et al, "Antioxidant Supplements for Prevention of Gastrointestinal Cancers: A Systematic Review and Meta-analysis," *Lancet* 364 (October 2–8, 2004): 1219–28.

171   *The study, published in the* Annals of Internal Medicine   See Edgar R. Miller, III, Roberto Pastor-Barriuso, Darshan Dalal, et al, "Meta-Analysis: High-Dosage Vitamin E Supplementation May Increase All-Cause Mortality," 142 (January 4, 2005): 37–46.

The Journal of the American Medical Association *published a study*   See Eva Lonn, Jackie Bosch, Salim Yusuf, et al, "Effects of Long-Term Vitamin E Supplementation on Cardiovascular Events and Cancer," *JAMA* 293 (March 16, 2005): 1338–1347.

But the Council for Responsible Nutrition   A press release from CRN, describing its advertising campaign, can be found at www.crnusa.org/prpdfs/CRNVitaminESafety112904.PDF.

172   *In July of 2005, a large national survey*   See Earl S. Ford, Umed A. Ajani, and Ali H. Mokdad, "Brief Communication: The Prevalence of High Intake of Vitamin E from the Use of Supplements Among U.S. Adults," *Annals of Internal Medicine* 114 (July 19, 2005): 116–20.

Many good studies do, however, show   By the time of Linus Pauling's death at the age of ninety-three in 1994, at least sixteen well-designed studies had shown no effect of vitamin C on preventing a cold. Four of the largest, involving thousands of patients overall, were conducted by Terence W. Anderson, professor of epidemiology at the University of Toronto. The only beneficial effect he ever found came in a 1975 study of 622 people. They were each given either a placebo or a weekly sustained-release dose of 500 milligrams of vitamin C; in addition, they were instructed to take an additional dose of 1,500 milligrams of vitamin C (or placebo) on the first day of any illness, followed by 1,000 milligrams on the next four days. Of the 448 people who completed fifteen weeks in the study, there was no difference in preventing colds due to the weekly pill. But compared to those taking the placebo, those who took vitamin C at the onset of their illness experienced less severe colds and 25 percent fewer days spent indoors because of them. Another trial published that same year in the *Journal of the American Medical Association,* led by Thomas R. Karlowski at the National Institutes of Health, suggested a possible reason why so many people fervently believed in vitamin C (and why many still do). He managed to persuade 311 employees of NIH to participate in a nine-month study, in which, three times a day, they would take a capsule containing either 1,000 milligrams of vitamin C or a placebo. At the onset of a cold, they were also given either 3,000 milligrams of vitamin C or a placebo. After 190 of the participants completed the study, it initially seemed as if the vitamin C had a modest but significant effect on reducing the duration and severity of colds. But then Karlowski discovered that about half of the study's participants had been able to figure out, by taste alone, whether they had been taking the tart vitamin C or the sweet lactose placebo. Among those who had figured out which they were taking, the vitamin C group said they had significantly shorter, less severe colds than those who realized they were taking a placebo. But among the other half of the participants who never figured out which they were taking, there was no difference between the vitamin C and placebo groups. Dr. Karlowski concluded that any apparent effect of the vitamin C was simply another example of the well-known and powerful placebo effect.

The National Institute of Allergy and Infectious Diseases' current position   See www.niaid .nih.gov/factsheets/cold.htm.

Researchers from the Netherlands sought   See Ruth M. Grant, Evert G. Schouten, Frans J. Kok, "Effect of Daily Vitamin E and Multivitamin-Mineral Supplementation on Acute Respiratory Tract Infection in Elderly Persons," *JAMA* 288 (August 14, 2002): 715–21.

In February of 2005, the journal   The full story of the discredited *Lancet* paper by Ranjit K. Chandra was reported in the *British Medical Journal* on January 10, 2004, at bmj.bmjjournals.com/cgi/content/full/328/7431/67.

173   *Vitamin B₃, better known as niacin*   An overview on the risks and benefits can be found online at Medline Plus, a service of NIH and the National Library of Medicine, at www.nlm .nih.gov/medlineplus/druginfo/natural/patient-niacin.html.

B₆ is widely promoted   An overview on the risks and benefits of vitamin B_6 can be found at www.nlm.nih.gov/medlineplus/druginfo/natural/patient-b6.html.

a 2004 study found tentative signs   See Deborah Charles, Andy R. Ness, Doris Campbell, et al, "Taking Folate in Pregnancy and Risk of Maternal Breast Cancer," *BMJ* 329 (December 11, 2004): 1375–76.

folic acid can worsen a B₁₂ deficiency   Dr. Robert M. Russell of Tufts University told me in an interview, "I think one of the big public health concerns right now is whether, by fortifying the food supply with folic acid, we're putting older people at risk of a vitamin B_{12} deficiency. In someone who's B_{12} borderline, folic acid can push them over the edge." And because a deficiency of either B_{12} or folic acid can cause anemia, doctors sometimes respond by simply prescribing a high-dose folic acid supplement without first checking to determine which vitamin is actually deficient. The folic acid will cure the anemia, making the doctor think that all is well. Meanwhile, the B_{12} deficiency will only get worse, causing irreversible brain damage.

The Women's Health Initiative   See Rebecca D. Jackson, Andrea Z. LaCroix, Margery Gass, et al, "Calcium Plus Vitamin D Supplementation and the Risk of Fractures," *NEJM* 354 (February 16, 2006): 669–83. An accompanying editorial was on pages 750–52.

175   *In July of 2004, the journal* Pediatrics   See Joshua D. Milner, Daniel M. Stein, Robert McCarter, et al, "Early Infant Multivitamin Supplementation Is Associated with Increased Risk for Food Allergy and Asthma," *Pediatrics* 114 (July 1, 2004): 27–32. I interviewed the lead author of the study, Dr. Milner, by telephone.

The strongest evidence to date comes from the Nurses Health Study   See Diane Feskanich, Vishwa Singh, Walter C. Willett, et al, "Vitamin A Intake and Hip Fractures Among Postmenopausal Women," *JAMA* 287 (January 2, 2002): 47–54.

176   *"Between supplements, fortified breakfast cereals and milk"*   Quoted in Susan J. Landers "Alphabet Overload: Which Dietary Supplements Are Effective?" *American Medical News,* September 6, 2004.

        the Centers for Disease Control and Prevention published an alarming article   See B. Weiss, E. Alkon, F. Weindlar, et al, "Toddler Deaths Resulting from Ingestion of Iron Supplements—Los Angeles, 1992–1993," in *MMWR* 42 (February 19, 1993): 111–13.

177   *the FDA . . . issued regulations*   The FDA published its "final rule" on labeling and packaging of iron supplements in the Federal Register on January 15, 1997 (62 FR 2218).

178   *Gerry Kessler and his Nutritional Health Alliance*   The lawsuit filed by Gerry Kessler's group was decided as *Nutritional Health Alliance v. FDA* (318 F.3d 92 [2d Cir.] 2003). In response to the ruling, the FDA published its revised rules in the Federal Register of October 17, 2003 (68 FR 59714). Gerry Kessler explained his motivation in filing the lawsuit during my interview with him in October of 2004.

        Chris Wermann, director of corporate affairs for Kellogg's in Europe   See James Meikle and Luke Harding, "Denmark Bans Kellogg's Vitamins," the *Guardian,* August 12, 2004. I interviewed both Mr. Drotsby and Dr. Salka E. Rasmussen.

180   *In February of 2005, the* Journal of the National Cancer Institute   See Kathleen M. Egan, Jeffrey A. Sosman, and William J. Blot, "Sunlight and Reduced Risk of Cancer: Is the Real Story Vitamin D?" 97 (February 2, 2005): 161–63.

        According to Michael F. Holick   I interviewed Dr. Holick by telephone.

        a 2004 study in the journal Neurology   See K. L. Munger, S. M. Zhang, E. O'Reilly, et al, "Vitamin D Intake and Incidence of Multiple Sclerosis," *Neurology* 62 (January 13, 2004): 60–65.

        And a December 2005 study in the journal CHEST   See Peter N. Black and Robert Scragg, "Relationship Between Serum 25-Hydroxyvitamin D and Pulmonary Function in the Third National Health and Nutrition Examination Survey," 128: 3792–98.

181   *a paper in the February 2006 issue*   See Cedric F. Garland, Frank C. Garland, Edward D. Gorham, et al, "The Role of Vitamin D in Cancer Prevention," 96: 252–61.

CHAPTER 8. WOMEN AND CHILDREN FIRST

182   *A mother had walked into a local health food store*   I was alerted to the case of the eighteen-month-old boy who suffered brain damage due to eucalyptus oil poisoning by a March 19, 2000, article in the *Washington Post* by Guy Gugliotta, "Alternative Medicines Promise Health, but Often Don't Deliver." I then interviewed Howard Mofenson, MD, a pediatrician with the Long Island Poison Control Center; the center's director, Tom Caraccio, PharmD; and Elaine Kang-Yum, who runs the center's Herb Watch program.

183   *Judy Robinson, a pediatric nurse practitioner*   I spoke with Judy Robinson, former executive director of the National Association of School Nurses, by telephone.

184   *dietary supplements are targeted at children everywhere*   I found these examples using Google.

        In the past decade, the Federal Trade Commission   See the press release from the FTC at www.ftc.gov/bcp/conline/features/kidsupp.pdf.

        The latest action came   See the FTC's index page describing its actions at www.ftc.gov/os/adjpro/d9317/index.htm.

a 1998 study in the Journal of the American Medical Association   See Steven B. Heymsfield, David B. Allison, Joseph R. Vasselli, et al, *"Garcinia cambogia* (Hydroxycitric Acid) as a Potential Antiobesity Agent," 280 (November 11, 1998): 1596–1600.

Says Hilary Perr   I spoke with Dr. Perr by telephone.

185   *A 2001 study by the Fred Hutchinson Cancer Research Center*   See M. L. Neuhouser, R. E. Patterson, S. Schwartz, et al, "Use of Alternative Medicine by Children with Cancer in Washington State," *Preventive Medicine* (November 2001): 347–54.

     Susan and Donald Pitzer   The death of Ryan Pitzer following his parents' reading of Adelle Davis's *Let's Have Healthy Children* was alleged in a complaint (case no. 79–6322) filed in the Circuit Court of the Seventeenth Judicial Circuit, in Broward County, Florida, on March 31, 1981, against Davis's estate and publisher. I contacted the lawyers who represented Ryan's parents, and searched phone directories around the United States, but was unable to track them down for an interview. My report is based on articles published at the time, including Doug Delp, "Mother Follows Book and Her Infant Dies," *Miami Herald,* April 22, 1978; Associated Press, "Book Blamed for Baby's Death," April 23, 1978; Patrick Malone, "Pompano Couple Sue Publisher, Say Book's Advice Fatal to Baby," *Miami Herald,* July 18, 1979; and John Latta "Mom Claims Her Baby Boy Killed by Colic Cure Published in a 'Child Care Bible,' " *Star,* May 23, 1978.

186   *Walked into the office of Tor A. Shwayder*   See Scott C. Wickless, Tor A. Shwayder, "A Medical Mystery," *NEJM* 351 (October 7, 2004): 1545, published with a photograph of the boy accompanying a challenge to other physicians to see if they could diagnose the cause. The "answer" was then published on November 25, 2004, (351: 2349–50). I interviewed Dr. Shwayder by telephone, as well as two other physicians familiar with the case.

187   *On February 13, 2004*   For my account of the Colorado Springs incident involving Green Hornet, I met with the young men involved and agreed to protect their confidentiality by not using their last names. I also met Kevin Schnitker and asked to interview him, but he declined my request. By telephone, I interviewed Dr. Mark James, the emergency room doctor who treated the boys.

189   *The FDA sent him its standard warning letter*   The FDA's warning letter, dated February 24, 2004, "FDA Warns Consumers Not to Purchase Green Hornet, Promoted as Herbal Version of 'Ecstasy,' " is online at www.fda.gov/bbs/topics/NEWS/2004/NEW01026.html.

     more than 45 deaths and 5,500 emergency room overdoses   Cited by Tamar Nordenberg, "The Death of the Party: All the Rave, GHB's Hazards Go Unheeded," *FDA Consumer,* March–April 2000.

     Brett Chidester, a seventeen-year-old straight-A student   See Oren Dorell, "Powerful but legal, hallucinogenic under scrutiny," *USA Today,* April 2, 2006.

     the FDA sent out a warning   The FDA's March 25, 2002, warning was titled "Kava-Containing Dietary Supplements May Be Associated with Severe Liver Injury." *Consumer Reports'* cover story on dangerous dietary supplements was published in May of 2004. Nakava's menu of kava offerings can be found at www.nakava.com.

190   *an unexpectedly important medical benefit*   The findings of apparent benefit for kava were reported on www.kavalive.com in the article "Kava Council Welcomes Cancer Cure News," on February 15, 2006.

     A study published in . . . the Journal of Adolescent Health   See Susan M. Yussman, J. C. West, K. M. Wilson, et al, "Complementary and Alternative Medicine Use by U.S. Adolescents with Special Health Care Needs," 38 (March 23, 2006): 395–400.

191   *recent surveys in both Iowa and Wisconsin*   See "Creatine Supplementation in Wisconsin High School Athletes," *Wisconsin Medical Journal* 101 (2002): 25–30. The Iowa survey was described in the September 2005 issue of *Coaching Management* at www.momentummedia .com/articles/cm/cm1308/bbsurvey.htm.

A 2004 study in the journal Neurology   See M. A. Tarnopolsky, D. J. Mahoney, J. Vasjar, et al, "Creatine Monohydrate Enhances Strength and Body Composition in Duchenne Muscular Dystrophy," *Neurology* 62 (2004): 1771–77.

A 1999 survey in the Journal of the American Dietetic Association   See Mark S. Juhn, John W. O'Kane and Debra M. Vinci, "Oral Creatine Supplementation in Male Collegiate Athletes: A Survey of Dosing Habits and Side Effects," 99 (1999): 593–96.

U.S. poison centers received   I tabulated these figures from reports published by AAPCC in the *American Journal of Emergency Medicine.*

"Because that's sixty percent"   I interviewed Dr. Arthur P. Grollman as well as Senator Durbin.

192   *A 2004 survey by the University of Michigan*   Results of the 2004 "Monitoring the Future" survey by the Institute of Social Research can be found at www.drugabuse.gov/News room/04/2004MTFDrug.pdf.

the News-Sentinel *conducted a survey*   See Ted Mero, "Survey Shows Widespread Use of Supplements Among Local Football Players," October 15, 2005.

Gary I. Wadler . . . blames DSHEA   I interviewed Dr. Wadler by telephone.

"Creatine is bodybuilding's ultimate supplement"   See www.bodybuilding.com/store/creatine.html.

193   *Schwarzenegger announced on July 15, 2005*   See Associated Press, "Schwarzenegger to End Ties to Magazines," July 15, 2005.

Jackie Speier   I interviewed her by telephone.

the most recent National Health and Nutrition Examination Survey   NHANES figures on use of supplements by men and women can be found at www.cdc.gov/nchs/data/nhanes/data briefs/dietary.pdf.

in April of 1998 an Australian company   See Jane L. Levere, "Campaigns for Supplements for That Midlife Event Contend That Mother Nature Knows Best," *New York Times*, August 18, 1998.

194   *What the ads failed to disclose*   See news report from the Australian Broadcasting Corp., "Menopause Research Misrepresented," July 29, 1999, at www.abc.net.au/science/news/stories/s39897.htm. Both of the studies were published in the June issue of *Climacteric*, the journal of the International Menopause Society, in Volume 2, June 1999.

Enzymatic Therapy   See Jane L. Levere, "Campaigns for Supplements."

"Dietary Supplement Use in Women"   A report on the meeting, coauthored by Dr. Coates, was published as "Dietary Supplement Use in Women: Current Status and Future Directions—Introduction and Conference Summary," in *Journal of Nutrition* 133 (June 2003): 1957S–60S.

195   *Novogen offered doctors $1,000*   See Associated Press, "Menopause Remedy Makers Get Tough," November 27, 2002.

A 2002 review in the Annals of Internal Medicine   See Fredi Kronenberg and Adriane Fugh-Berman, "Complementary and Alternative Medicine for Menopausal Symptoms: A Review of Randomized, Controlled Trials," 137 (November 19, 2002): 805–13.

In July 2003, the Journal of the American Medical Association   See Jeffrey A. Tice, Bruce Ettinger, Kris Ensrud, et al, "Phytoestrogen Supplements for the Treatment of Hot Flashes: The Isoflavone Clover Extract (ICE) Study," 290 (July 9, 2003): 207–14.

In April of 2003, Yale researchers reported   Sara Rockwell, Yanfeng Liu, and Susan Higgins presented the study at the ninety-fourth annual meeting of the American Association for Cancer Research, and later published it as "Alteration of the Effects of Cancer Therapy Agents on Breast Cancer Cells by the Herbal Medicine Black Cohosh," in *Breast Cancer Research and Treatment* (April 2005): 233–39.

woman who developed hepatitis   Stanley M. Cohen, MD, assistant professor of medicine at the University of Chicago in Illinois, reported this case at the American College of Gastroenterology meeting in Baltimore on October 12, 2003, as abstract 53.

In July of 2004   See Sanne Kreijkamp-Kaspers, Linda Kok, Diederick E. Grobbee, et al, "Effect of Soy Protein Containing Isoflavones on Cognitive Function, Bone Mineral Density, and Plasma Lipids in Postmenopausal Women," *JAMA* 292 (July 7, 2004): 65–74.

Susan Cruzan . . . cautions women   Ms. Cruzan made her comments to me in a telephone interview.

196   *A survey published in the December 2004* Journal of Clinical Oncology   See Grace K. Dy, Lishan Bekele, Lorelei J. Hanson, et al, "Complementary and Alternative Medicine Use by Patients Enrolled onto Phase I Clinical Trials," 22 (December 1, 2004): 4810–15.

a twenty-nine-year-old woman who had received a kidney-pancreas transplant   See G. W. Barone, B. J. Gurley, B. L. Ketel, et al, "Drug Interaction Between St. John's Wort and Cyclosporine," *Annals of Pharmacotherapy* 34 (September 2000): 1013–16.

197   *Johannes Wolf . . . estimates that about 5 percent of patients*   I interviewed Dr. Johannes Wolf by telephone.

Writing in Salon.com   Peter Kurth's article in Salon.com, "Quack Record," was published on May 21, 2002, at dir.salon.com/story/books/feature/2002/05/21/null/index.html.

a hearing on the decade-long aftermath of DSHEA   The June 8, 2004, hearing "Dietary Supplement Safety Act: How Is FDA Doing 10 Years Later?" was held before the Senate Subcommittee on Oversight of Government Management, the Federal Workforce, and the District of Columbia.

198   *Debbie Benson*   Her case was described in an article by Kenneth Spiker at www.quack watch.org/01QuackeryRelatedTopics/Victims/debbie.html.

Lucille Craven   Her case was described in an article by her husband, Richard Craven, at www.quackwatch.org/01QuackeryRelatedTopics/Victims/craven.html.

Megan Wilson   See Nina Shapiro, "Death by Natural Causes," *Seattle Weekly,* June 8, 2005, (Much as I admire the title of Ms. Shapiro's piece, I actually came up with the title of my book in 2004.)

Charlene Dorcy   See Associated Press, "Mother Accused of Killing Her Children," *Kitsap Sun,* June 20, 2004.

Jeanette Sliwinski   See "Defense Points to Sliwinski's Mental State," *Morton Grove Champion,* September 8, 2005.

199   *Bayer began airing television commercials*   See Barry Meier, "Industry's Next Growth Sector: Memory Lapses," the *New York Times,* April 4, 1999.

in August of 2002, the Journal of the American Medical Association   See Paul R. Solomon, Felicity Adams, Amanda Silver, et al, "Ginkgo for Memory Enhancement," 288 (August 21, 2002): 835–40.

the Journal of Arthroplasty *reported*   See A. Bebbington, R. Kulkarni, P. Roberts, "Persistent Bleeding After Total Hip Arthroplasty Caused by Herbal Self-Medication," 20 (January 2005): 125–26.

In November of 2004, the U.S. Agency for Healthcare   See "Melatonin for Treatment of Sleep Disorders," November 2004, at www.ahrq.gov/clinic/tp/melatntp.htm.

200   *no supplement tracked by U.S. poison center*   The numbers of adverse incidents involving melatonin were derived from AAPCC's annual reports published each September in the *American Journal of Emergency Medicine.*

CHAPTER 9. SHARK BAIT

201   *In an interview that Lane gave years later*   See "Shark Cartilage and Cancer, Revisited: A Follow-up Interview," www.healthy.net/scr/interview.asp?PageType=Interview&ID=182.

$30-million   Cited in "Shark Cartilage and Nutriceutical Update," *Journal of Alternative and Complementary Therapy* 1 (1995): 414–16.

more than 25 percent of some cancer patients   Cited in Edward R. Winstead, "Testing Shark Cartilage as a Cancer Drug," *NCI Cancer Bulletin*, July 26, 2005, at www.cancer.gov/ncicancerbulletin/NCI_Cancer_Bulletin_072605/page4.

203   *legitimate researchers began conducting well-designed studies*   A description of clinical trials of shark cartilage appears on the National Cancer Institute Web site at www.cancer.gov/cancertopics/pdq/cam/cartilage/HealthProfessional/page5.

204   *judge William Bassler . . . ordered it to destroy its inventory*   The legal decision against Lane Labs is described by the FDA in a July 13, 2004, press release, "U.S. District Judge Issues Permanent Injunction Against Lane Labs-USA, Inc. and Orders Firm to Refund Money to Purchasers of Illegally Marketed Unapproved Drugs," at www.fda.gov/bbs/topics/news/2004/NEW01086.html.

Dr. Loprinzi . . . reported his results   See Janet Raloff, "A Fishy Therapy," *Science News*, March 5, 2005.

205   *Mitchell Balbert, president of Natrol*   I interviewed Balbert at his office near Los Angeles, and toured his plant, in October of 2004.

206   *a national survey conducted in 1996 by Opinion Research Corporation*   See "Survey Indicates Increasing Herb Use," *HerbalGram* 37 (1996): 56.

207   *Richard Cleland, assistant director*   Cleland spoke with me both in person and by telephone.

the FDA and FTC   See "FDA Warns Distributors of Dietary Supplements Promoted Online for Weight Loss," April 1, 2004, at www.fda.gov/bbs/topics/news/2004/NEW01045.html.

208   *the FTC announced*   See news release, "FTC Targets Products Claiming to Affect the Stress Hormone Cortisol," at www.ftc.gov/opa/2004/10/windowrock.htm.

founded in a suburb of Cincinnati   See David Schardt, "Sex in a Bottle," *Nutrition Action Health Newsletter*, October 2004. Another excellent article on Enzyte, "Pill Company Thrives Despite Complaints," was written by Matt Crenson of the Associated Press and published on November 20, 2004.

a class-action suit was filed   A copy of the lawsuit filed by David Parker against Enzyte can be found at www.casewatch.org/cp/enzytecmp.pdf.

the Center for Science in the Public Interest filed a complaint   See www.cspinet.org/new/pdf/ftcenzyteletter.pdf.

209   *four of the company's former executives pleaded guilty*   See "Four Former Berkeley Execs Plead Guilty in Fraud," *Cincinnati Business Courier*, January 26, 2006.

"has changed [his] life and could change yours"   Quoted in Center for Science in the Public Interest, "Supplementing Their Income," *Nutrition Action Health Letter*, January/February 2006, at www.cspinet.org/new/200601241.html.

relieving scurvy in rats   See "Comparison of the Anti-Scorbutic Activity of L-ascorbic Acid and Ester C in the Non-Ascorbate Synthesizing Osteogenic Disorder Shionogi (ODS) Rat," *Life Sciences* 48 (1991): 2275–81.

another study . . . in dogs   See "Pharmacokinetics in Dogs After Oral Administration of

Two Different Forms of Ascorbic Acid," *Research in Veterinary Sciences* 71 (August 2001): 27–32.

a test-tube study from Norway   See L. Mathiesen, S. Wang, B. Halvorsen, "Inhibition of Lipid Peroxidation in Low-Density Lipoprotein by the Flavonoid Myrigalone B and Ascorbic Acid," *Biochemical Pharmacology* 51 (June 28, 1996): 1719–25.

But a 1998 study in the Journal of the American Medical Association   See Heiner K. Berthold, Thomas Sudhop, Klaus von Bergmann, "Effect of a Garlic Oil Preparation on Serum Lipoproteins and Cholesterol Metabolism: A Randomized Controlled Trial," *JAMA* 280 (June 17, 1998): 1900–02.

"Garlic preparation may have small"   AHRQ's report on garlic is online at www.ahrq.gov/clinic/epcsums/garlicsum.htm.

210   *"Either Larry King has a knack"*   Quoted in CSPI's "Supplementing Their Income."

the maker settled charges by the FTC   See "Seller of 'Ocular Nutrition' Dietary Supplement That Purports to Treat Eye Diseases Settles FTC Charges and Pays $450,000," at www.ftc.gov/opa/2005/02/hihealth.htm.

Harvey has since kept right on reading   As of May 30, 2006, Paul Harvey's Web site continued to list the maker of Ocular Nutrition as a sponsor, at www.paulharvey.com/sponsorspot.shtml.

Pamela Jones Harbour   A copy of her September 26, 2005, speech can be found at www.ftc.gov/speeches/harbour/050926selfreg.pdf.

211   *Herbalife has continued growing*   See Alex Veiga, Associated Press, "A New Life for Herbalife," March 26, 2006.

212   *"You can't assume it will work in people"*   Quoted in David Evans, "Nobel Prize Winner Didn't Disclose His Herbalife Contract," Bloomberg News, December 8, 2004.

Rakesh Amin . . . and Jay Jacobowitz   I heard their comments during their presentation at the NNFA meeting.

213   *A clerk named Rafi*   I encountered Rafi during a visit to the GNC at 1728 L Street, NW, in Washington, D.C., on September 30, 2004.

215   *"We are so much controlled by the context"*   Dr. Hantula spoke with me by telephone.

According to historian James Harvey Young   See Chapter 11, "The Pattern of Patent Medicine Appeals," *The Toadstool Millionaires: A Social History of Patent Medicines in America before Federal Regulation* (Princeton, New Jersey: Princeton University Press, 1961).

216   *"I'm not a medical doctor"*   Trudeau and Arthur Caplan are quoted in a CBS news story, "Is Trudeau a Charlatan or a Healer?" September 28, 2005, at www.cbsnews.com/stories/2005/09/28/earlyshow/leisure/books/main887681.shtml.

217   *"I submit that the best standard"*   Quoted in Ralph Nader *Unsafe at Any Speed: The Designed-In Dangers of the American Automobile* (New York: Grossman Publishers, 1965), 319.

That question has absorbed Wallace Sampson   I interviewed Dr. Sampson by telephone.

220   *"There's a lot more public mistrust"*   I interviewed Dr. Topol by telephone.

A poll published in November of 2005   See Harris Poll of November 2, 2005, "Majorities of U.S. Adults Think Oil Companies and Pharmaceuticals Should Be More Regulated," at www.harrisinteractive.com/harris_poll/index.asp?PID=611.

221   *A 1998 study of 303 men*   See Jayne E. Edwards and R. Andrew Moore, "Placebo Therapy of Benign Prostatic Hyperplasia: A 25-Month Study," *British Journal of Urology* 81 (March 1998): 383.

Another study, involving 340 severely depressed people   See Hypericum Depression Study Group, "Effect of *Hypericum perforatum* (St. John's Wort) in Major Depressive Disorder: A Randomized, Controlled Trial," *JAMA* 287 (April 10, 2002): 1807–14. A press release on the study from the National Center for Complementary and Alternative Medicine can be found at nccam.nih.gov/news/2002/stjohnswort/pressrelease.htm.

So pronounced is the placebo effect   See Franklin G. Miller, Ezekiel J. Emanuel, Donald L. Rosenstein, and Stephen E. Straus, "Ethical Issues Concerning Research in Complementary and Alternative Medicine," *JAMA* 291 (February 4, 2004): 599–604.

222   *even the book of Numbers*   See Numbers 21:9: "And Moses made a serpent of brass, and put it upon a pole, and it came to pass, that if a serpent had bitten any man, when he beheld the serpent of brass, he lived."

Tom Cruise's infamous harangue   On June 23, 2005, Cruise was asked by Matt Lauer, "Might not Brooke Shields be an example of someone who benefited from one of those drugs?" Cruise replied, "All it does is mask the problem, Matt. And if you understand the history of it, it masks the problem. That's what it does, that's all it does. You're not getting to the reason why. There is no such thing as a chemical imbalance." Lauer then asked, "But aren't there examples where it works?" Cruise answered, "Matt, Matt, Matt, you don't even—you're glib." Shields later issued a statement calling Cruise's remarks "outrageous," adding, "Tom should stick to saving the world from aliens and let women who are experiencing postpartum depression decide what treatment options are best for them."

223   *On September 17, 1997, the predictable outcome*   See Max J. Coppes, Ronald A. Anderson, R. Maarten Egeler, et al, "Alternative Remedies for the Treatment of Childhood Cancer," *NEJM* 339 (September 17, 1998): 846–47.

CHAPTER 10: LOOKING FOR MR. NATURAL

225   *the company's founder . . . settled unrelated charges*   The FTC's settlement with Garden of Life on March 9, 2006, was announced on the Commission's Web site at www.ftc.gov/opa/2006/03/gardenoflife.htm.

226   *Patient Heal Thyself,* by Jordan Rubin, was published in December 2002 by Freedom Press, Topanga, California.

Consider Valerie Saxion   After hearing her speak at the NNFA annual meeting in 2004, I interviewed her by telephone.

determined by the FDA in 2002   The FDA announced its final ruling that cascara sagrada is not generally recognized as safe in the Federal Register on May 9, 2002, volume 67, no. 90, pages 31125–27.

227   *"Pat's Age-Defying Shake"*   See Associated Press, "Televangelist's Diet Shake, Distributed by GNC, Draws Ire," August 22, 2005.

228   *And then there is Kevin Trudeau*   Trudeau's crimes have been widely reported, including by the New York State Consumer Protection Board, at www.consumer.state.ny.us/press releases/2005/august505.htm. The FTC's 1998 action against Trudeau is at www.ftc.gov/opa/1998/01/megasyst.htm. A news release from the FTC announcing its decision against Trudeau on September 7, 2004, was titled (ironically, given the many infomercials he subsequently did for his book) "Kevin Trudeau Banned from Infomercials."

229   *A. Glenn Braswell is far less well known*   Braswell was the primary subject of a hearing held by the Senate Special Committee on Aging on September 10, 2001, "Swindlers, Hucksters, and Snake Oil Salesmen: The Hype and Hope of Marketing Anti-Aging Products to Seniors." An excellent review of Braswell's record was written by Michael Isikoff for *Newsweek,* published as a Web exclusive on March 8, 2001: "The Bush Family and the Medicine Man." The $610,000 payment made to the FTC is described at www.ftc.gov/opa/predawn/F85/heafraud3.htm.

230   *Braswell . . . went on to donate*   See Lucy Morgan, "Bush Brothers Pop Up in Potion Peddler's Magazine," *St. Petersburg Times,* September 29, 2000.

Ponich and the company's number-three executive   Mike O'Neil testified about his and Ted Ponich's employment experience with Braswell, and about Braswell's illegal activities, during his testimony before the Senate Special Committee on Aging, "Swindlers, Hucksters."

Braswell fired Ponich   The details of how Mr. Ponich was fired, and how he subsequently died, were related to me by his son, Paul Ponich, in a series of telephone interviews from his home in Orange, California.

Hugh Rodham   See James V. Grimaldi and Peter Slevin, "Hillary Clinton's Brother Was Paid for Role in 2 Pardons," *Washington Post,* February 22, 2001.

231   *Braswell was sentenced*   See Associated Press, "Businessman Pardoned by Clinton Sentenced," September 13, 2004.

In 2006, he also agreed to pay $1 million   Braswell's FTC settlement was announced at www.ftc.gov/opa/2006/01/braswell.htm.

A window onto their world opened   I attended the CRN annual meeting at the Landsdowne Resort.

233   *assistant attorney general Joel Klein announced*   Klein's statement about the vitamin conspiracy, made on May 20, 1999, can be found at www.usdoj.gov/atr/public/press_releases/1999/2451.htm. I also learned a great deal about the conspiracy from John M. Conner, PhD, professor of agricultural economy at Purdue University, who kindly sent me a copy of his fantastic work-in-progress, "The Great Global Vitamins Conspiracy, 1989–1999."

Mitchell Balbert, president of Natrol   As noted above, I interviewed Balbert and toured the company's manufacturing facility near Los Angeles, October 2004.

234   *June Grell of California died*   I interviewed her husband, Christopher E. Grell. The *American Journal of Gastroenterology* published its report on the subject, "Laci LeBeau Syndrome," in volume 88, December 1993, pages 2140–41. A report on the FDA's investigation into stimulant-laxative teas appeared in the July–August 1997 *FDA Consumer,* "Dieter's Brews Make Tea Time a Dangerous Affair," by Paula Kurtzweil, at www.fda.gov/fdac/features/1997/597_tea.html.

235   *Balbert agreed to pay*   An announcement of Natrol's $250,000 settlement with district attorneys in Sonoma, Napa, and Solano counties is at www.sonoma-county.org/Da/press_releases/press_091404.htm.

236   *only one has inherited the mantle of prestige*   As noted in the notes for the Prologue, I made many attempts to seek an interview with Dr. Andrew Weil, but he declined my requests. He refused similar requests from the Center for Science in the Public Interest during its preparation of "Supplementing Their Income," ibid.

In a tiny study   Weil's study was published in *Science,* "Clinical and Psychological Effects of Marijuana in Man," 162 (December 13, 1968): 1234–42.

237   *Upon graduating from Harvard Medical School*   An extensive interview with Dr. Weil, in which he tells much about his early career, was published on May 22, 1998, on the Web site of the Academy of Achievement, appearing at www.achievement.org/autodoc/page/weilint-1.

"A Trip to Stonesville"   I was alerted to some of Dr. Weil's wilder writings by an extraordinary article, "A Trip to Stonesville" (the title of which was borrowed from Dr. Weil's book chapter) by Arnold S. Relman, MD, former editor in chief of the *New England Journal of Medicine,* in the December 14, 1998, issue of the *New Republic.* A copy of the article is available at www.quackwatch.org/11Ind/weil.html.

Dr. Weil insisted in an interview in 1998   See the Academy of Achievement interview.

238   *"so that young people could make up their own minds"*   Ibid.

"I really think I'm in the middle"   Quoted in Relman, "A Trip to Stonesville."

"I think that my voice is very much listened to"   See Academy of Achievement.

Eva Forrester   See *Spontaneous Healing: How to Discover and Enhance Your Body's Natural Ability to Maintain and Heal Itself* (New York, Knopf, 1995): 123–25.

239   *"manifestations of good and evil"*   From *Health and Healing* (New York, Random House, 1986).

"Virtually all of the well-designed scientific studies"   See "Supplementing Their Income," *Nutrition Action Healthletter.*

An adoring 1996 profile   See Anne Raver, "A Shaman's Tools: Ma Huang and Bloodroot Paste," the *New York Times,* October 16, 1996.

240   *despite signing a deal with Drugstore.com*   These figures were revealed in a civil lawsuit filed on August 26, 2005, by Drugstore.com against Dr. Weil in the U.S. District Court for the District of Colorado over his alleged failure to make "reasonable efforts" to fulfill the contract between them. A copy of the suit can be found at www.casewatch.org/civil/weil/complaint.shtml.

CSPI's senior nutritionist, David Schardt, remains critical   See "Supplementing Their Income."

CHAPTER 11: PROOF

241   *Growing up poor in rural Iowa*   As with Orrin Hatch and Dr. Andrew Weil, Senator Tom Harkin never spoke with me, despite months of repeated phone calls and e-mails to and from his press representatives. For background on him, I consulted many sources, including the *Almanac of American Politics* by Michael Barone and Richard E. Cohen (National Journal Group, 2003); an interview he conducted for an Herbalife distributor, "Sen. Tom Harkin Speaks in Support of Herbal Supplements," at health.wellness.edietstar.com/Healthy_Nutrition/Herbal_Supplements/index.html; an extensive interview with him for a *Frontline* report, "The Alternative Fix," that appeared on November 6, 2003; and "Unlikely Allies, Harkin and Hatch Aid Industry," by Guy Gugliotta in the *Washington Post,* December 25, 2000. An invaluable resource on the early history of NCCAM can be found in James Harvey Young's article, "The Development of the Office of Alternative Medicine in the National Institutes of Health, 1991–1996," *Bulletin of the History of Medicine* 72 (1998): 279–98. Another excellent article can be found in the July 17, 1995, issue of *Newsweek,* "Cures or 'Quackery': How Senator Harkin Shaped Federal Research on Alternative Medicine," by Stephen Budiansky.

"I went on this very tough regimen"   Quoted in "The Alternative Fix" on *Frontline.*

242   *Royden Brown, the man who provided him with the bee pollen*   See the FTC report at www.ftc.gov/opa/predawn/F93/ccpollen.6.htm.

He pushed through Public Law 102–170   See "Important Events in NCCAM's History" at nccam.nih.gov/about/ataglance/timeline.htm.

Joseph J. Jacobs   Dr. Jacobs spoke with me by telephone in May of 2006.

He wore a blue blazer and black loafers   These observations are drawn from a profile of Dr. Jacobs by Natalie Angier, "Where the Unorthodox Gets a Hearing at N.I.H.," *New York Times,* March 16, 1993.

"I describe my role as the captain"   Quoted in Natalie Angier, "U.S. Opens the Door Just a Crack to Alternative Forms of Medicine," *New York Times,* January 10, 1993.

"We're going where no one has gone before"   Quoted in Anastasia Toufexis, "Dr. Jacobs' Alternative Mission," *Time,* March 1, 1993.

243　Dr. Jacobs's joke about 1–800–PEYOTE was quoted in Angier, "Where the Unorthodox Gets a Hearing."

"the unbendable rules of randomized clinical trials"　From an article by Senator Harkin, "Public Policy: The Third Approach," in *Alternative Therapies in Health and Medicine* 1, no. 1 (1995).

Dr. Barrie Cassileth was quoted in Natalie Angier "U.S. Head of Alternative Medicine Quits," *New York Times,* August 1, 1994.

244　*"I took his therapy and became nauseous"*　Dr. Jacobs made his comments during a Senate hearing on alternative medicine on June 24, 1993.

Harkin then demanded　The Senate Appropriations Subcommittee on Labor, Health, and Human Services, chaired by Harkin, met on June 24, 1993.

245　*"I'm leaving this job"*　My account of Dr. Jacobs's resignation is based on the interview he gave me.

"The office is not only supposed to look at alternative ideas"　Quoted in Angier, "U.S. Head of Alternative Medicine Quits."

"There's a fear that the peer review"　Frist made his remarks during a Senate hearing on October 9, 1997, on the funding of studies of alternative medicine. See Paul Smaglik, "Office of Alternative Medicine Gets Unexpected Boost," *Scientist* 11 (November 10, 1997).

Moran testified at a House hearing　His testimony came before a February 1998 hearing of the House Committee on Government Reform and Oversight, quoted in a February 15, 1998, article at naturalhealthline.com/newsletter/HL980215.html.

246　*OAM's budget*　The yearly budgets of OAM and NCCAM, from 1992 through 1993, are listed in an article by Wallace I. Sampson, MD, "Why the National Center for Complementary and Alternative Medicine (NCCAM) Should Be Defunded," published on December 10, 2002, at www.quackwatch.org/01QuackeryRelatedTopics/nccam.html.

Paul Berg . . . wrote to Frist　Comments by prominent scientists against NCCAM were described in "Scientists Campaign Against NIH Alternative Medicine Office," in *Cancer Letter,* July 11, 1997, and in Lois R. Ember, "Alternative Medicine Slammed," *Chemical Engineering News,* August 4, 1997.

247　*Leon Jaroff . . . wrote an op-ed*　See "Bee Pollen Bureaucracy," in the *New York Times,* October 6, 1997.

"I think there's very little skepticism left"　Quoted in Eugene Russo and Brendan A. Maher, "A Conversation with Stephen E. Straus," *Scientist* 16 (December 9, 2002): 34.

the studies—more than 700 of them　According to Dr. Straus in his statement to the Senate Subcommittee on Labor-HHS-Education Appropriations on April 1, 2004, in which he presented NCCAM's FY 2005 Budget Request. The center's other activities were likewise described in that presentation.

Saul Green . . . published the results　See "Stated Goals and Grants of the Office of Alternative Medicine/National Center for Complementary and Alternative Medicine," *Scientific Review of Alternative Medicine* 5 (Fall 2001).

248　*NCCAM announced that it would permit*　See press release, "The Future of PC-SPES Research Funding by NCCAM," August 26, 2002.

the company that manufactured (and doctored) the PC-SPES　See Justin Gillis, "Herbal Remedies turn Deadly for Patients."

Sampson . . . called for Congress to shut down NCCAM　See Sampson, "Why the National Center for Complementary and Alternative Medicine (NCCAM) Should Be Defended."

On April 10, 2002　See Hypericum Depression Trial Study Group, "Effect of *Hypericum perforatum* (St John's Wort) in Major Depressive Disorder."

"Our commitment is to apply exacting scientific methods"　Dr. Straus's comments were made in

a NCCAM press release, "Study Shows St. John's Wort Ineffective for Major Depression of Moderate Severity."

249   *"it would be prudent for patients and their oncologists"*   These remarks appeared in an editorial coauthored by Dr. Straus, "St. John's Wort: More Implications for Cancer Patients," *Journal of the National Cancer Institute* 94 (August 21, 2002): 1187–88.

a large, randomized study was published   See Brian M. Berman, Lixing Lao, Patricia Langenberg, et al, "Effectiveness of Acupuncture as Adjunctive Therapy in Osteoarthritis of the Knee," *Annals of Internal Medicine* 141 (December 21, 2004): 901–10.

"the effect is almost so small"   Dr. Felson was quoted in Rob Stein, "Study Says Acupuncture Eases Arthritis Pain," *Washington Post*, December 21, 2004.

"Because NCCAM's early research demonstrated"   See NCCAM's budget for FY 2007 at nccam.nih.gov/about/congressional/2007.pdf.

hundreds of small studies of remedies   Each year, NCCAM releases a report on the research it is funding. The latest fiscal year for which the center has released a report is 2005, at nccam.nih.gov/research/extramural/awards/2005/.

Gonzalez Protocol   A description of NCCAM's study of the Gonzalez Protocol can be found at nccam.nih.gov/news/19972000/121599.htm.

250   *mistletoe*   A description of NCCAM's mistletoe study can be found at nccam.nih.gov/mistletoe/faq.htm.

harp music   The study is being carried out by Kathi J. Kemper, MD, who holds the Caryl J. Guth Chair for Holistic and Integrative Medicine at Wake Forrest University in North Carolina, where she is also professor of pediatrics and public health sciences.

With its budget for fiscal year 2007   See NCCAM's budget for FY 2007.

Meyer's Blood Purifier   See Wallace Sampson, MD, "Studying Herbal Remedies," *New England Journal of Medicine* 353 (July 28, 2005).

251   "Echinacea Considered Valueless: Report of the Council on Pharmacy and Chemistry," *JAMA* 53, February 27, 1908, 1836.

echinacea was by far the most popular   *Nutrition Business Journal* reported that echinacea was the most popular herb used in the United States in 2002. A national survey in 2004 of more than 31,000 Americans conducted by NCCAM also found echinacea to be the most popular herb used, by about 10 percent of adults.

JAMA published a study of 407 children   See James A. Taylor, Wendy Weber, Leanna Standish, "Efficacy and Safety of Echinacea in Treating Upper Respiratory Tract Infections in Children: A Randomized Controlled Trial," 290 (December 3, 2003): 2824–30.

Another major study   A press release of the March 15, 2005, study in the journal *Clinical Infectious Diseases* was issued by Stanford University, at news-service.stanford.edu/news/2005/march9/med-echinacea-030905. html.

NCCAM weighed in   See Ronald B. Turner, Rudolf Bauer, Karin Woelkart, et al, "An Evaluation of *Echinacea angustifolia* in Experimental Rhinovirus Infections," *New England Journal of Medicine* 353 (July 28, 2005): 341–48.

"We've got to stop attributing any efficacy to echinacea"   Quoted in Gina Kolata, "Study Says Echinacea Has No Effect on Colds," *New York Times*, July 28, 2005.

252   *"It is essential that all such communications"*   See press release from the American Herbal Products Association, dated October 12, 2005, "NCCAM Revises Report of Echinacea Study, Notes Criticism of Low Dose," at www.ahpa.org/Default.aspx?tabid=69&aId=192&zId=10.

the next major study funded by the center   See Stephen Bent, Christopher Kane, Katsuto Shinohara, et al, "Saw Palmetto for Benign Prostatic Hyperplasia," *NEJM* 354 (February 9, 2006): 557–66.

"If you look at the change in symptoms"   Quoted in a press release from the University of California, San Francisco, at pub.ucsf.edu/today/cache/news/200602085.html.

Dr. Andrew Shao   His comments appeared in a press release, "New Study on Saw Palmetto Demonstrates Puzzling Results," issued by the Council for Responsible Nutrition in February of 2006.

two other recent, well-designed trials   The study by Columbia researchers, "A Prospective, 1-Year Trial Using Saw Palmetto Versus Finasteride in the Treatment of Category III Prostatitis/Chronic Pelvic Pain Syndrome," was published in *Journal of Urology* 171 (January 2004): 284–88. The Australian study, "Serenoa Repens Extract for Benign Prostate Hyperplasia: A Randomized Controlled Trial," appeared in *BJU International* 92 (August 2003): 267–70.

253   *"Our goal is not to debunk things"*   Quoted in Sylvia Pagán Westphal, "Popular Herb Shows No Benefit for Prostate," *Wall Street Journal*, February 9, 2006.

President Bush was using it   His discontinuation of glucosamine and chondroitin was described in an Associated Press article, "Study: Supplements Fail to Ease Arthritis," February 22, 2006, which stated: "President Bush was among the customers for a while because of knee pain, but spokeswoman Dana Perino said Wednesday the president no longer takes the supplements."

The new study   See Daniel O. Clegg, Domenic J. Reda, Crystal L. Harris, et al, "Glucosamine, Chondroitin Sulfate, and the Two in Combination for Painful Knee Osteoarthritis," *NEJM* 354 (February 23, 2006): 795–808.

254   *the press was almost unanimous*   According to a search on Google, *USA Today*'s headline was "Study: No Overall Benefit for Mild Arthritis from Supplements"; the *Dallas Morning News,* "Study: Supplements Show Little Benefit for Mild Arthritis"; *Forbes,* "Glucosamine, Chondroitin Not Much Help for Arthritic Knees"; the *Seattle Post-Ingelligencer,* "Supplements Fail to Ease Arthritis"; and Reuters, "Supplements Fail to Help Mild Knee Arthritis: Study," all dated February 22, 2006.

But NCCAM's press release   Its announcement was released on February 22, 2006, at nccam.nih.gov/news/2006/022206.htm.

the audacious Council for Responsible Nutrition   CRN's news release can be found at www.crnusa.org/prpdfs/PR06_GAIT022206.pdf.

Between 1992 and 2006, Senator Hatch received   To come up with the figures on donations from the supplement industry to Senator Harkin, I first spoke with Steven Weiss, communications director of the Center for Responsive Politics, and then searched the center's database at www.opensecrets.org.

255   *"He's a politician who panders"*   Dr. Jacobs stated this during my interview.

Consumer Reports *published a cover story*   Its outstanding article on dangerous supplements can be found at www.consumerreports.org/co/supplements/.

256   Annals of Internal Medicine   See Ilene B. Anderson, Walter H. Mullen, James E. Meeker, et al, "Pennyroyal Toxicity: Measurement of Toxic Metabolite Levels in Two Cases and Review of the Literature," 124 (April 15, 1996): 726–34.

essential oils of all kinds   The AAPCC figures are compiled from the group's annual reports each September in the *American Journal of Emergency Medicine.*

A 2001 report in the Journal of Paediatrics and Child Health   See Zorina Flaman, Sandra Pellechia-Clarke, Benoit Bailey, "Unintentional Exposure of Young Children to Camphor and Eucalyptus Oils," 6 (February 2001) 80–83.

257   *forty-two-year-old African-American man*   See "Yohimbine-Induced Cutaneous Drug Eruption, Progressive Renal Failure and Lupus-Like Syndrome," *Urology* 41 (April 1993): 343–45.

an FDA study   See "Gas Chromatographic Determination of Yohimbine in Commercial Yohimbe Products," *Journal of AOAC International* 78 (1995): 1189–94.

two reports from Norway   The Norwegian reports of scullcap and liver damage are indexed on PubMed as appearing in *Tidsskr Nor Laegeforen* 112 (August 10, 1992): 2389–90; and *Tidsskr Nor Laegeforen* 112 (June 10, 1992): 2006. The Japanese report appeared in *Internal Medicine* 40 (August 2001): 764–68.

258   AHRQ's review of the effects of garlic can be found at www.ahrq.gov/clinic/epcsums/garlicsum.htm.

The review of ginseng and other supplements appeared in "The Risk-Benefit Profile of Commonly Used Herbal Therapies: *Ginkgo,* St. John's Wort, Ginseng, Echinacea, Saw Palmetto, and Kava," *Annals of Internal Medicine* 136 (January 1, 2002): 42–53.

ConsumerLab.com reported   Its report on pesticides in ginseng can be found at www.consumerlab.com/news/news_082803.asp.

In 2002, AHRQ published a review   AHRQ's findings on SAM-e can be found at www.ahrq.gov/clinic/epcsums/samesum.htm.

the FDA sent letters   A copy of the FDA's letter regarding SAM-e can be found at www.fda.gov/ohrms/dockets/DOCKETS/95s0316/rpt0092_01.pdf.

259   *an April 2002 study in the* Annals of Internal Medicine   See Meenakshi Khatta, Barbara S. Alexander, Cathy M. Krichten, "Effect of Coenzyme Q_{10} in Patients with Congestive Heart Failure," 132 (April 18, 2000): 636–40.

There is conjugated linoleic acid   See "Effects of Cis-9, Trans-11 Conjugated Linoleic Acid Supplementation on Insulin Sensitivity, Lipid Peroxidation, and Proinflammatory Markers in Obese Men," *American Journal of Clinical Nutrition* 80 (August 2004): 279–83; and "Supplementation with Conjugated Linoleic Acid Causes Isomer-Dependent Oxidative Stress and Elevated C-Reactive Protein: A Potential Link to Fatty Acid–Induced Insulin Resistance," *Circulation* 106 (October 8, 2002): 1925–29.

A press release from AHRQ summing up its findings on omega-3 fatty acids, fish oil, and ALA can be found at www.ahrq.gov/news/press/pr2004/omega3pr.htm.

There's guggul   See Philippe O. Szapary, Megan L. Wolfe, LeAnne T. Bloedon, et al, "Guggulipid for the Treatment of Hypercholesterolemia: A Randomized Controlled Trial," *JAMA* 290 (August 13, 2003): 765–72.

red yeast rice   A review of FDA's actions against red yeast rice can be found at www.fda.gov/ora/about/enf_story/archive/2001/ch4/cfsan4.htm.

policosanol   See Heiner K. Berthold, Susanne Unverdorben, Ralf Degenhardt, et al, "Effect of Policosanol on Lipid Levels Among Patients with Hypercholesterolemia or Combined Hyperlipidemia," *JAMA* 295 (May 17, 2006): 2262–69.

260   *In the journal* Nature Medicine   See "Problems with Over-the-Counter 5-Hydroxy-L-tryptophan," 4 (September 1998): 983.

Renee Kleemeier   Her injuries after taking 5-HTP are alleged in a complaint she filed against Nature's Bounty and Vitamin World in the U.S. District Court in Minnesota on November 20, 2002.

261   *Such was the state of knowledge*   FDA announced its decision to allow a qualified health claim for omega-3 fatty acids in a letter sent on October 31, 2000, to the attorney who brought the case, www.cfsan.fda.gov/~dms/ds-ltr11.html. On September 8, 2004, the FDA updated the claims it allows for omega-3 fatty acids, at www.fda.gov/bbs/topics/news/2004/NEW01115.html.

in April of 2004, AHRQ got into the act   AHRQ announced the findings of its review on April 22, 2004, in a press release, "Evidence Reports Confirm That Fish Oil Helps Fight Heart Disease."

the largest double-blind study of fish oil   See Ingeborg A. Brouwer, Peter L. Zock, A. John

Camm, et al, "Effect of Fish Oil on Ventricular Tachyarrhythmia and Death in Patients With Implantable Cardioverter Defibrillators," *JAMA* 295 (June 14, 2006): 2613–19.

CONCLUSION: WHAT WE CAN DO

262   *"misguided"*   See "Botanical Medicines—The Need for New Regulations," *NEJM* 347 (December 19, 2002): 2073–76.

"truly terrible federal law"   See "What Took So Long?" *Washington Post*, January 2, 2004.

"Snake Oil Protection Act"   See *New York Times*, October 5, 1993.

The Institute of Medicine   IOM released its report "Dietary Supplements: A Framework for Evaluating Safety" on April 1, 2004.

the Office of the Inspector General   A copy of the OIG's report, "An Inadequate Safety Valve," can be found at oig.hhs.gov/oei/reports/oei-01-00-00180.pdf.

263   *When Charles Bell*   His testimony on October 28, 2003, can be found at commerce.senate .gov/hearings/testimony.cfm?id=976&wit_id=2750.

the New York State Task Force on Life and Law urged   The task force's report on dietary supplements can be found at www.health.state.ny.us/press/releases/2005/2005-10-06_dietary_ supplements.htm.

According to Phil Waddington   I interviewed him in October of 2004.

264   *Commissioner Crawford promised*   He made his promise to implement GMPs for dietary supplements during his remarks at CRN's annual meeting in October of 2004.

Tod Cooperman of ConsumerLab.com   He made these remarks in the course of an interview I conducted with him.

In its 2005 report   See Institute of Medicine of the National Academies, *Complementary and Alternative Medicine in the United States,* 2005 National Academies Press, Washington, DC.

The Office of Inspector General analyzed   OIG, "An Inadequate Safety Valve."

265   New England Journal of Medicine *editorial*   See "The FDA, Regulation, and the Risk of Stroke," 343 (December 21, 2000): 1886–87.

Alexander M. Walker   See Walker, "The Relation Between Voluntary Notification and Material Risk in Dietary Supplement Safety," submitted to the FDA on March 9, 2000.

266   *The Star-Ledger of Jersey reported*   See Robert Cohen, "Bill Would Require Reports on Ill Effects of Supplement," August 2, 2006.

267   *The FDA has already contracted*   A brief history of how the National Academy of Sciences reviewed the evidence for drugs that had been approved prior to 1962 can be found at the FDA's Web site, at www.fda.gov/cder/about/history/Histext.htm.

268   *FDA's funding for all of its activities*   The FDA's $6 million budget and forty-six employees for regulating dietary supplements in 2001 was described in a statement by Joseph A. Levitt, who was then director of the FDA's Center for Food Safety and Applied Nutrition, before the House Committee on Government Reform, on March 20, 2001.

"the dietary supplement industry"   A copy of the FDA's report can be found at www.fda.gov/ ope/fy02plan/dietsupp.html.

When Cynthia T. Culmo   A copy of Dr. Culmo's testimony on July 31, 2002, can be found at www.afdo.org/afdo/position/3p2002.cfm.

269   *In January of 2003*   See Mary E. Palmer, Christine Haller, Patrick E. McKinney, et al, "Adverse Events Associated with Dietary Supplements: An Observational Study," *Lancet* 361 (January 11, 2003): 101–6.

A 2001 survey by the Blue Cross   See www.fepblue.org/toyourhealth/tyhhfsportsdrugs .html.

In 2002, a survey of high school and college coaches   A description of the 2002 survey conducted for GNC can be found at www.state.nj.us/steroids/final_report/finalreport.pdf.

the National Federation of State High School Associations   The group issued a statement, "Sports Medicine: NFHS Position Statement on Supplements," on November 7, 2002.

INDEX

A

Aane, Fritz, 160
AARP, 53, 94, 100, 229
Actra-Rx, 155
acupuncture, 139, 249
Adams, Samuel Hopkins, 31–32
Adamson, Raphiella, 112
adverse event reporting, 263, 264–65, 265–66
adverse reactions, 18, 19. *See also* safety *entries; specific supplements*
advertising. *See* deceptive advertising; health claims; marketing; supplement marketing
AIDS: A Second Opinion (Null), 197
AIDS, 93, 197. *See also* HIV
Airborne, 215
Ajinomoto, 161
ALA, 259
Albert, Eddie, 95
allergies, 97, 175, 241, 243, 244
Alliance U.S.A., 105
Alpha Omega Labs, 4–6, 7, 9–10, 12–13, 15
alpha tocopherol. *See* vitamin E

Alterman, Ruth, 56–57, 58
alternative medicine, 6, 17, 222–23. *See also* conventional medicine
    Andrew Weil as guru of, 238–40
    use statistics, 3, 16, 147
American Academy of Pediatrics, 53, 165
American Association of Retired Persons (AARP), 53, 94, 100, 229
American Botanical Council, 106–7, 142
American Dietetic Association, 165, 166
American Herbal Products Association, 251–52
American Medical Association, 165–66
Amerifit, 194
Ames, Bruce, 169
Amin, Rakesh, 212–13
amino acids, 68. *See also specific types*
amphetamines, 109
AMP II Pro Drops, 155
Andrade-Wheaton, Donna, 149
androstenedione, 191, 256
Angell, Marcia, 212, 219
anti-aging supplements, 198–99, 205, 227, 229

antibiotics, 35, 36, 70
antidepressants, 117, 221, 222. *See also* St.
    John's wort
antineoplastons, 244–45
antioxidants, 167–72, 185, 227, 259
antipsychotic drugs, 198
Archer, Bill, 112, 113
Archer, Douglas, 69, 70
Archer, William "Reyn," 112, 113, 114
Archer Daniels Midland, 231, 233
L-arginine, 211–12
argyria, 186–87
aristolochia, 142, 143–44, 148–51,
    161–62, 256
arnica, 148
arsenic, 152
arthritis, 250, 253–54, 258
asarum, 148
asthma, 175, 198
AST Sports Science, 116
athletes, 160–61, 191–93, 269–70
autism, 175
Avacor, 155
Ayurvedic medicines, 153–54, 154*n*

B

Baicalcumin, 144–45
Balbert, Mitchell, 205–6, 233–36
BASF Corp., 231, 233
Bass, Milton, 51, 81
Bass, Scott, 81, 91
Bassler, William, 204
Bayer HealthCare, 231
Beales, Howard, 184, 198
Bechler, Steve, 117–18
Bedell, Berkley, 243
bee pollen, 97, 241, 243, 244
Bell, Charles, 263
Bell, Charles E., 115
BeneFin, 203–4, 247
Bennett, William M., 146–48
Benson, Debbie, 198
Bent, Peter, 252
Berg, Paul, 246
beriberi, 38
Berkeley Premium Nutraceuticals, 208–9
beta-carotene, 169–71
Bilbray, Brian P., 255

Bingham, Fred, 93
Bionate International, 155
Bioterrorism Act of 2002, 265
birthwort. *See* aristolochia
Bishop, Katherine, 38
bitter orange, 126–27, 256
Black Beauty, 111, 122
black cohosh, 135, 194, 195
Blevins, Michael, 111, 114, 129, 228
Blizzard, Ed, 130
bloodletting, 28, 29
bloodroot, 3, 4, 6–7, 8, 9, 11, 13–15, 239
Blumberg, Jeffrey, 165
Blumenthal, Mark, 106–7
bone health, 174, 175–76, 180
Bonica, John, 140
Boozer, Carol, 123–24
Bork, Robert, 117
BotanicLab, 156, 158
Boxer, Barbara, 98–99
Braswell, A. Glenn, 229–31
breast cancer, 3, 173–74, 181, 194, 195,
    203
    refusals of conventional care, 198,
    238–39
Bromley, D. Allan, 246
Brown, Royden, 242, 244
Burkey, Cooper, 163–64, 225
Burton, Dan, 130, 156
Bush, George H. W., 72, 74, 246
Bush, George W., 116, 132, 253, 260
    supplement industry contributions,
    114, 230
    Texas ephedra investigation and, 110,
    112, 115
B vitamins, 166, 168, 173–74. *See also*
    specific types

C

Cadbury Adams, 231–32
caffeine, 105, 108, 109
calcium, 41, 45, 174, 179, 209, 228
calomel, 28, 29
Campbell, Tena, 128
Campbell, Walter, 39
cancer patients
    drug/supplement interactions, 185,
    195, 196, 249

supplement use statistics, 147, 185,
    196, 201
cancers. *See also specific types*
    antineoplastons for, 244–45
    antioxidants and, 169–71, 185
    aristolochia and, 148
    Chinese herbs claims, 144, 145
    kava and, 190
    laetrile for, 47, 218
    shark cartilage for, 201–4, 223, 246
    vitamin D and, 180, 181
Cansema, 5–6, 7, 13
Cantrell, Larry, 105
Caplan, Arthur, 216
Cargill, 232
Carmona, Richard H., 166
carotene, 168
Carson, Rachel, 36
cascada sagrada, 226
Cassileth, Barrie, 243–44
Caton, Gregory, 11–13, 228
Cavett, Dick, 45–46
CDC investigations, 63–65, 153,
    176–78
celebrity endorsements/ads, 86–87,
    94–96, 209–10, 214, 215–16
Center for Science in the Public Interest,
    92–93, 131, 208, 209, 210, 239,
    240
Centers for Disease Control and
    Prevention. *See* CDC
Chamomile Calm, 184
Chandra, Ranjit K., 172–73
Chao, Elaine L., 131
chaparral, 150, 256
chemotherapy, 6, 185, 195, 239, 249
Chen, K. K., 108
Chen, Sophie, 156–57, 248
Chidester, Brett, 189
children and supplement use, 164–65,
    166, 184
    ill children, 185, 197, 223, 245–46
    potential harm, 154, 175, 176–78,
    182–86
    teens, 186–93
children's nutrition, 179–80, 184–85
child-resistant packaging, 178, 268–69
Chinese herbs, 141–42, 143, 144–51, 257.
    See also Hames, Beverly

contaminants in, 143–44, 151–52,
    155
Chinese patent medicines, 139, 140, 148
Chin Koo Tieh Shang Wan, 148
chitosan, 235–36
cholesterol, 40, 168, 173, 209, 213,
    259–60, 261
chondroitin, 159, 250, 253–54
Chopra, Deepak, 153
Christensen, David, 231
Christian Broadcasting Network,
    227
Christian Science, 222
cinchona, 27
cinnabar, 151
L-citrulline, 211
Clark Stanley Snake Oil Liniment, 24–26,
    33–35
Cleland, Richard, 207
clerodendron, 148
Clinton, Bill, 88, 90, 101, 117, 230–31
Coates, Paul M., 194
Coca-Cola, 32
Coca-Cola Company, 232
cocaine, 32
Codex Alimentarius Commission, 263
coenzyme Q10, 159, 259
coffee, 27
coffee enemas, 243, 250
Coffey, Kendall, 230
Cohen, Marsha N., 52–53
colds, 168, 172, 251–52
colloidal silver, 186–87
comfrey, 150, 256
conjugated linoleic acid, 259
ConsumerLab.com, 158–59, 199, 264
Consumer Reports, 52, 189–90, 255–57,
    262–63
Consumers Union, 52, 94, 263
contamination issues, 137, 160–62. *See
    also* Hames, Beverly
    aristolochic acid, 143–44, 148–51,
    162
    heavy metals, 151–54, 199, 236
    pesticide residues, 154, 258
    pharmaceuticals, 154–58, 189, 245
    steroids, 160–61
conventional medicine, 221
    public views of, 35, 36, 216, 271

refusals of conventional care, 197–98, 217–18, 223, 238–39
supplement industry views of, 4–5
Cooke, Helena, 27–28
Cooperman, Tod, 158, 264
Coppes, Max J., 223
coral calcium, 209, 228
CortiSlim, 208
cortisol, 250
Council for Responsible Nutrition. *See* CRN
cow urine, 154*n*
Coyle, Mike, 231
Craven, Lucille, 198
Crawford, Lester, 159, 264
creatine, 191, 192–93
CRN (Council for Responsible Nutrition), 171, 231, 232, 252, 270–71
Cruise, Tom, 222
Cruzan, Susan, 195
Culmo, Cynthia, 105, 107, 110, 112–13, 114, 130, 268
CVS pharmacies, 215
cyclamates, 51–52
cyclosporine, 196–97

D

Davis, Adelle, 37–45, 46, 185
Davis, Gray, 115–16
Davis, Susan, 265
DEA, 111, 155
deceptive advertising, 207–10, 235–36, 270–71. *See also* health claims; supplement marketing
  FTC actions, 203–4, 207–9, 210, 225–26, 228
decongestants, 108, 112
DeGette, Diana, 123
DeLay, Tom, 132
de Merode, Prince Alexandre, 160
Denmark, 108–9, 178–80
DeNobel, Victor, 71
depression, 221, 222, 248, 258
Dern, Laura, 96
DES, 157–58
dextromethorphan, 189
Dharmananda, Subhuti, 142–45, 149, 161
DHEA, 191–92

Dietary Guidelines for Americans, 166, 174, 180–81
Dietary Supplement and Awareness Act, 265
Dietary Supplement Health and Education Act. *See* DSHEA
diethylstilbestrol (DES), 157–58
digitalis, 27–28
digoxin, 197
Dingell, John D., 100, 265
diphenhydramine, 189
dirt, 225–26
Dole, Bob, 50–51
Dorcy, Charlene, 198
Downs, Hugh, 205
dropsy, 27–28
Drotsby, Paolo, 178
Drug Enforcement Administration. *See* DEA
Drugstore.com, 240
DSHEA (Dietary Supplement Health and Education Act), 19, 89–103, 160–61
  health claims rules, 100, 102, 144, 203
  hearings, 90–94, 96–98
  Hollywood support, 94–96
  legacy/effects of, 102–3, 131, 153, 192, 197, 226, 264
  manufacturing standards, 159–60
  passage, 98–102
  reaction to passage, 262–63
  retailer recommendations and, 212–14
  safety standards/regulation, 102, 115, 125, 131
Durbin, Richard, 128, 192, 266
Dykstra, Gary, 78–79
Dynamic Health, 184

E

echinacea, 159, 250–52
Edita's Skinny Pill, 127
efficacy, 17–18, 19, 259–60. *See also* *specific supplements*
Eli Lilly & Co., 108
Elizondo, Hector, 199
Ellis, Michael, 111, 112, 114, 116, 117, 122
  criminal activities, 111, 129, 228
Elsinore pills, 108–9

Emerson, Gladys, 44
EMS. *See* L-tryptophan EMS
Enzymatic Therapy, 194
Enzyte, 208–9
E'ola, 116, 155
eosinophils, 55, 57, 58, 59–60. *See also*
    L-tryptophan EMS
ephedra, 19, 104–32
    adverse reactions, 19, 104–6, 110,
        115, 117–18, 121–23, 127, 128,
        130
    in China, 107–8
    Congressional hearings, 122–24
    early research, 107–8
    FDA ban, 19, 125–29, 131, 255
    FDA investigations, 110, 112, 114–15,
        117–18
    litigation over, 117, 127–29
    market/sales, 105, 106, 111–12, 115,
        125–26, 129
    maximum dose limits, 110, 112, 114,
        128, 129
    safety studies, 114–15, 122–24
    state bans, 115–16, 118, 193
    Texas investigation, 105–6, 107,
        109–10, 112–14, 115, 125
ephedra manufacturers, 110–12, 126–27,
    129–30, 131, 233–34
    lobbying efforts, 110–12, 113–14,
        115–16, 117
ephedrine, 105, 107, 108–9, 110, 111,
    155
ephedrine alkaloids, 108, 112, 114–15
essential oils, 18, 183, 256
essiac, 185
Ester-C, 209
Ester-E, 171
estrogen, 192. *See also* DES
estrogen alternatives, 194–96
Estroven, 194
eucalyptus oil, 182–83
Evans, Herbert, 38
evening primrose oil, 97, 239

F
FCC Products, 154
FDA, 6, 19, 35–36, 73, 116–17, 130
    adverse event report hotline, 266

adverse event reporting to, 264–65,
    265–66
DSHEA negotiations, 100–101
funding, 268
GRAS list, 69
Kessler as commissioner, 72–74,
    77–79, 84–86
manufacturing rules, 159–60, 264
public opinion about, 86, 87–88,
    94–96, 98–99
research summary development
    program, 267
subpoena/recall powers bill, 78, 80,
    88
supplement regulation powers, 19,
    48–49, 53, 78
FDA actions
    aristolochia, 148, 149, 154
    cascada sagrada, 226
    consumer warnings, 61, 153, 154, 155,
        189, 257
    cyclamates, 52
    DHEA, 191
    DSHEA's effect on, 102, 110, 153, 191
    ephedra ban, 19, 125–29, 131, 255
    ephedra/ephedrine investigation, 109,
        110, 114–15, 116, 117–18
    ephedrine-caffeine ban, 19, 109
    estrogen alternatives, 195
    evening primrose oil, 97
    food labeling, 77–78
    For Your Health Pharmacy raid,
        84–86
    iron supplements, 177
    litargirio, 153
    mind-altering supplements, 189
    omega-3 health claims, 260–61
    over deceptive health claims, 207–8
    SAM-e, 258–59
    senna, 235
    shark cartilage, 203–4
    L-tryptophan, 61, 63, 69–70, 84, 87
    vitamin regulation attempts, 47–53
FDA supplement rules (proposed 1992),
    77, 78–79, 81–84, 91, 98. *See also*
    DSHEA
    DSHEA as response to, 89
    Hatch-Richardson moratorium, 86, 88,
        98

industry opposition, 75, 79, 81–84,
86–88

public opinion/response, 86, 87–88
federal dietary guidelines, 166, 174,
180–81
Federal Trade Commission. *See* FTC
Felson, David, 249
fenfluramine, 155
Ferrier, Grant, 16
Finkelstein, Joel S., 174
Firestone, 217
fish oil supplements, 17, 259, 260–61
5HTP, 62, 260
flaxseed oil, 259
Fletcher, William, 38
Floberg, John, 217
flu, 215
Foley, Heather, 100
Foley, Tom, 99, 100
folic acid, 17, 166, 173
Folkman, Judah, 202
Food, Drug, Cosmetic, and Device
Enforcement Amendments, 78
Food, Drug, and Cosmetic Act of 1938,
35, 70
Proxmire Amendment, 48–53, 69, 70
food allergies, 175
Food and Drug Administration. *See* FDA
food labeling, 73, 74–77, 77–78
Formula One, 105, 106, 110
Forrester, Eva, 238–39
For Your Health Pharmacy, 84–85
foxglove, 27–28
Franklin, Ben, 28
free radicals, 167, 168
Frieden, Thomas R., 152, 153
Frist, Bill, 245, 246
From Chocolate to Morphine (Weil and
Rosen), 238
FTC actions, 184, 216, 228, 229, 231
bee pollen, 242
Enzyte, 208–9
estrogen alternatives, 195–96
Garden of Life, 225–26
shark cartilage, 203–4
weight-loss supplements, 207–8
FTC health claims standard, 75, 78–79,
91, 261

Funk, Casimir, 38
Furchgott, Robert, 212
Furcich, Steve, 231

G

garcinia, 184
Garden of Life, 163, 225–26
garlic, 209–10, 258
Garlique, 209
GB Data Systems, 229–30
"generally recognized as safe" list, 69
germander, 150, 256
Gero H3 Anti-Aging Pill, 229
Gerson Institute, 243
GHB, 189
Gibson, Mel, 94–95
Gilbert, Don A., 115
Gilliatt, Sue, 1–4, 6–11, 13, 15
Gingrich, Newt, 99
ginkgo biloba, 199, 205, 258
ginseng, 154, 258
Giordano, Mike, 125
glandular extracts, 256
Gleich, Gerald, 60
Global Vision Products, 155
glucosamine, 159, 250, 253–54
GMPs, 158, 159, 264
GNC stores, 161, 212, 213–14, 227
Gold, Lois Swirsky, 154
Goldberg, Whoopi, 95
Gonzalez Protocol, 249–50
Gooch, Sandy, 81
good manufacturing practices, 158, 159,
264
Goratna Ayurvedic medicines,
154*n*
GRAS list (FDA), 69
Green, Saul, 247–48
Greene, Doug, 82, 83
Green Hornet, 188–89
Greenwood, James C., 122, 124
Grell, Christopher, 235
Grell, June, 234
Grimm-Schaefer, Robin, 140
Grollman, Arthur P., 149–50, 150–51,
191–92
guggul, 259

H

H3O, 9–10, 12, 13
Hahnemann, Samuel, 29
hallucinogens, 187–89, 237–38
Hames, Beverly, 137–41, 145–48, 161–62
Hamill, Pete, 45–46
Hantula, Donald A., 215, 220, 221
Harbour, Pamela Jones, 210, 270
Hardy, Linda, 155–56
Hardy, Thomas, 155–56
Harkin, Tom, 97, 99, 100, 101, 241,
    254–55
    and OAM, 242–45, 246, 266–67
Harris, Michael R., 26–27, 30, 35, 70–71,
    98, 272
Harrison, Channing W., 33
Harvey, Paul, 210
Hatch, Orrin, 73, 252
    and DSHEA, 91, 97–98, 99, 100, 107,
    160
    FDA rules moratorium, 86, 88, 98
    and NLEA, 75, 77, 78, 81
    supplement industry ties, 75–77, 89,
    90, 254–55
Hatch, Scott, 77
Hathaway, William, 52
Hauser, Wings, 96
Health and Healing (Weil), 238
health claims. *See also* deceptive
    advertising; FDA actions; FDA
    supplement rules; FTC actions;
    specific supplements
    DSHEA rules, 100, 102, 144, 203,
    229
    evidence standards, 74–75, 77, 78–79,
    91, 92, 261
    FDA surveys of, 92, 97
    on food labels, 74–75
    made by retailers, 212–14, 239
    misleading, 74, 92, 97, 220
    premarket review issue, 74–75, 92
    in third-party literature, 102, 213, 214,
    215
Health Research Group, 51, 73
heart attack, 127, 194, 257
    ephedra and, 104, 114–15, 121–22,
    123
heart disease, 259–60, 261

vitamins/minerals and, 169–71, 173,
    179, 239
heart problems, 27–28, 185, 234–35,
    260. *See also* heart attack; heart
    disease
heavy metals, 151–54, 199, 236
Hein, Sarah A., 147
Helphrey, Debbie, 234
Hemingway, Mariel, 86
Henney, Jane E., 117
hepatitis, 195
herbal enemas, 226
Herbalife International, 76, 211–12, 255
herbs, herbal supplements, 18, 19, 29–30.
    See also Chinese herbs; *specific herbs*
    contamination issues, 143–44,
    151–58, 189
    estrogen alternatives, 194–96
    liver injury and, 150, 155
    manufacturing process, 136–37
    media coverage, 205–7
    mind-altering supplements, 187–91
Hertzman, Phillip, 59, 60
Hildenbrand, Gar, 243
Hines, Kenneth, 129
hip fractures, 174, 175–76
Hippocrates, 28
HIV, 144–45, 197, 214. *See also* AIDS
Hoffman-LaRoche, 233
Holick, Michael F., 180
Holt, Stephen, 214
homeopathy, 16, 18, 29, 139, 148, 215
hoodia gordonii, 126, 207
hormone replacement therapy, 174, 194
Houts, Paul L., 54–55, 63, 64, 66, 67
Howry, Julie Puett, 104–5
Howry, Phil, 104–5, 113
HRx, 9, 10
Huenemann, Ruth, 44
Hughes, Mark, 211
Hutt, Peter B., 73
hydroxycitrate, 184

I

IdeaSphere, 129
Ignarro, Louis, 211–12
illegal drugs, 190–91

illness, supplement use and, 185, 195,
    196–98. *See also specific illnesses*
    refusals of conventional care, 197–98,
    217–18, 223, 238–39
indinavir, 197
insomnia, 62, 199–200, 260. *See also*
    L-tryptophan
Institute for Traditional Medicine,
    142–43, 148, 161
Institute of Medicine, 262, 263, 264, 266
Insulin Amendment, 35–36
irinotecan, 249
iron, 17, 18, 29, 176–78, 179
Israelson, Loren, 91
Istook, Ernest J., 255

J

Jacobowitz, Jay, 212
Jacobs, Joseph J., 242–45, 255
James, Mark, 189
Jaroff, Leon, 247
Jarrow Formulas, 199
Javaan Corporation, 173
Jesuit bark, 27
Jin Bu Huan, 148
Johnson, Anita, 51–52
Johnson, Earvin "Magic," 214
Johnson, Michael, 212
Jonas, James, III, 114
Jones, Jenny, 95–96
Jones, W. P., 33
Journal of Longevity, 229
Jovanovic, Pavle, 161
The Jungle (Sinclair), 32

K

Kalo-Vita, 227
Kamil, Harvey, 232
Kang-Yum, Elaine, 182
Kapoor, Sam, 125–26
Karny, Rona, 43–44
kava, 150, 189–90, 205, 256
Kefauver-Harris Amendments, 36, 70
Keith, Kathryn, 60
Kellogg's, 178
Kennedy, Edward, 48–49, 72, 73, 131
    and DSHEA, 89, 90–91, 98

Kessler, Craig, 80, 81
Kessler, David, 72–74, 77–78, 89, 117,
    148–49
    at DSHEA hearings, 91–92, 97–98
    For Your Health Pharmacy raid,
    84–86
Kessler, Gerald A., 79–80, 81, 110, 178
    and DSHEA, 89–91, 92, 98, 99–101,
    125
    and NLEA opposition, 80–84, 86–87
Khudagulyan, Genia, 234
kidney impairment, 185, 191, 257, 259
    Chinese herbs and, 141–42, 143,
    145–51
kidney transplants, 196–97
King, Larry, 171, 209–10
Klausner, Richard, 170
Kleemeier, Renee, 260
Klein, Joel, 233
Knapp, Nicholas, 28
Knight, Patricia, 81, 91
Ko, Richard, 149
kola nuts, 105, 106
Koss, Johann Olav, 160–61
Krebs, Ernst T., Jr., 47, 218
Kurth, Peter, 197

L

labels, labeling regulation, 73, 74–77,
    100, 101, 158–59
    patent medicines, 32–33
    proposed reforms, 265
Laci LeBeau teas, 234–35
laetrile, 47, 218
Lane, Bill, 201–2, 203, 204
Lane Labs—USA, 203–4
laxative teas, 234–35
LDL cholesterol, 168, 259
lead, lead poisoning, 152–54, 199, 236
Lee, Camille, 119, 121, 122
Lee, Sharon, 12
Lee, Shayna, 119, 120, 121
Lee, Todd, 118–22
Lee, William Martens, 150
legislation, 35–36, 70. *See also* DSHEA
    adverse events reporting, 232
    ephedra bans, 115–16, 118, 193
    FDA rules moratorium, 86, 88, 98

FDA subpoena/recall powers, 78, 80, 88

Food, Drug, Cosmetic, and Device Enforcement Amendments, 78

manufacturer registration/reporting, 265

mind-altering supplement bans, 190

NLEA, 73, 74–77

proposed reforms, 265, 266

Proxmire Amendment, 48–53, 69, 70

Pure Food and Drugs Act (Wiley Act), 32–33, 35

state supplement regulation, 263

steroid precursor ban, 191–92

teen supplement use/sales, 193, 269

Let's Cook It Right (Davis), 39–40

Let's Eat Right to Keep Fit (Davis), 40–42

Let's Get Well (Davis), 43–44

Let's Have Healthy Children (Davis), 40, 43, 45, 185

leukemia, 145, 190

Li, Xiaomei, 151

Li'l Critters Gummi Vites, 154

Lind, James, 38

Lindsey, Ron, 114

Li Shih-chin, 150

litargirio, 152–53

litigation, 45, 130, 158, 178, 211, 230, 233

ephedra, 117, 127–29

steroid contamination, 160, 161

L-tryptophan, 64, 65–66, 69, 70

liver injury, 150, 155, 173, 189, 257

lobelia, 29–30, 256

Loeffler, Jonas & Tuggey, 114, 115

Loprinzi, Charles L., 203

Lormel, Dennis M., 198–99

lovastatin, 259

Lumen Foods, 12

lupus, 257

Lutwak, Leo, 44

lymphoma, 180

Lynn, Marcy, 163, 164

M

mad cow disease, 200, 256

Madis Botanicals, 135

magnesium, 41–42

magnolia bark, 142–43

ma huang. *See* ephedra

Malchow-Moller, Axel, 109

Male Power Plus, 155

manic depression, 198, 258–59

March, Lois, 13–14

marijuana, 236–37

marketing, 215–16, 219. *See also* deceptive advertising; supplement marketing

Martin, Jack, 77, 81, 91

Martinez, Tony, 90, 99

Mayer, James W., 59

McClellan, Mark, 125

McGuiness, Kevin, 77

McGwire, Mark, 191

Mead, Margaret, 83

media, media coverage, 55–56, 85–86, 254, 262

supplement sales/marketing and, 201, 205–7, 216, 270–71

Melancon, Tucker, 13

melanoma, 180

melatonin, 199–200

Menendez, Jose, 202

mercury, 151

mercury chloride (calomel), 28, 29

Metabolife 365, 111–12, 115, 117

Metabolife International, 18, 76, 111–12, 123, 228

ephedra litigation, 117, 129

political activities, 113–14, 115–16, 132, 255

methamphetamine, 111, 228

methyl sulphonyl methane, 9

Metzenbaum, Howard, 73, 96–97

Mevacor, 259

Meyer, John, 157

MII Liquidation, 129

Milner, Joshua D., 175

mind-altering drugs/supplements, 187–89, 237–38

Mind Excursions, 187–88

minerals. *See* vitamin and mineral supplements; vitamins and minerals; *specific minerals*

mistletoe, 250

MLM, 105, 111, 210–12

MLM Fraud: A Practical Handbook for the Network Marketing Professional (Caton), 11–12
Mooney, Patrick, 95
Moore, Carolyn E., 232
Moran, Dorothy, 245–46
Moran, James, 245–46
Morgan, Francis P., 33
Moss, Ralph W., 243
Mrs. Gooch's, 81
multilevel marketing, 105, 111, 210–12
multiple-ingredient supplements, 269
multiple sclerosis, 180
multivitamins, 17–18, 154, 159, 160, 165–66. *See also* vitamin and mineral supplements
  potential harm, 175, 177
  supposed benefits, 172–73
My Defense, 214
Myer, Julius, 136

N

Nader, Ralph, 42, 51, 217
Nagai, Nagajoshi, 107, 108
nandrolone, 160
narcotics, 35
National Academy of Sciences, 267
National Cancer Institute. See NCI
National Center for Complementary and Alternative Medicine. *See* NCCAM
National Health Federation, 47
National Institute of Mental Health, 61, 71
National Institutes of Health. *See* NIH
National Nutritional Foods Association. *See* NNFA
Natrol High, 234
Natrol Inc., 205, 214, 233–36
Natural Cures "They" Don't Want You to Know About (Trudeau), 12, 19, 216, 228–29
The Natural Mind (Weil), 237–38
Nature's Plus, 80, 93. *See also* Kessler, Gerald
Nawalowalo, Ratu Josateki, 190
NBTY, 81, 232

NCCAM (National Center for Complementary and Alternative Medicine), 16–17, 222, 246–50
  abolishment proposal, 266–67
  dubious studies, 203–4, 247, 248, 249–50, 257, 258–60, 267
  recent study results, 250–54
  research standards/criticism, 246–50
NCI (National Cancer Institute), 170, 203, 204, 244
nephropathy. *See* kidney impairment
Neuhouser, Marian L., 185
NexProtein, 116
NHA (Nutritional Health Alliance), 81–83, 178
niacin. *See* vitamin B$_3$
NIH (National Institutes of Health), 166, 194, 237, 242, 267. *See also specific institutes*
  Office of Alternative Medicine, 242–46
  PC-SPES study, 157
  L-tryptophan EMS investigation, 63, 64–65
Niteworks, 211–12
nitric acid, 211
Nitro-Tech, 161
Nixon, Richard M., 48
NLEA (Nutrition Labeling and Education Act), 73, 74–77
NNFA (National Nutritional Foods Association), 51, 77, 81, 82, 91
19-norandrostenedione, 161
19-norandrosterone, 160
Novogen Ltd., 194, 195
Null, Gary, 197
Nu Skin International, 76
nutrition, 39, 42. *See also* Davis, Adelle
  children's, 179–80, 184–85
  federal dietary guidelines, 166, 174, 180–81
Nutritional Health Alliance (NHA), 81–83, 178
Nutrition for Life, 11–12, 228
Nutrition Labeling and Education Act (NLEA), 73, 74–77
nux vomica, 29
NVE Pharmaceuticals, 111, 129–30, 155

O

OAM (Office of Alternative Medicine),
242–46, 247–48, 266–67. *See also*
NCCAM
Occhifinto, Robert, 111, 122, 127, 129,
228
Office of Alternative Medicine. *See*
OAM
Oliveras, Jerry, 151–52
Olsen, Dean, 189
Olympian Labs, 199
Olympic athletes, 160–61
omega-3 fatty acids, 259, 260–61
opiates, 32
Optimum Health (Davis), 38
organ extracts, 256
osteoarthritis. *See* arthritis
osteoporosis, 174. *See also* bone health
ovarian cancer, 181, 190

P

packaging. *See also* labels
child-resistant, 178, 268–69
Packer, Lester, 169
pancreatic cancer, 249–50
pancreatic enzymes, 9
panic disorder, 257
ParaCease, 226
parasites, 226
Parker, Cory, 14
Parnes, Lydia, 231
Parry, Romani, 77
Parry, Thomas, 77
patent medicines, 28, 30–35, 215–16. *See
also* snake oil
Chinese, 139, 140, 148
Patient Heal Thyself (Rubin), 225–26
Pat's Age-Defying Antioxidants, 227
Pat's Age-Defying Shake, 227
Pauling, Linus, 47, 52, 168, 172
PC-SPES, 156–58, 248, 257
Pedia Loss, 184
Penicillin Amendment, 36
pennyroyal, 150, 256
People Against Cancer, 243
Perfect Food Super Green Formula,
163–64

performance-enhancing supplements
for athletes, 160–61, 191–93, 269–70
sexual enhancement, 155–56, 207,
208–9, 257
Perr, Hilary, 184–85, 186
pesticides, 36, 154, 258
petroleum, 216
Pfizer, 117
pharmaceutical industry, 6, 19, 88,
219–20. *See also specific companies*
pharmaceuticals. *See also specific drugs*
in supplements, 154–58, 189, 245,
248
supplement use and, 185, 196–97,
200, 249
pharmacy supplement sales, 214–15, 270
Pharmics, 76–77
phenobarbitol, 108–9
Pisano, Joel, 127–28
Pitzer, Donald, 185
Pitzer, Ryan, 185
Pitzer, Susan, 185
placebo effect, 221–22, 253
Podesta, John, 90
Podesta, Tony, 90, 100, 101
poisonings, 18, 176–78, 256, 268–69
policosanol, 259–60
Pollack, Randy, 232
Pond's Extract, 31, 32
Ponich, Ted, 230, 231
Porter, Donna V., 99
Porter, John, 246
potassium chloride, 185
Potts, Annie, 199
Pound, Dick, 161
prescription drugs. *See* pharmaceuticals;
specific drugs
price-fixing, 233
Probert, Greg, 212
Procter & Gamble, 77
progesterone, natural, 17
Promensil, 194, 195
prostate cancer, 156, 157, 248, 253
prostate health supplements
PC-SPES, 156–58, 248, 257
saw palmetto, 76, 250, 252–53
Proxmire, William, 48, 49–50
Proxmire Amendment, 48–53, 69, 70

pseudoephedrine, 108
Public Citizen Health Research Group,
    51, 73
Public Law 102–170, 242
pukeweed. *See* lobelia
Pure Food and Drugs Act (Wiley Act),
    32–33, 35
Pure World, 135–37
Puziss, Paul M., 140

Q

Quanterra Mental Sharpness Product,
    199
quinine, 27, 29

R

Raber, Dan, 6, 8, 9, 11, 13–15
radiation therapy, 239
Radol, 216
Randall, Russell, 44
Rasmussen, Salka E., 179
red clover, 135, 194, 195
red yeast rice, 213, 259
Rehme, Christopher G., 9
religion, 222–23, 225–27
Remifermin, 194
retailers, retail stores, 87, 214–15, 270
    advice from, 212–14, 239
    third-party literature, 102, 213, 214,
        215
retinol, 175–76. *See also* vitamin A
Rexall Sundown, 76, 81, 232
Richardson, Bill, 89–90, 93, 99, 100
    FDA rules moratorium, 86, 88, 98
Rimostil, 195
Robbins, Mark, 88
Robbins, Tony, 129
Robertson, Pat, 226–27
Robinson, Judy, 183
Rodale, J. I., 45–46
Rodham, Hugh, 230–31
Rogovin, Jarrow L., 88
Roosevelt, Theodore, 24, 32
Rosen, Winifred, 238
Rosenbloom, Chris, 165
Rubin, Jordan S., 225–26
Rudolph, Scott, 81, 101

Runion, Kristie, 119, 120, 122
Rush, Benjamin, 28–29
Russell, Robert M., 167
Rynerson, Edward, 44

S

safety, 17–18, 19. *See also* contamination
    issues; safety review/regulation;
    specific supplements
    most dangerous supplements, 255–57
safety review/regulation. *See also specific*
    supplements
    drugs, 35–36, 70–71
    in DSHEA hearings, 91–92, 98
    proposed reforms, 266–67
    in Proxmire Amendment hearings,
        48–49, 51–52
    in L-tryptophan hearing, 66–70
    under DSHEA, 102, 115, 125, 131
safety warnings, 101, 265
    FDA consumer warnings, 153, 154,
        155, 189, 257
salvia, 189
SAM-e, 258–59
Sampson, Wallace, 217–19, 248
Sandoz, 80
sanjivani ark, 154*n*
saw palmetto, 76, 250, 252–53
Saxion, Valerie, 226
Schardt, David, 210, 240
Schectman, Gordon, 43
Schiff Vitamins, 69
Schiller, Lawrence R., 155
schizophrenia, 42, 198
Schmidt, Alexander M., 50, 51
Schmidt, Carl Frederic, 107
Schnitker, Kevin, 189
Schreck, Russell, 123
Schultz, Bill, 77, 100
Schwarzenegger, Arnold, 193
Scientific Review of Alternative Medicine,
    218–19
Scientology, 222
scleroderma, 62
scurvy, 38
selenium, 168
seniors' supplement use, 198–200
senna, 234, 235

serotonin, 54, 68
Seven Forests Chinese herbs, 143–44,
    145, 148
sexual enhancement supplements,
    155–56, 207, 208–9, 257
Shalala, Donna, 243
Shao, Andrew, 252
shark cartilage, 201–4, 223, 246
Sharks Don't Get Cancer (Lane), 201
Shields, Brooke, 222
Showa Denko KK, 64, 65–66, 67
Shuren, Jeffrey, 128
Shwayder, Tor A., 186, 187
Silent Spring (Carson), 36
silver, colloidal, 186–87
Silver, Richard, 62, 63
Silver Creek Laboratories, 226
Silverglade, Bruce, 92–93, 131
Simone, Charles, 203
Sinclair, Upton, 32
60 Minutes, 201–3, 205, 206
skin cancers, 5–6, 7, 180
    bloodroot for, 4, 6–7, 14, 15, 239
skin problems, 239. *See also* Gilliatt,
    Sue
Skolnick, Allen, 81, 83, 101
Skolnick, Connie, 101
Skolnik, Norma, 231–32
skullcap, 257
Sleeping Buddha, 155
Sliwinski, Jeanette, 198
Small, Eric, 157
Smith, Anna Nicole, 126
Smith, David R., 106, 109–10, 112
Smith, Harry, 216
snake oil, 23
Snake Oil Liniment, Clark Stanley's,
    23–26, 33–35
snakeroot. *See* aristolochia
Snare, Jonathan L., 131–32
soil microorganisms, 225–26
Solgar Vitamin and Herb Company, 81,
    231
Soller, R. William, 87
soy, 194, 195
Spacek, Sissy, 86
Specter, Arlen, 246
Speier, Jackie, 193
spina bifida, 173

Spontaneous Healing (Weil), 238–39
sports supplements, 160–61, 191–93,
    269–70
Stackers, 111, 120, 127, 129–30
Stampfer, Meir, 176
Stanley, Clark, 23–26, 33–35
Stargrove, Mitchell, 138–40, 161
Starlight International, 76, 255
stephania, 142–44, 145, 148
Sternberg, Esther, 61–63, 63–66, 67,
    71
steroids, steroid precursors, 160–61, 190,
    191–92, 256
Stieber, Tamar, 58–61, 66, 71
St. John's wort, 196–97, 198, 205–6, 221,
    248, 249
Straus, Stephen, 222, 247, 248–49,
    251–52, 253
stroke, 130, 194
strychnine, 29
sugar, 40, 41
sulfanilamide, 35, 70
sunlight, 180, 181
Super Complete, 160
Super Slimming Tea, 234
supplement industry, 19, 223–24. *See also*
    DSHEA; *specific companies,*
    organizations, and individuals
    Andrew Weil's role, 240
    ephedra manufacturers, 110–12
    ephedra regulation attempts and,
        113–14
    felons in, 11, 47, 111–12, 129, 227–31
    labeling rules opposition, 75, 79,
        80–84, 86–88
    lobbying by, 77, 89–90, 114, 115–16,
        117, 132, 232
    mega-corporations in, 231–33
    NLEA and, 75–77
    political contributions/influence, 75,
        114, 115–16, 230, 254–55
    price-fixing in, 232–33
    Proxmire Amendment and, 47, 51
    public image, 219
    public opinion campaigns, 86–88,
        94–96
    religion in, 225–27
    role in DHEA, 89–91
    in Utah, 75–76, 191–92

supplement manufacturing, 136–37, 264.
  See also contamination issues
  proposed reforms, 264–65, 266
  standards/quality control, 137, 158,
    159–60, 234, 236, 264
  unreliable purity/potency, 158–59,
    199, 264
supplement marketing. *See also* deceptive
    advertising
  celebrity endorsements, 209–10, 214,
    215–16
  children's products, 184
  media's role, 201, 205–7, 216, 270–71
  multilevel marketing, 105, 111, 210–12
  proposed reforms, 269–70
  retailer advice, 212–14, 239
  retailing strategies, 214–17
  to seniors, 198–200
  shark cartilage, 201, 203
  to teen athletes, 192–93, 269–70
  to women, 193–94
supplement regulation, 19, 263. *See also*
    DSHEA; FDA *entries*; safety
    review/regulation
  proposed reforms, 264–71
supplement research, 16–18, 247, 267. *See
    also specific herbs and supplements*
  standards and criticism, 243–44, 245,
    246–50
supplement sales, 259. *See also specific
    types and companies*
  figures and trends, 16, 130–31, 240,
    260
  media coverage and, 201, 205–7, 216
supplement use
  consumer confidence about, 16,
    18–19, 164
  psychological reasons for, 220–21, 272
  reticence about, 8, 147, 196
  statistics, 16, 147, 164–65, 193, 198,
    199, 268
Synar, Mike, 90
synephrine, 126

T

Taising Trading, 143–44
tea, 27
teas, for weight loss, 234–35

teen supplement use, 186–93, 269–70
thalidomide, 36, 70
thiamine. *See* vitamin B_1
Thies, Greg, 231
Thompson, Frances L., 56, 58, 63, 66–67
Thompson, Tommy G., 115, 125
Thomson, Samuel, 29–30
Tibetan herbal vitamins, 152
Timpone, Walter P., 127
Ting, Mai, 60
The Toadstool Millionaires (Young), 30, 216
tobacco, 26, 27
Topol, Eric, 219–20
Toshniwal, Purushottam, 154n
traditional Chinese medicine, 139. *See
    also* acupuncture; Chinese herbs
Travis, Clay, 227
Travis, Randy, 96
triglycerides, 259, 261
TrimSpa, 126
Trinity Foundation, 227
Troy, Dan, 116–17, 130
Troy, Tevi, 116
Trudeau, Kevin, 11, 12, 19, 216, 228–29
The Truth About the Drug Companies
    (Angell), 219
L-tryptophan, 54, 62, 68–69, 94, 189
  ban/recalls, 61, 84, 87
  media coverage, 55–56
L-tryptophan EMS, 63–64, 93–94
  Congressional hearing, 66–70
  indications and investigation, 55,
    57–58, 59–65
  manufacturer's response, 64–66
L-Tryptophan-Rest, 69–70
20/20, 205, 206
TwinLab Corporation, 77, 129

U

Ulbricht, Catherine, 147, 196
Ultimate Nutrition, 160
Ultra Health Laboratories, 155
Ultra Male, 93
Unilever, 78
Unsafe at Any Speed (Nader), 217
Utah Natural Products Alliance, 76
Utah supplement industry, 75–76,
    191–92

V

Valium, 155
Vanherweghem, Jean-Louis, 142, 143
Vencill, Kicker, 160
Viagra, 155, 257
Viga for Women, 155
Vinerol, 155
Vioxx, 219, 220
Vitality Through Planned Nutrition (Davis), 39, 44–45
vitamin and mineral supplements, 17–18, 163–81. *See also specific vitamins and minerals*
    advice concerning, 165–67, 170
    antioxidant supplements, 167–72, 185
    manufacturing/contamination issues, 154, 159, 160, 164
    maximum safe doses, 48–53, 179, 181, 268
    multivitamins, 17–18, 165–66, 172–73, 175
    popularity, 164–65, 169, 171–72, 173, 181
    potential benefits, 180–81
    potential harm, 175–80, 181
    price-fixing, 233
    sales statistics, 164, 169, 172, 173
    supposed benefits, 164, 169–71, 172–74
vitamin A, 38, 44–45, 168, 169, 211–12
    potential harm, 175–76, 186
vitamin B, 38
vitamin B$_1$, 38
vitamin B$_3$, 41, 42, 173
vitamin B$_6$, 173
vitamin B$_9$. *See* folic acid
vitamin B$_{12}$, 166, 174
vitamin "B$_{17}$," 47
vitamin C, 38, 52, 185, 209
    supposed benefits, 47, 168, 169, 172, 211–12
Vitamin C and the Common Cold (Pauling), 168
vitamin D, 17, 44, 45, 174
    potential benefits, 180–81, 260, 261
vitamin E, 38, 172
    potential harm, 17, 44, 185
    supposed benefits, 168–71, 239

vitamin K, 166
vitamins and minerals, 38–39, 41–42, 49, 178–79. *See also* vitamin and mineral supplements; *specific types*
    antioxidant claims, 167–72
    safe upper limits, 48–53, 179, 181, 268
Vitamin Shoppe, 212, 214
Voinovich, George V., 197
Voorhees, Ron, 60, 61

W

Waddington, Phil, 263, 267
Wadler, Gary I., 161, 192
Walden, Greg, 123–24
Walker, Alexander M., 18, 265
Wallace, Mike, 201, 202–3
Walters, Barbara, 205
warfarin, 158
warning statements. *See* safety warnings
Warren, Lesley Ann, 96
warts, 239
Washington, George, 28
Watergate scandal, 48
Waxman, Henry, 265
    and DSHEA, 89, 91, 99, 100
    and FDA rules moratorium, 98
    FDA subpoena/recall powers bill, 78, 80, 88
    and NHA lobbying, 87–88, 90
    NLEA and proposed FDA rules, 74, 75, 77, 78–79
weight-loss supplements, 108–9, 126–27, 207–8, 214, 234–36, 256. *See also* ephedra
Weil, Andrew, 3–4, 15, 236–40
Weinstein, Ralph, 141
Weiss, Ted, 66
Weisskopf, Michael, 114
Wentworth, Jeff, 114, 115
Wermann, Chris, 178
Whisenant, Barbara, 106
White, Jeffrey, 203
Whitmore, George, 159
Whittekin, Martie, 81, 82
Whole Foods, 81, 219
Wiewel, Frank, 243, 245
Wiley, Harvey W., 32

Wiley Act, 32–33, 35
Wilson, Dorothy, 56, 57–58, 66, 93–94
Wilson, Megan, 198
Winter, Wallace, 116
Withering, William, 27–28
Wolf, Johannes, 197
Wolfe, Sidney, 51, 73
Wolnik, Karen A., 148
Women's Health Initiative, 174, 194
women's supplements/supplement use,
 193–96
Wright, Jonathan V., 84–85
Wurtman, Richard J., 67–68
Wyeth, 231

X
X32, 126
Xenadrine, 117–18, 126

Y
Yellow Jacket, 111
yew needle, 185
yohimbe, yohimbine, 257
You Can Stay Well (Davis), 39
Young, Eliza, 45
Young, Frank E., 73
Young, James Harvey, 30, 215, 216
Young, Katherine, 45
Yussman, Susan, 190–91

Z
Zeller, Mitchell, 67, 74, 75
Zheng, Qun Yi, 137
zinc, 50
zinc chloride, 5
Zoloft, 117, 221